Good Nutrition: Perspectives for the 21st Century

Editors

Manfred Eggersdorfer

Klaus Kraemer

John B Cordaro

Jess Fanzo

Mike Gibney

Eileen Kennedy

Alain Labrique

Jonathan Steffen
(Technical Editor)

Kaiseraugust

79 figures and 19 tables, 2016

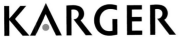
Basel · Freiburg · Paris · London · New York · New Delhi · Bangkok
Beijing · Tokyo · Kuala Lumpur · Singapore · Sydney

Manfred Eggersdorfer
DSM Nutritional Products Ltd
Wurmisweg 576, 4303 Kaiseraugst, Switzerland

Klaus Kraemer
Sight and Life
PO Box 2116, Basel, CH-4002, Switzerland

John B Cordaro
Mars, Incorporated – Consultant
Food Security, Nutrition and Safety, 6885 Elm Street,
McLean, VA 22101, USA

Jess Fanzo
*Berman Institute of Bioethics and Nitze School
of Advanced International Studies*
The Johns Hopkins University, 1809 Ashland Avenue,
Baltimore, MD 21205, USA

Mike Gibney
Institute of Food and Health
University College Dublin, Stillorgan Rd, Belfield,
Dublin 4, Ireland

Eileen Kennedy
Tufts University
Friedman School of Nutrition Science and Policy,
150 Harrison Avenue, Boston MA, 02111, USA

Alain Labrique
*Johns Hopkins University Bloomberg School
of Public Health*
615 N Wolfe St, Baltimore, MD, 21205, USA

Jonathan Steffen
Jonathan Steffen Limited
Suite C, 153 St Neots Road, Hardwick, Cambridge,
CB23 7QJ, UK

Library of Congress Cataloging-in-Publication Data

Good Nutrition: Perspectives for the 21st century / editors, Manfred Eggersdorfer, Klaus Kraemer, John B Cordaro, Jess Fanzo, Mike Gibney, Eileen Kennedy, Alain Labrique, Jonathan Steffen.
Basel; New York: Karger, 2016.
Includes bibliographical references and index.
LCCN 2016039583| ISBN 9783318059649 (hard cover: alk. paper)
ISBN 9783318059656 (e-ISBN)
Eggersdorfer, Manfred, editor.
MESH: Nutrition Policy | Global Health | Nutrition Disorders--prevention & control | Food Supply |
Conservation of Natural Resources
362.1--dc23   2016039583
LCC RA427.8 | NLM QU 145.72 | DDC 362.1--dc23 LC record available at https://lccn.loc.gov/2016039583

Printed in Germany on acid-free and non-aging paper (ISO 9706) by Kraft Druck, Ettlingen
ISBN 9783318059649
e-ISBN 9783318059656

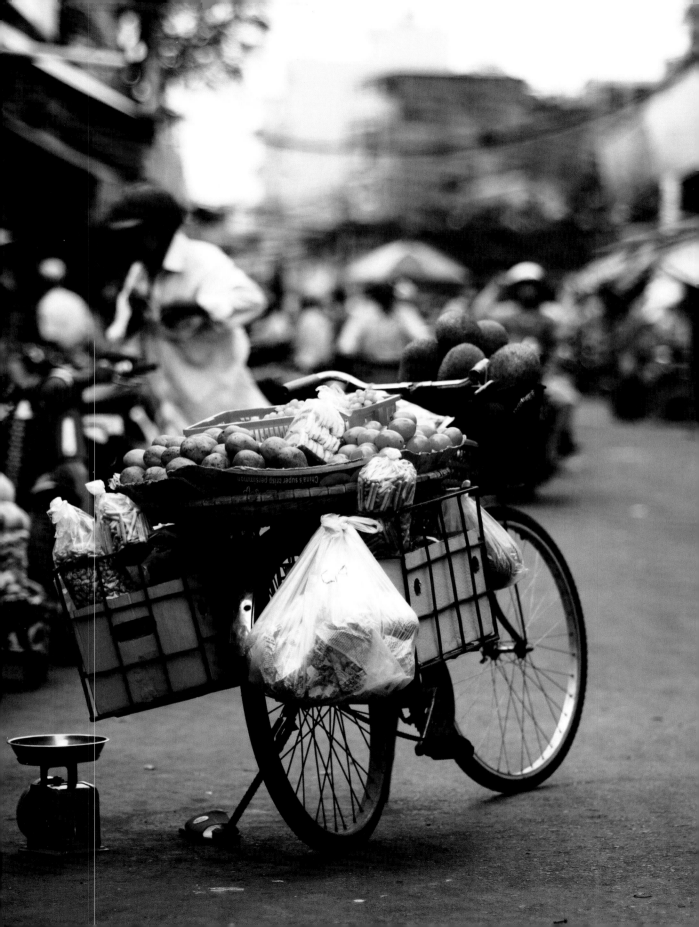

Foreword

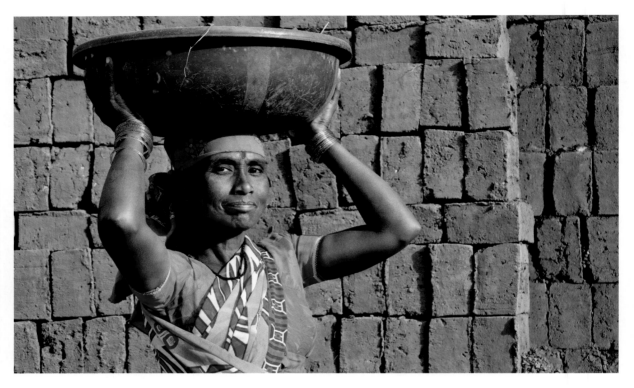

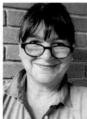

Prof. Hilal Elver
UN Special Rapporteur
on the Right to Food

Embedding nutrition in a human rights agenda

Good Nutrition: Perspectives for the 21ˢᵗ century offers a wide-ranging view of the challenges and opportunities for nutrition in the era of the Sustainable Development Goals (SDGs). Nutrition has a role to play in all 17 goals. If nutrition is accepted as a human right, then its potential to bring about positive change on a global scale is vast. If it is not, however, even our best efforts to implement the SDGs will be very limited in their effect.

International law instruments provide a normative and legal foundation for the human right to adequate food and nutrition. Subsequent to Article 25 of the Universal Declaration on Human Rights, Article 11 of the International Covenant on Economic, Social and Cultural Rights (ESCR) recognizes the right to adequate food and the fundamental right of everyone to be free from hunger.

Yet, nearly 800 million people worldwide remain chronically undernourished, and over 2 billion suffer from micronutrient deficiencies, also known as hidden hunger. Another 2 billion are overweight, with 600 million of these being obese. Meanwhile some 159 million children under 5 years of age are stunted, approximately 50 million children from this same age bracket are wasted, and 42 million are obese. For the first time in human history, there are more obese than underweight adults in the world. As a result, non-communicable diseases (NCDs) associated with obesity have surpassed undernutrition as the leading cause of death in low-income countries.

These figures indicate that the challenges of malnutrition in all its forms are daunting. Nevertheless, in many developing and least developed countries (LDCs), policies against hunger receive more attention than does the prevention of malnutrition in general, or the stunting and wasting of children. Therefore it is important to emphasize that the right to adequate food includes nutrition. Adequacy with respect to food simply embraces nutritional value. This means that the quality of the food we consume has to become as important as the quantity. It is not enough to provide quantities of food as measured by caloric intake to eliminate hunger. This caloric intake must include the necessary ingredients for human health.

Like access to food in general, access to nutritious food is often a key indicator of economic inequalities, as well as of discrimination. Therefore including nutrition in a rightsbased framework is critical to ensuring that marginalized and vulnerable segments of the population are able to access adequate, healthy, and nutritious food.

Dealing with global nutrition challenges through a rights-based perspective is not only desirable, but also obligatory, since several key principles recognize nutrition as an inherent element of the right to food. The human-rights-based approach to nutrition enables the implementation of procedural rights. These include participation, accountability, non-discrimination, transparency, empowerment and rule of law – each a demonstration of respect for human dignity. At the International Conference on Nutrition 2 (ICN2), in Rome in November 2014, the implications of a human-rights- based approach to nutrition were explained as follows: "[e]mbedding nutrition in a human rights agenda makes issues of governance and accountability central to effective implementation."

There are several human rights documents that support the claim that the right to adequate food and nutrition is not only legitimate but constitutes a legal duty. The clear inclusion of a nutrition dimension of the right to food reveals that the right to food, properly conceived, is closely linked to the right to health. The Covenant of the ESCR Article 12.1 recognizes "the right of everyone to the enjoyment of the highest attainable standard of physical and mental health." If there is insufficient nutritious food available and accessible, there will be adverse consequences for physical and mental health.

In its General Comment 12, the Committee on Economic, Social and Cultural Rights (CESCR) Paragraph 8 interpreted the right to adequate food as follows: "Every State is obliged to ensure for everyone under its jurisdiction access to the minimum essential food which is sufficient, nutritionally adequate and safe, to ensure their freedom from hunger." Furthermore, General Comment 14 Paragraph 43 (b) reiterates that one of the core State obligations under the right to health includes ensuring "access to the minimum essential food which is nutritionally adequate and safe, to ensure freedom from hunger to everyone."

The Voluntary Guidelines to Support the Progressive Realization of the Right to Adequate Food in the Context of National Food Security (Voluntary Guidelines) of 2004 notes that "States should take measures to maintain, adapt or strengthen dietary diversity and healthy eating habits and food preparation, as well as feeding patterns, including breastfeeding, while ensuring that changes in availability and access to food supply do not negatively affect dietary composition and intake."

Malnutrition does more harm to vulnerable populations, particularly to poor women and children. Therefore, besides the universally protected right to food and nutrition for all, children, pregnant and lactating women are selected for further protection in universally accepted human rights conventions. The Convention on the Rights of the Child (CRC) in Article 24 acknowledges that "to pursue the full implementation of the right of the child to the enjoyment of the highest attainable standard of health… States shall take appropriate measures to (c) combat disease and malnutrition… through, *inter alia*, the provision of adequate nutritious foods." Article 27(3) states that: "Parties… shall take appropriate measures to assist parents and others responsible for the child to implement this right and shall in case of need provide material assistance and support programs, particularly with regard to nutrition, clothing and housing."

III The Committee of the CRC in its General Comment on Article 24 calls on States to ensure that all segments of society are informed of the advantages of breastfeeding. The CRC further states that "exclusive breastfeeding for infants up to 6 months of age should be protected and promoted and breastfeeding should continue alongside appropriate complementary foods preferably until two years of age, where feasible."

The protection and promotion of breastfeeding is also enshrined in the International Code on Marketing of Breast-milk Substitutes, which was adopted by the World Health Assembly in 1981. The Global Strategy for Infant and Young Child Feeding, adopted in 2002, sets out the obligations of States to develop, implement, monitor and evaluate comprehensive national policies addressing infant and young child feeding, accompanied by a detailed action plan.

The 1979 Convention on the Elimination of All Forms of Discrimination Against Women (CEDAW) highlights the importance of children, as well as the importance of lactating and pregnant women. Article 12 stipulates that all states shall ensure to women appropriate services in connection with pregnancy, confinement and the postnatal period, granting free services where necessary, as well as adequate nutrition during pregnancy and lactation. Unfortunately, CEDAW fails to fully protect a woman's right to adequate food and nutrition as an individual, but only provides protection within the parameters of pregnancy and breastfeeding. Despite scientific evidence demonstrating that women have special needs due to physiological differences from men, CEDAW surprisingly does not provide special protection of the right to adequate food and nutrition for women as individuals. It is vitally important to correct this protection gap as soon as possible.

Considering the pivotal role of the private sector in the provision of adequate food and nutrition, it is appropriate that the primary role of regulating and monitoring the private sector should be given to the governments of sovereign states. A human rights framework underlines the responsibility of corporations that produce food and shape nutritional standards to respect human rights and to contribute to equitable access for all persons to nutritious foods. Such responsibility is implied in the Universal Declaration on Human Rights, which clearly asserts that "everyone has duties to the community" (Art. 29), and that groups and persons must refrain from activities causing encroachment on the rights enshrined within the Declaration (Art. 30).

In 2011 the UN Human Rights Council endorsed the UN Guiding Principles on Business and Human Rights, formally recognizing the responsibility of enterprises to avoid infringing on the human rights of others and to address adverse human rights impacts arising from their commercial activities. This responsibility extends to the adverse impacts caused by the food industry in relation to the right to adequate food.

Although there is no significant resistance opposing a human rights approach to adequate food and nutrition, several potential barriers exist that affect proper implementation. Corporations greatly prefer voluntary commitments to regulatory frameworks. We see this resistance at domestic levels. There are corporate initiatives against several states dealing with such issues as labeling, taxing, limiting excessive advertisements of junk foods, which covers highly processed foods high in salt, sugar and saturated fats. Secondly, there is a governance problem, since nutrition poses a multifaceted challenge that needs to be coordinated through the cooperative effort of several separate parts of government machinery. Finally, the complex character and long-term impacts of malnutrition on human health, as well as the absence of indicators and lack of proper data, creates difficulties when it comes to establishing workable monitoring, accountability and transparency mechanisms.

The role of nutrition within the Sustainable Development Goals (SDGs)

In September 2015, 170 world leaders gathered at the UN Sustainable Development Summit in New York to adopt a 2030 Agenda. The new Agenda covers a broad set of 17 Goals and 167 targets and will serve as the overall framework to guide global and national development action for the next 15 years. The SDGs are universal, transformative, comprehensive, and inclusive.

If we evaluate the SDGs from the perspective of nutrition policies, we notice that nutrition is relevant to all 17 goals. As with all SDGs, nutrition also has a universal character. Without achieving nutrition targets, development policies cannot be successful. The present burden of malnutrition on public health and the national budget has become staggering. At the ICN2, world leaders recognized that a key action for improving nutrition governance is to anchor nutrition targets in the SDGs. While Goal #2 explicitly references "nutrition" ("end hunger, achieve food security, improved nutrition, and promote sustainable agriculture") and Goal # 3 refers to non-communicable diseases, nutrition is arguably "interwoven" in relation to all 17 SDGs, as at least 50 of the indicators set forth in the 17 SDGs pertain to nutrition. The root causes of malnutrition are more complex than the lack of sufficient and adequate food,

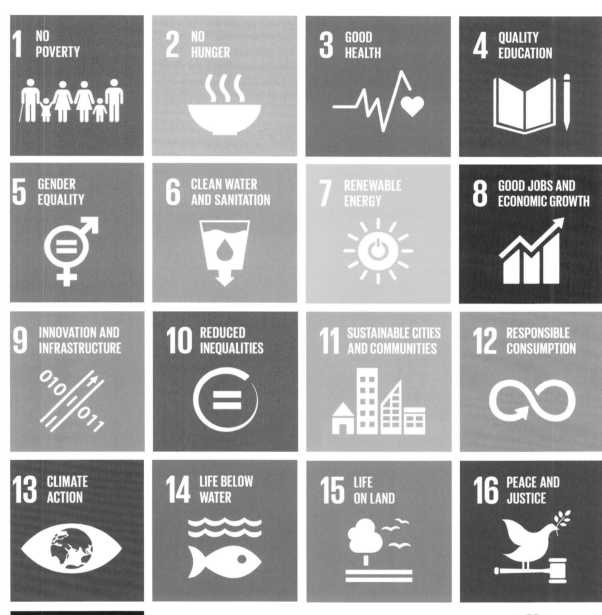

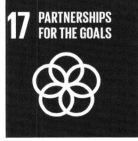

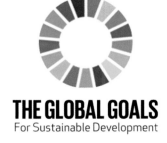

THE GLOBAL GOALS
For Sustainable Development

V reflecting as they do a variety of interrelated conditions addressed in the SDGs with respect to health, care, education, sanitation and hygiene, access to resources, environmental degradation, climate change and women's empowerment. All of these conditions are directly related to development policies. The underlying reality is this: the SDGs cannot be achieved without special attention to nutrition, and the nutrition Goals cannot be met without the fulfilment of other SDGs.

We conclude that despite the potential success of the SDGs on account of their inclusion of nutrition (in contrast to the antecedent Millennium Development Goals [MDGs]), they still arguably fail to establish a framework that will facilitate the development of sustainable food systems – something which is crucial in the fight against malnutrition. Moreover, some SDG targets lack the focus to enable effective implementation, and a number are not quantified. Many targets are associated with several goals, and some goals and targets may be in conflict with one another. Action to meet one target could have unintended consequences for others if the pursuit of all is not coordinated. Among the 169 targets, only one is dedicated specifically to nutrition; and obesity is not even mentioned. So the indefiniteness of the SDG framework seems to create gaps between the ambition of the goals and the likely performance of states, which gives cause for concern.

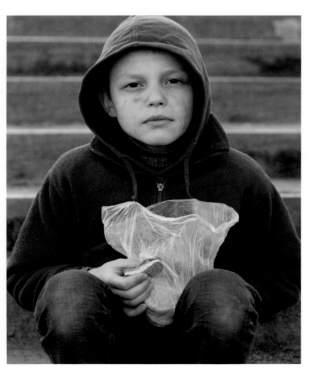

Furthermore, the lack of an effective accountability and monitoring system is a major obstacle to realizing the SDGs. Voluntary national reporting and reviewing mechanisms through the High Level Political Forum of the UN General Assembly are unlikely to be effective enough to reach the nutrition targets in a timely and sufficiently thorough fashion. The multisectoral nature of nutrition, its long-term impact on human rights and development, and the invisibility of some of its consequences together make accountability a complex and difficult challenge. Meeting such a challenge requires a clear understanding of data collection. This calls for an understanding what is needed to improve nutrition coverage, as well as developing a systematic tracking system for monitoring investment and accountability at country and global levels.

Although significant progress has occurred vis-à-vis the Millennium Development Goals, the 2030 Sustainable Development Goals still avoid directly articulating a human-rights-based approach. We cannot find anywhere in the text of the SDGs a direct affirmation of the "right to adequate food," or language imposing on states the duty to "respect, protect, and fulfil" human rights, despite the fact earlier noted that all 17 goals are directly or indirectly relevant to the fulfilling the 2030 Agenda for the

Sustainable Development Goals.

Overcoming barriers in the "Decade of Nutrition"? It is true that even if the human rights approach to nutrition were recognized, several barriers would still stand in the way of the adoption of effective nutrition policies and their implementation in pursuit of the various targets. At the height of the global food price crises in 2008, The Lancet Series on Maternal and Child Undernutrition warned that the international nutrition system was fragmented, dysfunctional and desperately in need of reform. Since then, significant initiatives have taken place at the global level. On April 1, 2016, following the recommendation of the ICN2, the UN general Assembly declared the Decade of Action on Nutrition that will run from 2016 to 2025. The Decade presents a unique opportunity to centralize globally agreed targets, align actors around implementation, and address the shortcomings identified in the current forms of nutrition governance. While ambitious targets have been set to ensure the global governance of nutrition, much more is needed to meet the challenge of providing each person with enough nutritious food to live a healthy and productive life, while at the same time protecting the environment and natural resources, including with regard to climate change.

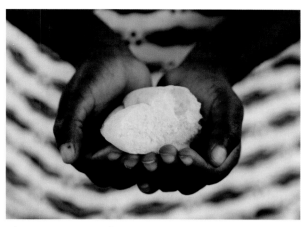

The ICN2 Rome Declaration on Nutrition acknowledged that "current food systems are being increasingly challenged to provide adequate, safe and diversified and nutrient-rich food for all that contribute to healthy diets due to, inter alia, constraints posed by resource scarcity and environmental degradation, as well as by unsustainable production and consumption patterns, food losses and waste, and unbalanced distribution."

Starting from the observation of the ICN2, the first barrier is the industrial food systems, including production, processing, transport and consumption of food, that are currently dominant in many parts of the world. Food systems have a direct impact on overall diet and in determining what food is available in the market place. Industrial food systems focus on increasing production and maximizing efficiency at the lowest possible economic (and consumer) cost. This type of system relies on industrialized agriculture, including mono-cropping and factory farming, industrial food processing, mass distribution, and marketing. Due to considerations of affordability, availability and palatability, as well as marketing and promotion strategies, food produced from industrialized food systems constitutes a significant portion of global food sales. The adverse impact of industrial food systems on nutrition and public health is widely acknowledged. It is now obvious that excessive food production neither eliminates hunger nor remedies malnutrition. Removing these barriers depends on the appropriate transformation of current food systems into "nutrition-sensitive" food systems. Reflecting the various conditions of specific countries, nutrition-sensitive food systems need to be diverse, but the general principles should be sensitive to global nutrition policies and the human rights approach that gives a high priority to nutritionally deprived groups and vulnerable peoples.

The second barrier is a set of factors relating to political, environmental and socioeconomic conditions that have direct and indirect impacts on nutrition in any given society. These conditions include economic development without inclusive growth; population increase, poverty as well as vertical and horizontal inequality; rural urban migration and urbanization; trade and investment policies as well as economic globalization; equal access to natural resources, sustainable resource management, environmental degradation, and climate change.

These conditions are interrelated and give rise to negative or positive effects on nutrition depending on policy interventions. Therefore each country should create a "national master plan for good nutrition." Addressing global nutrition challenges and ensuring that every individual is guaranteed a right to nutrition requires significant reforms in several areas: agriculture, education, health, social protection, water, sanitation and hygiene, gender, trade relations, socioeconomic conditions, environmental degradation, and climate change.

To meet the Decade of Nutrition and 2030 Sustainable Development Targets, political will is vital first and foremost. National governments should take these global targets seriously and dedicate substantive financial resources to reaching the targets. Governments should also establish effective, transparent, and independent accountability mechanisms to follow up and review the progress and detect obstacles. Without such monitoring mechanisms and financial resources, there will be little progress, and few nutrition targets will be reached. Needless to say, effective monitoring and accountability systems, as well as inclusive decision-making processes, would be realized if a human-rights- based approach were to be credibly applied to nutrition policies.

Perspectives for the 21st century

Good Nutrition: Perspectives for the 21st century showcases the thinking of some of today's most influential and respected scientists from a wide range of fields. With clear presentation and accessible argumentation, it offers a composite view of where global nutrition stands today and outlines a wide range of evidence-based approaches for bringing about positive change. The fact that its scope covers the developed as well as the developing world makes it all the more powerful, for there are no countries in the world today, however affluent they might be, that are not faced with significant malnutrition challenges. I am confident that scientists and policy-makers working in nutrition, food, agriculture and public health, as well as non-specialists, will find this publication informative, useful, and thought provoking, and that it will inspire everyone who reads it to help build a world in which nutrition is indeed recognized as a fundamental human right.

Prof. Hilal Elver
UN Special Rapporteur on the Right to Food

Preface

A moment for concerted thought – and action

Nutrition brings the world together. All human beings, everywhere in the world, have broadly the same nutritional needs. Nutrition also divides the world – into those who have enough to eat and those who have not, those who enjoy safe, quality foods and those who do not, and those who have highly specific nutritional requirements and those who do not. The food we eat is a potent symbol of both the unity and the division of the world we live in.

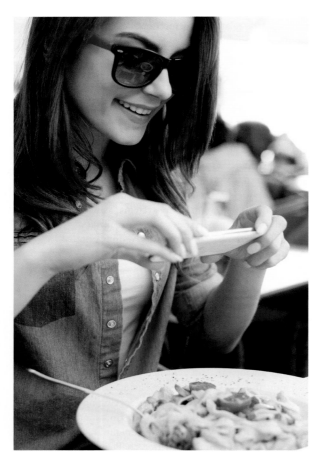

Next to breathing and hydrating, eating is the most essential of all bodily requirements. For this reason, it is sometimes considered a simple matter. Nothing could in fact be further from the truth. Continuing advances in nutrition science, genetics and genomics show how complex the many biochemical processes involved in nutrition are, while the dramatically increasing rate of population growth is placing unprecedented strains on natural and man-made food systems alike. Nutrition is anything but simple.

The world's population is growing at an unprecedented rate, and is due to pass the 7.5 billion mark as this book is just about to go to press. It is also ageing, with people living longer than ever, especially in the developed world. Yet even as we consider the age-related nutritional needs of our growing populations of senior citizens, we have to recognize that the trend towards ever-increasing life expectancies may not continue, even in the supposedly affluent developed world. We are at a potential tipping point in history.

Not only are poverty and deprivation widespread in some of our most affluent societies; non-communicable diseases (NCDs) also are growing at an unprecedented rate, placing a massive strain on current healthcare and social protection systems and promising a level of demand in years to come that will be patently unsustainable. NCDs have replaced communicable diseases as the greatest threat to human life. Yet – irony of ironies – many of these NCDs are directly attributable to changing lifestyles and, in particular, changing dietary habits.

The trend towards highly processed foods and beverages containing high levels of sugar, salt and saturated fats is leading to an epidemic growth in cardiovascular disease, obesity and type 2 diabetes. This has happened in the course of a generation, in most parts of the world. It will take much longer than a generation to bring under control. At the same time, the nutritional inadequacy of many contemporary diets has led to the reappearance in the developed worlds of dietary deficiency diseases that not long ago were considered to have been eliminated, with cases of rickets (vitamin D deficiency) and scurvy (vitamin C deficiency), for example, making the headlines in the countries of the developed world. One thing is clear: the traditional division between the "developed" and the "developing" world is not as neat as it used to be. While the developing world still carries a massive burden of poverty and nutritional deprivation, many nutritional problems are shared across the globe: the same challenges present themselves not only on the streets of ever-more crowded cities but also in increasingly depopulated rural areas. Changes in food habits around the world are creating populations whose health status will place unprecedented burdens on health systems. Unless something is done to reverse current trends, the world's ever-growing population will also be increasingly ill-equipped to help solve the planet's problems. Whether we have a lot or a little on our plate, literally or metaphorically, we are staring at a ticking time bomb.

Defusing that time bomb will call for a concerted effort – not just from governments, but also from non-governmental organizations, the private sector, and civil society, working across sectors, regions, cultures and religions. There has arguably never been a time when the individual has had such potential to shape his or her own future, and the future of the world with it, through his or her dietary choices. Nor has there ever been a moment when concerted "systems" thinking about nutrition has been so necessary – and concerted action, even more so.

The global nutrition community has become both more interdisciplinary and closer-knit in recent years, as the effects of globalization have made themselves felt in every corner of the world. If there is much to alarm us in the spread of industrialized eating patterns, massive food wastage and the state of chronic micronutrient deficiency known as "hidden hunger," there is also reason for hope. The Millennium Development goals brought us closer to one another. The Sustainable Development Goals will bring us closer still, as we strive to work together across sectors, frontiers and cultures to provide better nutritional solutions for the world.

As the Editorial Board that has overseen the development of this book, it is our hope that Good Nutrition: Perspectives for the 21st century will help show that we do indeed all share one world, and that poor nutrition has an impact far beyond its effect on the individual who suffers from an inadequate diet, wherever he or she may be. We also hope that this book will help point the way towards practical solutions based on trusted science and robust programming – multisector and multidisciplinary solutions that offer improved nutritional value while at the same time helping to protect the fragile ecological balance of our planet. Our thanks go to all the distinguished experts who have graciously made themselves available to contribute to this important work, and to everyone else who has helped to make it happen.

Nutritious, accessible, affordable and sustainable food for all is possible – if we all work together to make it a reality.

Manfred Eggersdorfer

Senior Vice President, DSM Nutritional Products (Member of the Leadership Council DSM Nutritional Products); Head of DSM Nutrition Science & Advocacy, Kaiseraugst, Switzerland; Honorary Professor Healthy Ageing at the University Groningen, the Netherlands

John B Cordaro

Global Food Security, Nutrition and Safety Consultant, Mars, Incorporated

Mike Gibney

Emeritus Professor of Food and Health at University College Dublin, Institute of Food and Health

Alain B Labrique

Director, Johns Hopkins University Global mHealth Initiative & Associate Professor Department of International Health/ Epidemiology (jt) Johns Hopkins Bloomberg School of Public Health Baltimore, MA, USA; Department of Community-Public Health, Johns Hopkins School of Nursing (jt); Division of Health Sciences Informatics, Johns Hopkins School of Medicine (jt)

Klaus Kraemer

Managing Director of *Sight and Life* Foundation, and Adjunct Associate Professor in the Department of International Health of Johns Hopkins Bloomberg School of Public Health, Baltimore, MA, USA

Jess Fanzo

Bloomberg Distinguished Associate Professor of Global Food and Agriculture Policy and Ethics at the Berman Institute of Bioethics and the Nitze School of Advanced International Studies at the Johns Hopkins University, Baltimore, MA, USA, and Director of the Global Food Ethics and Policy Program

Eileen Kennedy

Professor of Nutrition and former Dean of the Tufts University, Friedman School of Nutrition Science and Policy, Medford, MA, USA

Jonathan Steffen

Managing Director, Jonathan Steffen Limited, Cambridge, UK (Technical Editor)

How to Use this Book

Good Nutrition: Perspectives for the 21st century builds upon *The Road to Good Nutrition: A global perspective*, which was published by Karger in 2013 and which won First Prize in the Health and Social Care category of the British Medical Association Book Awards 2014.

Apart from its obviously greater length and greater number of contributors, the current volume differs from its predecessor in two essential respects. First, it is set firmly within the context of the United Nations Sustainable Development Goals (SDGs), which were officially ushered in on January 1, 2016. Second, it gives its attention to both the developed and the developing worlds, juxtaposing the nutrition challenges of different regions of the globe in order to highlight not only the gulf that separates the "haves" from the "have-nots" but also the many problems that are now common to all societies worldwide.

Like its predecessor, *Good Nutrition: Perspectives for the 21st century* is written with the general reader in mind, and offers insights and opinions from some of the world's most influential and respected experts in the field. Although such a book can never aim to be definitive, or even comprehensive, we are pleased to present here the expertise of specialists drawn from five continents, and from a wide range of nutrition-related disciplines.

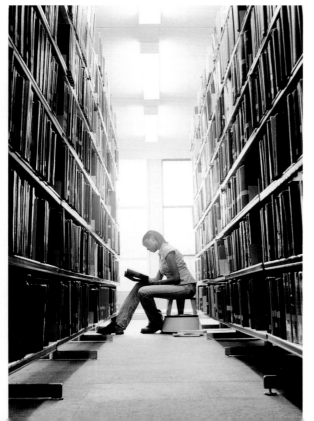

Good Nutrition: Perspectives for the 21st century is written in five sections, each divided into numbered chapters. Commencing with a view of "a world hungry for nutrition", the narrative explores the economics of nutrition and malnutrition and moves on to discuss a wide range of tried and tested, evidence-based approaches and interventions that can improve the nutritional status of at-risk groups. And there are virtually no groups in today's world that are not exposed to risks in some way, whether in the light of broken food systems, faddish diets or rampant consumerism.

There is a strong case, therefore, for reading the chapters in sequential order. Nevertheless each chapter is fully self-contained and offers recommendations for further reading, thus inviting the reader to dive deeper into the individual topic, beyond the parameters of the present publication. We hope the book will appeal to the general reader seeking a coherent panorama of a complex and rapidly evolving field, and that it will also provide inspiration for the specialist wishing to pursue a specific avenue of investigation with the help of an experienced and trustworthy guide.

Each chapter follows approximately the same format, opening with key messages and ending with a personal conclusion from the author(s). Graphics from a wide variety of sources have been used to interpret and enrich the flow of the narrative. These have been recreated in the house style of the book and their source acknowledged. Case studies, stories and thought pieces have likewise been quoted from a variety of sources and their original publication details provided. Where necessary in view of the constraints of space, these have been abridged, but they have not been otherwise re-edited or re-formulated. The Editorial Board gratefully acknowledges the use of all material drawn from the public realm and re-presented in this volume. In furnishing such a wide variety of graphic, and also photographic, material to complement the main argumentation of the book, we hope to provide the reader with a powerful impression of the global nature of (mal-) nutrition and of the pressing need for multisectoral solutions worldwide.

Good Nutrition: Perspectives for the 21st century moves a significant step beyond its predecessor volume, *The Road to Good Nutrition*. The case for good nutrition for all people, in all parts of the globe, throughout the entire life-cycle, is growing stronger all the time. And the means to deliver it at scale are available as never before.

Contents

Key Definitions

Acute malnutrition (also known as wasting)
Reflects a recent and severe process that has led to substantial weight loss, usually associated with starvation and/or disease. Acute malnutrition is calculated by comparing the weight-for-height (WFH) of a child with a reference population of well-nourished and healthy children. Often used to assess the severity of emergencies because it is strongly related to mortality.[1]

Aflatoxin
A toxin produced by mold that can damage the liver and may lead to liver cancer. Aflatoxins cause cancer in some animals. The fungi that produce aflatoxin grow on crops such as peanuts (especially) and wheat, corn, beans and rice. Aflatoxin is a problem particularly in undeveloped and developing countries.[2]

Anemia
A medical condition in which the red blood cell count or hemoglobin is less than normal. For men, anemia is typically defined as hemoglobin level of less than 13.5 gram/100 ml and in women as hemoglobin of less than 12.0 gram/100 ml. Anemia is caused by either a decrease in production of red blood cells or hemoglobin, or an increase in loss (usually due to bleeding) or destruction of red blood cells.[3]

Anorexia
A psychiatric condition, which is part of a group of eating disorders. The cause of anorexia has not been definitively established, but self-esteem and body-image issues, societal pressures, and genetic factors likely each play a role. Anorexia affects females far more often than males and is most common in adolescent females.[4]

Benefit corporation
Also known as B corp. A type of corporate structure recognized by some state governments in the United States. In addition to being profitable, a benefit corporation assumes the legal responsibility of considering its impact on society and the environment. The goal of the corporate structure is to encourage for-profit companies to identify social missions and demonstrate corporate sustainability efforts. In exchange, the corporation may be eligible for certain types of legal protection, bidding protection or tax benefits.[5]

Biofortification
The practice of deliberately increasing the content of an essential micronutrient, i.e., vitamins and minerals (including trace elements) in a food, so as to improve the nutritional quality of the food supply and provide a public health benefit with minimal risk to health. Biofortification differs from conventional fortification in that biofortification aims to increase nutrient levels in crops during plant growth rather than through manual means during processing of the crops.[6]

Birth rate
The proportion of births in a defined population.

Body mass index (BMI)
A nutritional index based on anthropometry, used for the assessment of acute malnutrition in adults. It is measured using weight/height^2 (kg/m^2).[7]

Centers for Disease Control and Prevention (CDC)
CDC works 24/7 to protect America from health, safety and security threats, both foreign and in the US. Whether diseases start at home or abroad, are chronic or acute, curable or preventable, human error or deliberate attack, CDC fights disease and supports communities and citizens to do the same.[8]

Chronic malnutrition
Chronic malnutrition, also known as stunting, is a sign of "shortness" and develops over a long period of time. In children and adults, it is measured through the height-for-age nutritional index.[9]

Committee on World Food Security
The foremost inclusive international and intergovernmental platform for all stakeholders to work together to ensure food security and nutrition for all. The Committee reports to the UN General Assembly through the Economic and Social Council (ECOSOC) and to the FAO Conference.[10]

Common results framework
Government ministries and other stakeholders in SUN countries are aligning their efforts to scale up nutrition using Common Results Frameworks (CRFs). These frameworks ensure that all share the same goals and implement effective and aligned actions to achieve these goals. Country CRFs include both specific nutrition interventions and nutrition-sensitive approaches to development.[11]

Complementary feeding

The transition from exclusive breastfeeding to complementary feeding typically covers the period from 6 to 24 months of age. This is a critical period of growth during which nutrient deficiencies and illnesses contribute globally to higher rates of undernutrition among children under five years of age. The SUN Movement aligns with the WHO recommendation that infants should be exclusively breastfed for the first six months of life to achieve optimal growth, development and health. Thereafter, infants should receive nutritionally adequate and safe complementary foods, while continuing to breastfeed for up to two years or more.[12]

Convergent innovation

A pragmatic, solution-oriented framework to help decision-makers incorporate the social objectives of nutrition into the economic mission of business, while ensuring that economic viability is better integrated into organizations focused on social benefit.

COP 21 (the United Nations Climate Change Conference)

The international political response to climate change began at the Rio Earth Summit in 1992, where the "Rio Convention" included the adoption of the UN Framework Convention on Climate Change (UNFCCC). This convention set out a framework for action aimed at stabilizing atmospheric concentrations of greenhouse gases (GHGs) to avoid "dangerous anthropogenic interference with the climate system." The UNFCCC which entered into force on 21 March 1994 now has a near-universal membership of 195 parties. The main objective of the annual Conference of Parties (COP) is to review the Convention's implementation. The first COP took place in Berlin in 1995.[13]

Coronary heart disease (CHD)

A narrowing of the small blood vessels that supply blood and oxygen to the heart. CHD is also called coronary artery disease. Coronary heart disease is the leading cause of death in the United States for men and women. Coronary heart disease is caused by the buildup of plaque in the arteries to [the] heart. This may also be called hardening of the arteries.[14]

Coverage

The proportion of the target population reached by an intervention. Coverage is a key indicator for monitoring and evaluating interventions.[15]

Creutzfeldt-Jakob disease (CJD)

A rare, degenerative brain disorder. Symptoms usually start around age 60. Memory problems, behavior changes, vision problems, and poor muscle coordination progress quickly to dementia, coma, and death. Most patients die within a year.[16]

Cardiovascular disease (CVD)

CVD includes all the diseases of the heart and circulation including coronary heart disease, angina, heart attack, congenital heart disease and stroke. It is also known as heart and circulatory disease. Other types of cardiovascular disease include heart valve disease and cardiomyopathy.[17]

Demographic and health surveys (DHS)

The DHS project, funded primarily by the US Agency for International Development (USAID) with support from other donors and host countries, has conducted over 230 nationally representative and internationally comparable household surveys in more than 80 countries since its inception in 1984. DHS evolved from World Fertility Surveys and Contraceptive Prevalence Surveys implemented in the 1970s and 1980s.[18]

Developmental origins of health and disease (DOHaD) paradigm

A conceptual paradigm used to describe a cluster of phenomena and processes that link the environmental conditions of the early life with the state of health and risk of disease in later life.[19]

Diabetes

Type 1 diabetes, also sometimes called juvenile-onset diabetes or insulin-dependent diabetes, is a chronic condition in which the pancreas produces little or no insulin. Type 2 diabetes, also sometimes called adult-onset or non-insulin-dependent diabetes, is a chronic condition that affects the way the body metabolizes sugars. With type 2 diabetes, the body either resists the effects of insulin or else does not produce enough insulin. "Diabesity" is a term coined by Dr Francine Kaufman to indicate a combination of diabetes and obesity.

Diarrhea

The presence of three or more loose or fluid stools over a 24-hour period, accompanied or not by blood, mucous or fever. Diarrhea is caused by various bacteria or by viruses, or may be a symptom of other infections. Diarrhea is one of the major killers of young children in developing countries and in emergencies.[20]

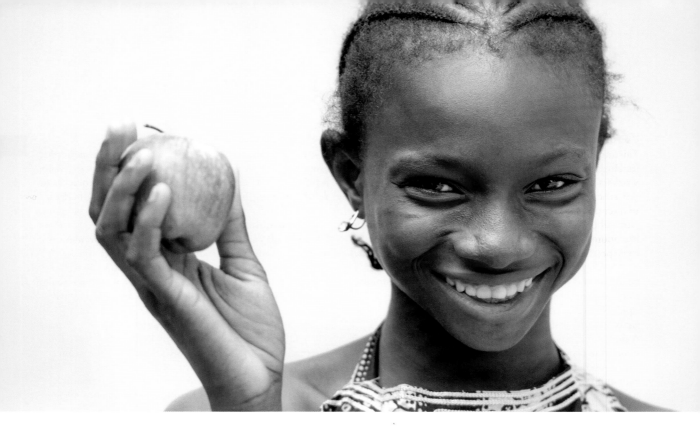

Disability-adjusted life years(DALYs)
A measure of overall disease burden expressed as the number of years lost due to ill-health disability or early death.[21]

Doha
The Doha Round of world trade negotiations – also known as the Doha Development Agenda – was launched in Doha, Qatar in November 2001. The talks aimed at further liberalizing trade, whilst making it easier for developing countries, particularly Least Developed Countries (LDCs), to integrate into the WTO multilateral system.[22]

Double burden of malnutrition[23]
The "double burden of malnutrition" is defined as the coexistence of undernutrition and overweight in the same community or even the same household.

Early warning system
An information system designed to monitor indicators that may predict or forewarn of impending food shortages or famine.[24]

El Niño
A warm ocean current of variable intensity that develops after late December along the coast of Ecuador and Peru and sometimes causes catastrophic weather conditions.[25]

Endemic disease
An infectious disease that occurs throughout the year in a population, such as malaria, worms or chest infections.[26]

Enrichment
When micronutrients lost or removed during food processing are added back or restored in the final product (e.g., wheat flour is enriched with vitamin B_1, niacin and iron).[27]

ENSO
El Niño / Southern Oscillation.

Essential fatty acids (EFAs)
Fatty acids that cannot be constructed within an organism from other components by any known chemical pathways, and therefore must be obtained from food sources, such as flaxseed oil and sunflower oil.[28]

Exclusive breastfeeding (adapted from WHO definition)
Breast milk contains all the nutrients an infant needs in the first six months of life. It protects against common childhood diseases such as diarrhea and pneumonia, and may also have longer-term benefits such as lowering mean blood pressure and cholesterol, and reducing the prevalence of obesity and type-2 diabetes. The SUN Movement aligns with the WHO recommendation on exclusive breastfeeding whereby infants receive only breast milk, no other liquids or solids – not even water – for the first six months of life, to achieve optimal growth, development and health. Thereafter, infants should receive nutritionally adequate and safe complementary foods, while continuing to breastfeed for up to two years or more.[29]

Fairtrade

Fairtrade is about better prices, decent working conditions, local sustainability, and fair terms of trade for farmers and workers in the developing world. By requiring companies to pay sustainable prices (which must never fall lower than the market price), Fairtrade addresses the injustices of conventional trade, which traditionally discriminates against the poorest, weakest producers. It enables them to improve their position and have more control over their lives.[30]

Food4Me

An EU-funded project whose aims are to determine the application of personalized nutrition, through the development of suitable business models, research on technological advances, and validation of delivery methods for personalized nutrition advice, and to compile current scientific knowledge and consumer understanding of personalized nutrition – including best practice communication strategies and ethical boundaries – to be shared with the EU institutions, the food industry, and other stakeholders.[31]

Food access

Income or other resources are adequate to obtain sufficient and appropriate food through home production, buying, barter, gathering, etc. Food may be available but not accessible to people who do not have adequate land to cultivate or enough money to buy it.[32]

Food aid

In-kind rations of food, which can be sourced locally, regionally or internationally.[33]

Food dollar

The food dollar series measures annual expenditures by US consumers on domestically produced food. This data series is composed of three primary series – the marketing bill series, the industry group series, and the primary factor series – that shed light on different aspects of the food supply chain. The three series show three different ways to split up the same food dollar.[34]

Food fortification

The addition of one or more essential nutrients to a food, whether or not it is normally contained in the food, for the purpose of preventing or correcting a demonstrated deficiency of one or more nutrients in the population or specific population groups (FAO/WHO 1994).[35]

Food loss

The decrease in edible food mass at the production, post-harvest, processing and distribution stages in the food supply chain. These losses are mainly caused by inefficiencies in the food supply chains, like poor infrastructure and logistics, lack of technology, insufficient skills, knowledge and management capacity of supply chain actors, no access to markets. In addition, natural disasters play a role.

Food miles

The distance between the place where food is grown or made and the place where it is eaten.[36]

Food wastage

Any food lost by wear or waste. Thus, the wastage is here used to cover both food loss and food waste.[37]

Food waste

Food which is fit for consumption being discarded, usually at retail and consumer level. This is a major problem in industrialized nations, where throwing away is often cheaper than using or re-using, and consumers can afford to waste food. Accordingly, food waste is usually avoidable.

Food assistance

The set of interventions designed to provide access to food to vulnerable and food insecure populations. Generally included are instruments like food transfers, vouchers and cash transfers to ensure access to food of a given quantity, quality or value.[38]

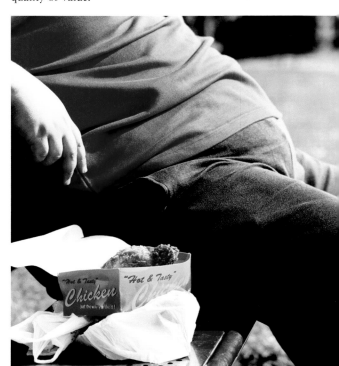

Food security

Food security exists when all people, at all times, have physical and economic access to sufficient safe and nutritious food that meets their dietary needs and food preferences for an active and healthy life.

Fortificant

The vitamins and minerals added to fortified foods.[39]

Genetically modified organisms (GMOs)

Genetically modified organisms (GMOs) can be defined as organisms (i.e., plants, animals or microorganisms) in which the genetic material (DNA) has been altered in a way that does not occur naturally by mating and/or natural recombination. The technology is often called "modern biotechnology" or "gene technology", sometimes also "recombinant DNA technology" or "genetic engineering." It allows selected individual genes to be transferred from one organism into another, also between nonrelated species. Foods produced from or using GM organisms are often referred to as GM foods.[40]

GINI index

A measurement of the income distribution of a country's residents. This number, which ranges between 0 and 1 and is based on residents' net income, helps define the gap between the rich and the poor, with 0 representing perfect equality and 1 representing perfect inequality. It is typically expressed as a percentage, referred to as the Gini coefficient.[41]

Global Nutrition Report

The *Global Nutrition Report 2015* is a report card on the world's nutrition – globally, regionally, and country by country – and on efforts to improve it. It assesses countries' progress in meeting global nutrition targets established by the World Health Assembly. It documents how well countries, aid donors, NGOs, businesses, and others are meeting the commitments they made at the major Nutrition for Growth summit in 2013. And it spells out the actions that have proven effective in combating malnutrition in all its forms.[42]

Governance

"The manner in which power is exercised in the management of a country's economic and social resources for development."[43]

GPS

A navigational system using satellite signals to fix the location of a radio receiver on or above the earth's surface; also: the radio receiver so used.[44]

Greenhouse gases (GHG)

Gases that trap heat in the atmosphere: carbon dioxide (CO_2), methane (CH_4), nitrous oxide (N_2O), and fluorinated gases (hydrofluorocarbons, perfluorocarbons, sulfur hexafluoride, and nitrogen trifluoride).[45]

Growth standard

Nutritional indices are compared to expected anthropometric values for an individual of the same sex and age. A growth standard is based on prescriptive criteria and involves value or normative judgments.[46]

Healthcare system

All organizations and institutions involved in the delivery of health services, including governmental, non-governmental, private organizations and institutions.[47]

Heavy metals

Arsenic, beryllium, cadmium, chromium, lead, manganese, mercury, nickel, and selenium are some of the metals (called "heavy" because of their high relative atomic mass) which persist in nature and can cause damage or death in animals, humans, and plants even at very low concentrations (1 or 2 micrograms in some cases). Used in industrial processes, they are carried by air and water when discharged in the environment. Since heavy metals have a propensity to accumulate in selective body organs (such as brain and liver) their prescribed average safety levels in food or water are often misleadingly high.[48]

Hidden hunger

Occurs when a population that may be consuming enough calories is not receiving enough micronutrients (vitamins and minerals), negatively impacting the health, cognitive development and economic development of over 2 billion people worldwide.[49]

High density lipoprotein (HDL) cholesterol

Lipoproteins, which are combinations of fats (lipids) and proteins, are the form in which lipids are transported in the blood. HDLs transport cholesterol from the tissues of the body to the liver, so the cholesterol can be eliminated in the bile. HDL cholesterol is therefore considered the "good" cholesterol: The higher the HDL cholesterol level, the lower the risk of coronary artery disease.[50]

Hunger

A weakened condition brought about by prolonged lack of food. Hunger can lead to malnutrition.[51]

Human genome

All the genetic information in a person. The human genome is made up of the DNA in chromosomes as well as the DNA in mitochondria.[52]

Hypertension

Abnormally high blood pressure and especially arterial blood pressure; also the systemic condition accompanying high blood pressure.[53]

Industrial fortification

Fortification involves the addition of nutrients to foods irrespective of whether or not the nutrients were originally present in the food. Fortification is a means of improving the nutritional status of a population (or potentially a sub-population). Some foods are fortified by law (e.g., white bread), others voluntarily (e.g., breakfast cereals, fat spreads).[54]

Infant

A child less than 12 months old.[55]

Infant formula

A breast milk substitute formulated industrially in accordance with applicable Codex Alimentarius standards to satisfy the normal nutritional requirements of infants up to six months of age.[56]

Information, education and communication (IEC)

Methods of providing people with an informed base for making choices. Nutrition information refers to knowledge, such as information about new foods that are being introduced in an emergency situation. Nutrition education refers to training or orientation for a particular purpose such as support for breastfeeding. Nutrition communication refers to the method by which information is imparted.[57]

IPCC

The Intergovernmental Panel on Climate Change (IPCC) is the leading international body for the assessment of climate change. It was established by the United Nations Environment Programme (UNEP) and the World Meteorological Organization (WMO) in 1988 to provide the world with a clear scientific view on the current state of knowledge about climate change and its potential environmental and socioeconomic impacts. In the same year, the UN General Assembly endorsed the action by WMO and UNEP in jointly establishing the IPCC.[58]

Ischemic heart disease

Ischemic cardiomyopathy (IC) is a condition that occurs when the heart muscle is weakened. In this condition, the left ventricle, which is the main heart muscle, is usually enlarged and dilated. This condition can be a result of a heart attack or coronary artery disease, a narrowing of the arteries. These narrowed arteries keep blood from reaching portions of the heart. The weakened heart muscle inhibits the heart's ability to pump blood and can lead to heart failure.[59]

Kyoto Protocol

The Kyoto Protocol treaty was negotiated in December 1997 at the city of Kyoto, Japan and came into force February 16th, 2005. The Kyoto Protocol is a legally binding agreement under which industrialized countries will reduce their collective emissions of greenhouse gases by 5.2% compared to the year 1990. The goal is to lower overall emissions from six greenhouse gases – carbon dioxide, methane, nitrous oxide, sulfur hexafluoride, HFCs, and PFCs – calculated as an average over the five-year period of 2008–12. National targets range from 8% reductions for the European Union and some others to 7% for the US, 6% for Japan, 0% for Russia, and permitted increases of 8% for Australia and 10% for Iceland."[60]

La Niña

El Niño and La Niña are opposite phases of what is known as the El Niño-Southern Oscillation (ENSO) cycle. The ENSO cycle is a scientific term that describes the fluctuations in temperature between the ocean and atmosphere in the east-central Equatorial Pacific (approximately between the International Date Line and 120 degrees West). La Niña is sometimes referred to as the cold phase of ENSO and El Niño as the warm phase of ENSO. These deviations from normal surface temperatures can have large-scale impacts not only on ocean processes, but also on global weather and climate.[60]

Life cycle assessment (LCA)

Life Cycle Assessment (LCA) is a tool for the systematic evaluation of the environmental aspects of a product or service system through all stages of its life cycle. LCA provides an adequate instrument for environmental decision support. Reliable LCA performance is crucial to achieve a life-cycle economy. The International Organization for Standardization (ISO), a world-wide federation of national standards bodies, has standardized this framework within the series ISO 14040 on LCA.[62]

Lipid-based nutrient supplement (SQ-LNS)

The term "lipid-based nutrient supplements" (LNS) refers generically to a range of fortified, lipid-based products, including products like Ready-to-Use Therapeutic Foods (RUTF) (a large daily ration with relatively low micronutrient concentration) as well as highly concentrated supplements (1-4 teaspoons/day, providing < 100 kcal/day) to be used for "point-of-use" fortification. RUTF have been successfully used for the management of severe acute malnutrition (SAM) among children in emergency settings.[63]

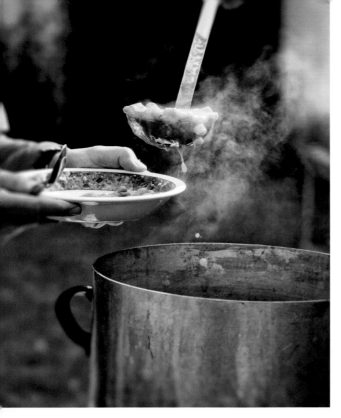

Listeriosis

A serious infection usually caused by eating food contaminated with the bacterium Listeria monocytogenes. The disease primarily affects older adults, pregnant women, newborns, and adults with weakened immune systems. However, rarely, people without these risk factors can also be affected.[64]

LMICs

Lower- and middle-income countries. WHO Member States are grouped into four income groups (low, lower-middle, upper-middle, and high) based on the World Bank list of analytical income classification of economies for fiscal year 2014, which is based on the 2012 Atlas gross national income per capita estimates (released July 2013). See the Notes sheet in each spreadsheet for more information.[65]

Low density lipoprotein (LDL) cholesterol

Low-density lipoprotein cholesterol [is] commonly referred to as "bad" cholesterol. Elevated LDL levels are associated with an increased risk of heart disease. Lipoproteins, which are combinations of fats (lipids) and proteins, are the form in which lipids are transported in the blood. Low-density lipoproteins transport cholesterol from the liver to the tissues of the body.[66]

Macronutrients

Nutrients that humans consume in the largest quantities which provide bulk energy and are needed for a wide range of body functions and processes. The three macronutrients are fat, protein and carbohydrate.[67]

Malnutrition

A condition resulting when a person's diet does not provide adequate nutrients for growth and maintenance or if they are unable to fully utilize the food they eat due to illness.[68]

mHealth

A general term for the use of mobile phones and other wireless technology in medical care.[69]

Micronutrient deficiency (MND)

A lack or shortage of a micronutrient, such as a vitamin or mineral, that is essential in small amounts for the proper growth and metabolism of a human or other living organism.[70]

Micronutrient powder (MNP)

Single-dose packets of vitamins and minerals in powder form that can be sprinkled onto any ready to eat semi-solid food consumed at home, school or any other point of use. The powders are used to increase the micronutrient content of a child's diet without changing their usual dietary habits.[71]

Micronutrients

Essential vitamins and minerals required by the body throughout the lifecycle in miniscule amounts.[72]

Millennium Development Goals (MDGs)

At the Millennium Summit in September 2000 the largest gathering of world leaders in history adopted the UN Millennium Declaration, committing their nations to a new global partnership to reduce extreme poverty and setting out a series of time-bound targets, with a deadline of 2015, that have become known as the Millennium Development Goals. The Millennium Development Goals (MDGs) are quantified targets for addressing extreme poverty in its many dimensions – income poverty, hunger, disease, lack of adequate shelter, and exclusion – while promoting gender equality, education, and environmental sustainability. They are also basic human rights – the rights of each person on the planet to health, education, shelter, and security.[73]

Moderate acute malnutrition (MAM)

Acute malnutrition, also known as wasting, develops as a result of recent rapid weight loss or a failure to gain weight. The degree of acute malnutrition is classified as either moderate or severe. Moderate malnutrition is defined by a mid-upper arm circumference (MUAC) between 115 mm and <125 mm or a WFH between -3 z-score and <-2 z-score of the median (WHO standards) or WFH as a percentage of the median 70% and <80% (National Center for Health Statistics [NCHS] references).[74]

Multiple Indicator Cluster Surveys (MICS)

An international household survey initiative developed by UNICEF to assist countries in filling data gaps for monitoring human development in general and the situation of children and women in particular.[75]

Multistakeholder platform

A shared space for cross-sector stakeholders – including government representatives, civil society, UN agencies, donors, businesses and the research and technical community – to come together within a SUN country to align activities and take joint responsibility for scaling up nutrition, including setting shared targets and coordinated, costed plans of action.[76]

Mycotoxins

A group of naturally occurring chemicals produced by certain molds. They can grow on a variety of different crops and foodstuffs including cereals, nuts, spices, dried fruits, apple juice and coffee, often under warm and humid conditions. The mycotoxins of most concern from a food safety perspective include the aflatoxins (B_1, B_2, G_1, G_2 and M_1), ochratoxin A, patulin and toxins produced by Fusarium molds, including fumonisins (B_1, B_2 and B_3), trichothecenes (principally nivalenol, deoxynivalenol, T-2 and HT-2 toxin) and zearalenone.[77]

Non-communicable diseases (NCDs)[6]

Non-communicable diseases (NCDs) – also known as chronic diseases – are not transmitted from person to person. NCDs can progress slowly and persist in the body for decades. The main types of NCDs include cardiovascular disease, cancers, respiratory diseases and diabetes.

Non-profits (NPOs)

Associations, charities, cooperatives, and other voluntary organizations formed to further cultural, educational, religious, professional, or public service objectives. Their startup funding is provided by their members, trustees, or others who do not expect repayment, and who do not share in the organization's profits or losses which are retained or absorbed. Approved, incorporated, or registered NPOs are usually granted tax exemptions, and contributions to them are often tax deductible. Most non-governmental organizations (NGOs) are NPOs.[78]

Nutrient use efficiency (NUE)

Nutrient use efficiency (NUE) is a measure of how well plants use the available mineral nutrients. It can be defined as yield (biomass) per unit input (fertilizer, nutrient content). NUE is a complex trait: it depends on the ability to take up the nutrients from the soil, but also on transport, storage, mobilization, usage within the plant, and even on the environment. NUE is of particular interest as a major target for crop improvement.[79]

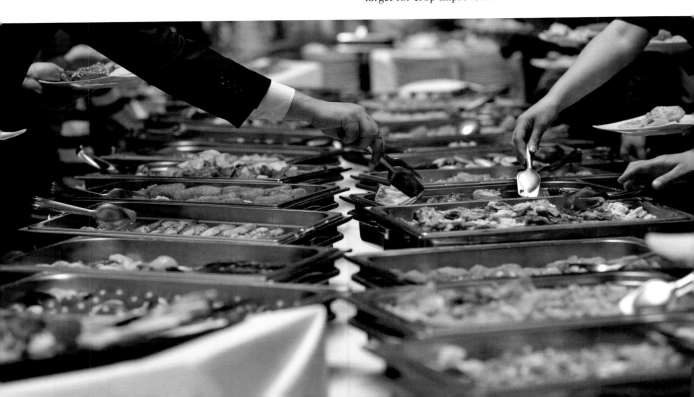

Nutrient-rich foods (NRF) score

A formal scoring system that ranks foods on the basis of their nutrient content. When used in conjunction with a food prices database, it can help identify foods that are both nutritious and affordable.[80]

Nutrition security

Achieved when secure access to an appropriately nutritious diet is coupled with a sanitary environment, adequate health services and care.[81] Nutrition security exists when, in addition to having access to a healthy and balanced diet, people also have access to adequate caregiving practices and to a safe and healthy environment that allows them to stay healthy and utilize the foods they eat effectively.

Nutrition-sensitive interventions and programs

Interventions or programs that address the immediate determinants of fetal and child nutrition and development – adequate food and nutrient intake, feeding, caregiving and parenting practices, and low burden of infectious diseases Examples [include] adolescent, preconception, and maternal health and nutrition; maternal dietary or micronutrient supplementation; promotion of optimum breastfeeding; complementary feeding and responsive feeding practices and stimulation; dietary supplementation; diversification and micronutrient supplementation or fortification for children; treatment of severe acute malnutrition; disease prevention and management; nutrition in emergencies.[82]

Nutrition-specific interventions and programs

Interventions or programs that address the underlying determinants of fetal and child nutrition and development – food security; adequate caregiving resources at the maternal, household and community levels; and access to health services and a safe and hygienic environment – and incorporate specific nutrition goals and actions. Nutrition-sensitive programs can serve as delivery platforms for nutrition-specific interventions, potentially increasing their scale, coverage, and effectiveness. Examples [include] agriculture and food security; social safety nets; early child development; maternal mental health; women's empowerment; child protection; schooling; water, sanitation, and hygiene; health and family planning services.[83]

Nutritional status

The internal state of an individual as it relates to the availability and utilization of nutrients at the cellular level.[84]

Obesity

Obesity for adults is a BMI 30 to 39.99. Morbidly obese for adults is BMI of 40 or greater.

Obesogenic

Promoting excessive weight gain; producing obesity.[85]

Overweight

Overweight for adults is a BMI between 25 and 29.

Personalized nutrition

A conceptual analog to personalized medicine. While there are food products available that address requirements or preferences of specific consumer groups, these products are based on empirical consumer science rather than on nutrigenomics and nutrigenetics. The latter two build the science foundation for understanding human variability in preferences, requirements and responses to diet, and may become the future tools for consumer assessment motivated by personalized nutritional counseling for health maintenance and disease prevention.[86]

Ready-to-use supplementary foods (RUSF)

Energy-dense, mineral- and vitamin-fortified foods that are designed to provide the quantities of macro- and micronutrients needed for the treatment or prevention of moderate acute malnutrition. RUSFs can be eaten without further preparation or cooking and are given as a supplement to the ordinary diet. They have very low moisture content and so can be stored without refrigeration.[87]

Ready-to-use therapeutic foods (RUTF)

Specialized ready-to-eat, portable, shelf-stable products, available as pastes, spreads or biscuits, that are used in a prescribed manner to treat children with severe acute malnutrition.[88]

Recommended dietary allowance (RDA)

The average daily dietary intake level that is sufficient to meet the nutrient requirement of nearly all (97 to 98 percent) healthy individuals in a group.[89]

Salmonella

A bacterial disease of the intestinal tract. Salmonella is a group of bacteria that causes typhoid fever, food poisoning, gastroenteritis, enteric fever and other illnesses. People become infected mostly through contaminated water or foods, especially meat, poultry and eggs.[90]

School feeding
Provision of meals or snacks to schoolchildren to improve nutrition and promote education.[91]

Severe acute malnutrition (SAM)
Acute malnutrition, also known as wasting, develops as a result of recent rapid weight loss or a failure to gain weight. The degree of acute malnutrition is classified as either moderate or severe. A child with severe acute malnutrition is highly vulnerable and has a high mortality risk. Severe acute malnutrition is defined by the presence of bilateral pitting edema or severe wasting, defined by MUAC <115 mm or a WFH <-3 z-score (WHO standards) or WFH <70% of the median [NCHS references]).[92]

Stunting
Low height-for-age measurement used as an indicator of chronic malnutrition, calculated by comparing the height-for-age of a child with a reference population of well-nourished and healthy children.[93]

Supplementation
Provision of nutrients either via a food or as a tablet, capsule, syrup, or powder to boost the nutritional content of the diet.

UN REACH (Renewed Effort Against Child Hunger and Undernutrition)
Established in 2008 by the Food and Agriculture Organization (FAO), the United Nations Children's Fund (UNICEF), the World Food Program (WFP), and the World Health Organization (WHO) to assist governments of countries with a high burden of child and maternal undernutrition to accelerate the scale-up of food and nutrition actions. The International Fund for Agricultural Development (IFAD) joined REACH later on with an advisory role. REACH operates at country level as a facilitating mechanism in the coordination of UN and other partners' support to national nutrition scale-up plans.[1]

Undernutrition
An insufficient intake of energy, protein or micronutrients, that in turn leads to nutritional deficiency. Undernutrition encompasses stunting, wasting and micronutrient deficiencies.[94]

Underweight
Wasting or stunting or a combination of both, defined by weight-for-age below the -2 z-score line.[95]

Value chain
A value chain is the whole series of activities that create and build value at every step. The total value delivered by the company is the sum total of the value built up all throughout the company. Michael Porter developed this concept in his 1980 book "Competitive Advantage."[96]

Vulnerability
The characteristics of a person or group in terms of their capacity to anticipate, cope with, resist and recover from the impact of a natural (or human-made) hazard.[97]

Wasting (also known as acute malnutrition)
Reflects a recent and severe process that has led to substantial weight loss, usually associated with starvation and/or disease. Wasting is calculated by comparing the weight-for-height of a child with a reference population of well-nourished and healthy children. Often used to assessthe severity of emergencies because it is strongly related to mortality.[98]

Z-score
An indicator of how far a measurement is from the median, also known as a standard deviation (SD) score. The reference lines on the growth charts (labeled 1, 2, 3, -1, -2, -3) are called z-score lines; they indicate how far points are above or below the median z-score = 0).[99] Severely wasted is below the -3 z-score line.[100]

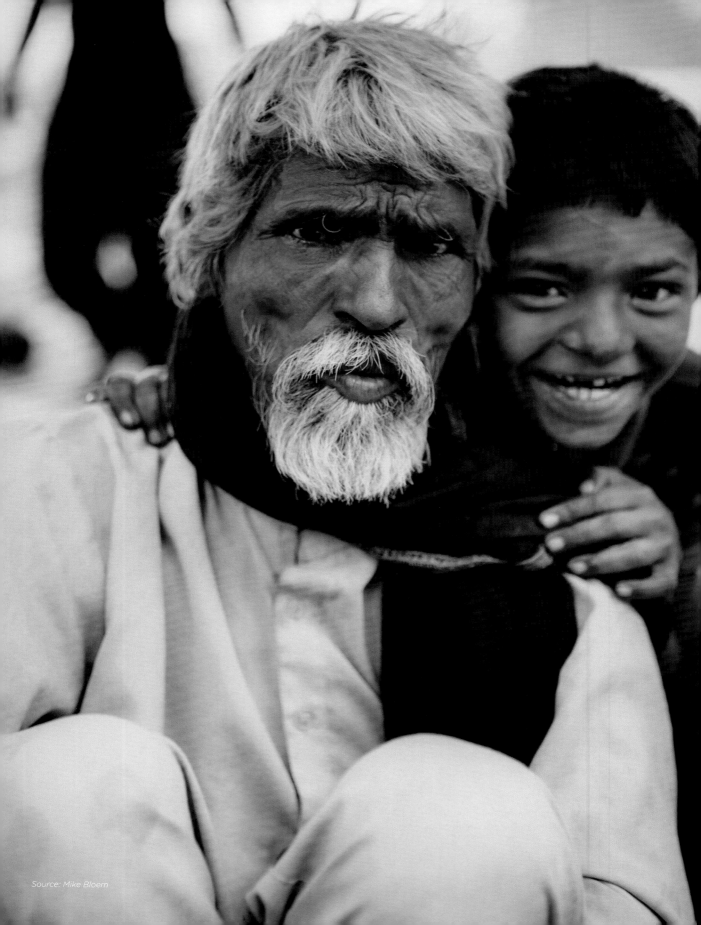

This glossary draws on a variety of sources. The provenance of individual definitions is indicated by a reference as follows:

1 UNICEF SUN 2012.

2 *http://www.medicinenet.com/script/main/art.asp?articlekey=10796.*

3 *http://www.medicinenet.com/script/main/art.asp?articlekey=10796.*

4 *http://www.medicinenet.com/anorexia_nervosa/article.htm.*

5 *http://searchcio.techtarget.com/definition/B-Corporation-Benefit-Corporation.*

6 *http://www.who.int/elena/titles/biofortification/en/.*

7 *UNICEF Training on Nutrition in Emergencies, Glossary of Terms.*

8 *http://www.cdc.gov/about/organization/mission.htm.*

9 *UNICEF Training on Nutrition in Emergencies, Glossary of Terms.*

10 *http://www.fao.org/cfs/en/.*

11 UNICEF SUN 2012.

12 UNICEF SUN 2012.

13 *http://www.cop21paris.org/about/cop21/.*

14 *https://medlineplus.gov/ency/article/007115.htm.*

15 *UNICEF Training on Nutrition in Emergencies, Glossary of Terms.*

16 *https://vsearch.nlm.nih.gov/vivisimo/cgi-bin/query-meta?v%3Aproject=medlineplus&v%3Asources=medlineplus-bundle&query=Creutzfeldt-Jakob&_ga=1.222425627.1811378850.1470854676.*

17 *https://www.bhf.org.uk/heart-health/conditions/cardiovascular-disease.*

18 *http://www.who.int/bulletin/volumes/90/8/11-095513/en/.*

19 *https://www.novapublishers.com/catalog/product_info.php?products_id=51866&osCsid=5e9a553a1b1129fed10cc0ad3598a587.*

20 *UNICEF Training on Nutrition in Emergencies, Glossary of Terms.*

21 *http://www.disabled-world.com/definitions/daly.php.*

22 *http://ec.europa.eu/trade/policy/eu-and-wto/doha-development-agenda/index_en.htm.*

23 *The Lancet 2013 Series on Maternal and Child Nutrition, adapted from Scaling Up Nutrition and Shekar and colleagues, 2013.*

24 *UNICEF Training on Nutrition in Emergencies, Glossary of Terms.*

25 *http://www.dictionary.com/browse/el-nino.*

26 *UNICEF Training on Nutrition in Emergencies, Glossary of Terms.*

27 *UNICEF Training on Nutrition in Emergencies, Glossary of Terms.*

28 *UNICEF Training on Nutrition in Emergencies, Glossary of Terms.*

29 UNICEF SUN 2012.

30 *http://www.fairtrade.org.uk/en/what-is-fairtrade/faqs.*

31 *http://www.food4me.org/about/aims-and-objectives.*

32 *UNICEF Training on Nutrition in Emergencies, Glossary of Terms.*

33 *Omamo SW, Gentilini U, Sandström S (eds). Revolution: From food aid to food assistance. Innovations in overcoming hunger. Rome: WFP, 2010.*

34 *http://www.ers.usda.gov/data-products/food-dollar-series.aspx.*

35 *http://www.fao.org/docrep/W2840E/w2840e0b.htm.*

36 *http://dictionary.cambridge.org/dictionary/english/food-miles.*

37 *Food Wastage Footprint and Environmental Accounting of Food Loss and Waste. Concept Note. Natural Resources Management and Environment Department Food and Agriculture Organization of the United Nations. March 2012.*

38 *Omamo SW, Gentilini U, Sandström S (eds). Revolution: From food aid to food assistance. Innovations in overcoming hunger. Rome: WFP, 2010.*

39 *UNICEF Training on Nutrition in Emergencies, Glossary of Terms.*

40 *http://www.who.int/foodsafety/areas_work/food-technology/faq-genetically-modified-food/en/.*

41 *http://www.investopedia.com/terms/g/gini-index.asp.*

42 *https://www.ifpri.org/publication/global-nutrition-report-2015.*

43 *World Bank, Governance and Development. Washington, DC: World Bank Publications, 1992. http://documents.worldbank.org/curated/en/1992/04/440582/governance-development.*

44 *http://www.merriam-webster.com/dictionary/GPS.*

45 *https://www.epa.gov/ghgemissions/overview-greenhouse-gases.*

46 *UNICEF Training on Nutrition in Emergencies, Glossary of Terms.*

47 *UNICEF Training on Nutrition in Emergencies, Glossary of Terms.*

48 *http://www.businessdictionary.com/definition/heavy-metal.html.*

49 UNICEF SUN 2012.

50 *http://www.medicinenet.com/script/main/art.asp?articlekey=3662*

51 UNICEF SUN 2012.

52 *http://www.medicinenet.com/script/main/art.asp?articlekey=3818.*

53 *http://www.merriam-webster.com/dictionary/hypertension.*

54 *https://www.nutrition.org.uk/nutritionscience/foodfacts/fortification.html.*

55 *UNICEF Training on Nutrition in Emergencies, Glossary of Terms.*

56 *UNICEF Training on Nutrition in Emergencies, Glossary of Terms.*

57 *UNICEF Training on Nutrition in Emergencies, Glossary of Terms.*

58 *http://www.ipcc.ch/organization/organization.shtml.*

59 *http://www.healthline.com/health/ischemic-cardiomyopathy#Overview1.*

60 *http://www.kyotoprotocol.com/.*

61 *http://oceanservice.noaa.gov/facts/ninonina.html.*

62 *http://www.unep.org/resourceefficiency/Consumption/StandardsandLabels/MeasuringSustainability/LifeCycleAssessment/tabid/101348/Default.aspx.*

63 *http://www.ncbi.nlm.nih.gov/pubmed/20055936.*

64 *http://www.cdc.gov/listeria/definition.html.*

65 *http://www.who.int/healthinfo/global_burden_disease/definition_regions/en/.*

66 *http://www.medicinenet.com/script/main/art.asp?articlekey=6233.*

67 *UNICEF Training on Nutrition in Emergencies, Glossary of Terms.*

68 UNICEF SUN 2012.

69 *http://searchhealthit.techtarget.com/definition/mHealth.*

70 *UNICEF Training on Nutrition in Emergencies, Glossary of Terms.*

71 *http://www.who.int/elena/titles/micronutrientpowder_infants/en/.*

72 UNICEF SUN 2012.

73 UNICEF SUN 2012.

74 *UNICEF Training on Nutrition in Emergencies, Glossary of Terms.*

75 *http://www.ceecis.org/mics/printed_material/User_Guide_to_MICS_eng.pdf*

76 UNICEF SUN 2012.

77 *https://www.food.gov.uk/business-industry/farmingfood/mycotoxins.*

78 *http://www.businessdictionary.com/definition/non-profit-organization-NPO.html.*

79 *http://www.springer.com/gp/book/9783319106342.*

80 *http://www.ncbi.nlm.nih.gov/pubmed/20181811.*

81 *UNICEF Training on Nutrition in Emergencies, Glossary of Terms.*

82 *http://www.unicef.org/ethiopia/3_Nutrition-sensitive_interventions_and_programmes_how_can.pdf.*

83 *http://www.unicef.org/ethiopia/3_Nutrition-sensitive_interventions_and_programmes_how_can.pdf.*

84 *UNICEF Training on Nutrition in Emergencies, Glossary of Terms.*

85 *http://www.merriam-webster.com/dictionary/obesogenic.*

86 *http://www.medscape.com/viewarticle/583041.*

87 *UNICEF Training on Nutrition in Emergencies, Glossary of Terms.*

88 UNICEF SUN 2012.

89 *http://www.ncbi.nlm.nih.gov/books/NBK45182/.*

90 *http://www.medicalnewstoday.com/articles/160942.php.*

91 *UNICEF Training on Nutrition in Emergencies, Glossary of Terms.*

92 *UNICEF Training on Nutrition in Emergencies, Glossary of Terms.*

93 UNICEF SUN 2012.

94 *UNICEF Training on Nutrition in Emergencies, Glossary of Terms.*

95 *UNICEF Training on Nutrition in Emergencies, Glossary of Terms.*

96 *http://economictimes.indiatimes.com/definition/value-chain.*

97 *UNICEF Training on Nutrition in Emergencies, Glossary of Terms.*

98 UNICEF SUN 2012.

99 *UNICEF Training on Nutrition in Emergencies, Glossary of Terms.*

100 *UNICEF Training on Nutrition in Emergencies, Glossary of Terms.*

Executive Summary

Good Nutrition: Perspectives for the 21ˢᵗ century is written in five sections.

Section 1: A World Hungry for Nutrition

Section 1 opens with a discussion by Profs. Glenn Denning of Columbia University and Jess Fanzo of Johns Hopkins University of *ten of the key forces shaping the global food system*. This chapter provides a general introduction to this book as a whole, and adumbrates many topics that are discussed in greater detail in the pages that follow. The ten key forces considered by Profs. Denning and Fanzo are: the degradation of natural resources; climate change; urbanization; globalization; consumer behavior; culture and tradition; government policies; conflict and fragile states: technology innovation; and sustainability. The authors argue that in spite of the many challenges facing the planet, there has never been a better time to think and act with sustainable development as our vision. They conclude by observing that the Sustainable Development Goals have the potential to set the global food system on a more sustainable path.

This broad introduction is followed by an in-depth analysis of *the relationship between population growth and malnutrition* presented by Profs. Michael Klag and Parul Christian, both of Johns Hopkins. The authors argue that the speed at which the world's population is increasing poses a wide range of complex challenges for nutritionists, agriculturalists and public health professionals alike – the authors note that there will be a third more mouths to feed by 2050 and that overall population growth will fuel the expansion of urban areas and the rise of urban populations. These developments will impact poor countries more severely than wealthy ones. The chapter concludes with the strong recommendation that family planning is essential to curb population growth.

Dr Shauna Downs of Columbia University and Prof. Jess Fanzo then offer a discussion of *how to manage value chains in order to make them deliver better nutrition*. The authors argue that the nutrition community needs to start thinking in terms of "adding value" in order to improve the quality of the food supply. Making value chains more nutrition-sensitive can help improve the quality of the foods that are available, affordable and acceptable. The chapter explains the merits of value chain analysis, arguing that it can help shape policies that will reorient the incentives in the food system toward the production and consumption of nutritious foods. Applying a "business lens" to tackle food system problems has the potential to lead to real change for the better.

In the next chapter, Prof. Ricardo Uauy of the Universities of London and Chile examines *dietary approaches that can deliver better nutrition*. Observing that changes in diet and physical activity levels are chiefly responsible for the recent increase in nutrition-related chronic diseases, Prof. Uauy puts forward the view the problems of diet-related diseases cannot be addressed by the traditional model of single-nutrient deficiency or excess. Believing that consumers will make healthier dietary choices if they have a practical option to do so, Prof. Uauy makes a strong plea for a return to diets based predominantly on plant foods, with limited processing and a restricted proportion of refined carbohydrates.

Underlining the key role played by the consumer in influencing dietary behaviors, Prof. Adam Drewnowski of the University of Washington concludes this opening review of the big themes in nutrition today with a chapter which argues that there are very practical limits to the freedom of choice available to consumers. *Consumer food choices* are driven by purchasing power and socioeconomic status, and while calories have become cheap, nutrients remain expensive. Eating more calories once used to mean obtaining more nutrients, but this is no longer the case. As empty calories sweep the globe, hidden hunger and obesity are no longer mutually exclusive: it is quite possible to be both undernourished and overweight. Prof. Drewnowski argues that the food industry has an increased responsibility to ensure that the world food supply remains affordable, sustainable, and nutrient-rich.

Section 2: Nutrition, Health and Economic Status

Section 2 considers the economic drivers of malnutrition, and the relationship between good and bad nutrition on the one hand and good and bad health on the other. In two closely twinned chapters, Prof. Susan Horton of the University of Waterloo and Prof. William A Masters of Tufts University present respectively *the costs and the causes of malnutrition*. Prof. Horton points out that nutritional status can no longer automatically be expected to improve with increased income and that targeted public health investments are essential to enhance the nutritional status of many populations around the world. Even high-income countries face issues of "hidden hunger", and the growing rate of obesity is a "one world" issue facing rich and poor countries alike. Prof. Masters points out that for most people, nutritious foods are more widely available and affordable than ever before, yet malnutrition remains the world's leading cause of death and disability. Malnutrition is hard to eradicate, but by identifying the causes of malnutrition, economic analysis

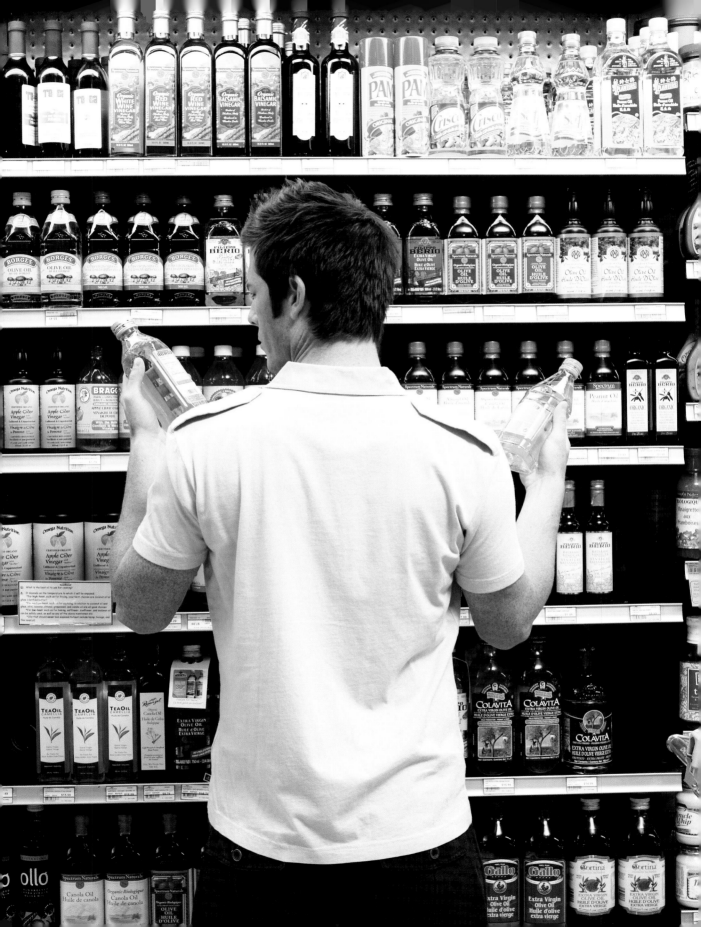

can help guide interventions and support changes that foster better nutrition.

Turning the focus away from economics and towards public health policy, Dr Henry Greenberg and Prof. Richard J Deckelbaum, both of Columbia University Medical Center, argue that there is an urgent need for *new paradigms in the treatment and management of non-communicable diseases* (NCDs). These diseases, which include, for instance, type 2 diabetes and cardiovascular disease, have many risk factors, and lifestyle-altering interventions are necessary to mitigate them. NCDs are very difficult to manage with traditional health measures, but innovative interventions do exist, and can be effectively implemented. The authors argue that, in order to reduce the prevalence of NCDs, public health professionals should engage more actively in the shaping of policies that influence health, while the food industry should be encouraged to offer a portfolio of nutritious food products and food supplements to fill the nutrient gaps.

The concluding chapter of section 2 is dedicated to *the Mediterranean diet.* The benefits of the Mediterranean diet were first attested in the "Seven Countries Study", an epidemiological longitudinal study directed by the American scientist Ancel Keys during the 1950s. The Mediterranean diet offers a range of potential health benefits, reducing susceptibility to cardiovascular disease and supporting the prevention and/or treatment of a variety of non-communicable diseases. Although the Mediterranean diet is a today a convenience phrase, this form of diet occurs in various parts of the globe characterized by a Mediterranean-type climate. No other dietary pattern has such a strong evidential base as the Mediterranean diet to support its benefits on cardiovascular disease, diabetes and other major chronic diseases.

Section 3: Sustainable Food Systems

Section 3 examines ways in which the world's food systems can be made more sustainable. In a chapter entitled *Approaches to Fixing Broken Food Systems,* co-authors Robyn Alders, Mike Nunn, Brigitte Bagnol, Julian Cribb, Richard Kock and Jonathan Rushton (all of the University of Sydney) put forward the view that everyone on the planet belongs to one and the same ecosystem, and that improved health and wellbeing for the world's population and better stewardship of the planet can be achieved by recognizing that adequate food and nutrition is a human right. Stating that food has to regain center stage in our attention, they present a variety of

means for improving nutrition and envisage a future in which consumers will purchase food that has been grown sustainably by farmers who are treated ethically and paid a fair price for their labor, enabling them to tend their land and sustain natural ecosystems.

The following chapter – penned by Madeleine Thomson (International Research Institute for Climate and Society and Columbia University), Lawrence Haddad (formerly at International Food Policy Research Institute and now director of the Global Alliance for Improved Nutrition) and Jess Fanzo – considers the *requirements for mitigating the influence of climate change.* Identifying climate change as one of the biggest global health and food security threats of the 21st century, the authors argue that improved management of seasonal and year-to-year changes in climate today may help future policy-makers to better address the climate-related nutrition and health risks of tomorrow. They plead for the creation of an evidence-based advocacy and public health movement to encourage decision-makers from governments, business and civil society to support new policies and personal actions to reduce greenhouse gas emissions from food systems while adapting to the effects of climate change on nutrition.

Continuing the theme of environmental health, Prof. Jess Fanzo follows with a contribution on *the impact of food choices, dietary patterns and consumerism on the planet.* Current food production methods are contributing to severe environmental problems, and we are starting to recognize that the health of human beings cannot be isolated from the health of ecosystems and the environment. Outlining the concept of sustainable food systems and diets, Prof. Fanzo calls for the development of incentives that encourage farmers to grow food in a more sustainable way. At the same time, she argues, consumers should be educated to make informed choices about what foods are healthy both for themselves and for the planet.

This section concludes with reflections by Dr Jenifer Baxter of the UK Institution of Mechanical Engineers on *the potential benefits of engineering food waste out of the world's current production, distribution, and retail systems.* Some 30–50% of all food produced is either lost or wasted, and levels of wasted food lead to overproduction in both the developed and the developing world. Engineering solutions can reduce food waste and protect the food-growing environment, and can also use food waste for heat, power and fertilizer, while changes in the behavior of consumers can reduce food waste in developed countries. Meanwhile, less food waste in combination with good engineering practices can lead to better access to food for those in developing countries. Dr Baxter argues that we could feed the projected population of 2075 today, but that it will be necessary to change our attitudes, behaviors and technologies to ensure that everyone in the world benefits.

Section 4: From Science to Solutions

Section 4 shifts the focus of the book from science to solutions. The first chapter of this section, co-written by Profs. Zulfiqar A Bhutta and Jai K Das, both of the Aga Khan University, examines *the potential of science to improve nutrition and nutrition-related policy-making at international, national and local levels.* Although a great deal of progress is being made in reducing malnutrition, this is still too slow and uneven, while some forms of malnutrition – namely adult overweight and obesity – are actually increasing. The authors argue that a concerted effort is required from both the nutrition-specific and nutrition-sensitive sectors for addressing both kinds of malnutrition synergistically. They also call for a more enabling political and financial environment, along with nutrition-friendly systems, in order to drive sustainable development forward.

The success of any policy or program is ineluctably dependent on the people who implement it, and thus the following chapter explores *the power of people-centered nutrition interventions.* Jointly penned by Prof. Sera Young of Northwestern University, Dr Rolf Klemm of Helen Keller International, and Shawn Baker of the Bill & Melinda Gates Foundation, this contribution argues that nutrition problems are often more complex than they appear, and that people-centered design can effectively inform nutrition interventions and help ensure that the needs of end-users are better served. People-centered design is based on design thinking, which includes end-users in the selection and design of services, products and behaviors. Putting people at the heart of nutrition interventions often requires hard work and creativity, but delivers better results in the long run.

Likewise the joint effort of three authors – Prof. Alain B. Labrique of JHU Global mHealth Initiative, Prof. Sucheta Mehra of Johns Hopkins Bloomberg School of Public Health, and Dr Marc Mitchell of the Harvard T.H. Chan School of Public Health – this chapter explores *the use of new and existing tools and technologies to support the global nutrition agenda.* The pace of information, communication and digital services continues to accelerate globally, and governments and NGOs are harnessing this

infrastructure to test and scale innovative new solutions. The global nutrition community has been at the forefront of many such innovations, although further innovation is still needed to achieve Universal Health Coverage. Continued measurement and reporting of results will therefore be critical in making the case for continued mHealth and mNutrition scale-up and integration, and for harnessing of the full potential of these developments.

Another production from a triumvirate of authors concludes this section. Prof. Laurette Dubé, Dr T. Nana Mokoah Ackatia-Armah and Dr Nii Antiaye Addy, all of McGill University, present *the potential of Convergent Innovation to address malnutrition* by scaling up cross-sector solutions from the social economy. Business principles of innovation, entrepreneurship, and financing have been increasingly adopted in addressing malnutrition, leading to the formation of enterprises and financing schemes of various types whose object is to simultaneously create social and economic value and increase the impact of efforts to address malnutrition. Convergent Innovation is a pragmatic, solution-oriented framework to help decision-makers incorporate the social objectives of nutrition into the economic mission of business, while ensuring that economic viability is better integrated into organizations focused on social benefit.

Section 5: Transforming the Nutrition Landscape

Section 5, which concludes this book, introduces a range of proven solutions that have the power to generate positive change. It opens with a discussion of *how personalized nutrition can pave the way to better population health.* Written by Prof. Michael Gibney and Marianne Walsh, both of University College Dublin, together with Jo Goosens on behalf of the Food4Me Consortium, this contribution argues that one of our biggest current challenges is how to change eating and behavior patterns so as to produce better health in any given individual. The essence of personalized nutrition is to assist individuals in achieving a lasting dietary behavior change that is beneficial for health. Personalized nutrition will represent an opportunity to achieve optimal health and will support self-realization, both within the realm of health and beyond it.

This chapter is followed by an account of *how to provide access to nutrient-rich diets for vulnerable groups in low- & middle-income settings.* Written jointly by Saskia de Pee, Lynnda Kiess, Regina Moench-Pfanner and Martin Bloem (all of the World Food Programme), this chapter explains how nutrient requirements are frequently not met due to the limited availability and affordability of an adequately diverse diet that includes plant-source, animal-source, and fortified foods. Foods fortified for the general population "piggy-back" on already existing distribution systems and consumption practices. Special nutritious foods, by contrast, are designed to meet the requirements of specific groups. While a wealth of evidence already exists about the need to meet nutrient requirements and how to do so, more information should be collected on the magnitude of the impact of a combination of nutrition-specific and nutrient-sensitive interventions in a particular context and at a particular cost.

Ensuring good nutrition for other vulnerable population groups such as elderly and hospitalized individuals in affluent societies is the theme of the ensuing chapter. Written by Prof. Peter Weber of the University of Stuttgart-Hohenheim, this contribution demonstrates how a growing body of evidence indicates that micronutrient deficiencies exist in the developed world as well as the developing world. Life expectancy continues to grow, but the last decade of life is often compromised by the burden of partially preventable health issues. Healthy ageing is essential if the elderly are to remain independent and play an integral role in society. Prof. Weber concludes that the same level of attention that is currently given to overnutrition in the developed world should be given to undernutrition and appropriate changes made to public health policies and programs.

Tom Arnold, recently retired *ad interim* Co-ordinator of the Scaling Up Nutrition (SUN) Movement, follows with a consideration of *nutrition-specific and nutrition-sensitive interventions*. SUN Countries are proving that tackling malnutrition is a multifaceted challenge that requires a genuine partnership driven by passionate leadership at the highest levels. Defeating malnutrition is the new normal, and SUN Countries are proving that alliances comprising critical sectors and committed stakeholders are transforming nutrition. How these alliances share, learn and build a culture of effective partnering is a stepping-stone toward achieving the vision of the SUN Movement. The tremendous energy and enthusiasm that drive the SUN Movement bodes well for the future. Nutrition is in the spotlight – more now than ever before.

Prof. Eileen Kennedy of Tufts University and Dr Habtamu Fekadu of Save the Children team up next for a consideration of *the role of good governance in delivering good nutrition*. Good governance is essential for effective policy and program development and implementation. Although there is no such thing as a formulaic approach to governance that can be applied universally, there are a

number of factors that contribute to effective governance, including leadership, advocacy, a legal framework, stakeholder involvement, and enduring commitment. Capacity development at all levels is essential, as are evidence and research, but advocacy is key, and the authors conclude with the observation that leadership at all levels is a prerequisite for sustaining the momentum of effective nutrition policies and programs.

Maria Elena D Jefferds and Prof. Rafael Flores-Ayala, both of the Centers for Disease Control and Prevention, next provide their thoughts on *the importance of measurement*. Most countries are currently not on track to meet the global nutrition targets agreed by the World Health Assembly (WHA) in 2013. The release of the WHA 2025 global nutrition targets and the Global Nutrition Report can, however, represent strategic opportunities for improving nutrition worldwide. Various monitoring, evaluation and surveillance frameworks exist to guide the development, implementation and evaluation of nutrition programs and systems. The authors explain how countries and nutrition programs benefit from nutrition monitoring and surveillance systems, which are used for decision-making, program improvement, accountability and policy development. Focusing on capacity building, innovation, and investing to support a "nutrition data revolution" are strategic opportunities to improve nutrition and health worldwide.

The critical role of food safety in ensuring food security is next discussed by Dr Dave Crean of Mars, Incorporated and Dr Amare Ayalew of the Partnership for Aflatoxin Control in Africa. Today's global food supply chains make the food safety landscape more complex and challenging than ever before. Food safety management has not kept pace with this development. Unsafe food cannot sustain human health and has tragic social and economic consequences. New food safety threats are emerging. Improving levels of food safety globally requires the development of new technologies, sustainable commitments, and human and institutional capacity, especially among farmers. Drs Crean and Ayalew make the case that collaboration among all stakeholders is necessary to leverage the right food safety knowledge, risk management methods and interventions across the global food supply. Without safe food, the world will not achieve global food security and improved nutrition.

The book concludes with the thoughts of Dr Achim Dobermann of Rothamsted Research on *putting the Sustainable Development Goals (SDGs) into practice*. Dr Doberman makes it clear that the new SDGs and their Targets provide a framework for all countries to develop roadmaps for sustainable development in all its dimensions. Agriculture contributes to many of the new SDGs and Targets, and therefore needs to receive particular attention. SDG 2 on sustainable agriculture is, however, among the most challenging goals to achieve. Transformative changes will be required regarding how food is produced, processed and consumed in order to meet multiple needs. Dr Doberman argues that agro-food systems need to be managed with greater precision and that long-term investment in public R&D is required to ensure that ground-breaking innovations continue to be developed and are widely accessible to all farmers, processors and other businesses.

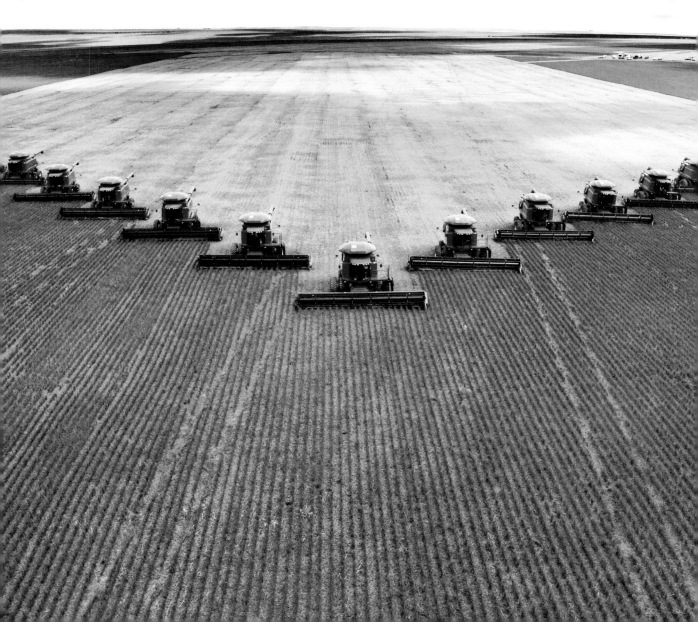

Ten Forces Shaping the Global Food System

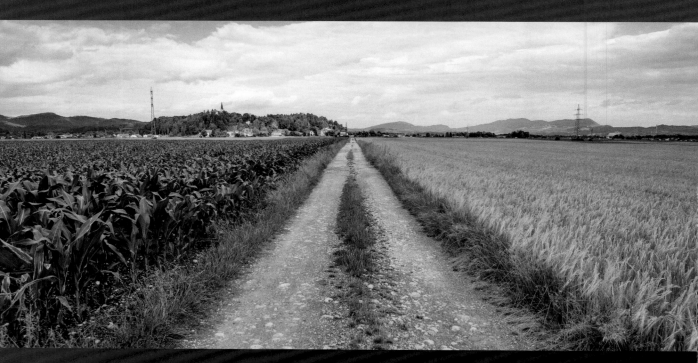

Source: Columbia SIPA

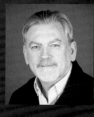

Glenn Denning
Professor of Professional
Practice in International and
Public Affairs, School of
International and Public Affairs,
Columbia University, New York,
NY, USA; Senior Policy Advisor,
Sustainable Development
Solutions Network (SDSN),
Earth Institute, Columbia
University, New York, NY, USA

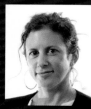

Jess Fanzo
Bloomberg Distinguished
Associate Professor of Ethics
and Global Food and
Agriculture Policy in the Berman
Institute of Bioethics and the
School of Advanced International
Studies at Johns Hopkins
University, Baltimore, MD, USA

"The wealth of the nation is its air, water, soil, forests, minerals, lakes, oceans, scenic beauty, wildlife habitats and biodiversity… that's all there is."

Gaylord Nelson (1916– 2005) Governor of Wisconsin, *United States Senator and founder of Earth Day*

Key messages

This chapter provides a general introduction to this book, and adumbrates many topics that are found in the following pages. It focuses on ten forces which have a pivotal influence on the global food system. These may be summarized as follows.

- **The degradation of natural resources:** Sustainable intensification of *existing* agricultural land will be essential if we are to meet growing population demands for food and better nutrition.

- **Climate change:** Climate-Smart Agriculture (CSA) is essential for managing landscapes in order to achieve increased productivity, enhanced resilience and reduced greenhouse gas emissions. Climate Smart *Food Systems* goes beyond CSA to incorporate dietary choices, food losses and waste, processing and packaging, and transport infrastructure.

- **Urbanization:** In the face of growing urbanization, our food system networks will have to change to ensure that food is accessed in an equitable way that crosses geopolitical boundaries.

- **Globalization:** Food commodities are moving across international borders at unprecedented levels and are changing food consumption patterns all over the world.

- **Consumer behavior:** Consumers are increasingly being asked to make complex choices about the food they eat. Providing them with useful information and better skills can shift consumer demand in the direction of healthier eating patterns.

- **Culture and tradition:** Food systems continually shape our culture and traditions and vice versa. The food environment around us is altering how we make food choices and how we access, prepare and consume food.

- **Government policies:** Sound government policies are necessary to enable a productive, sustainable and equitable food system, and getting policies right involves a tricky balance.

- **Conflict and fragile states:** Conflict creates unstable food systems. There is a critical need to enhance food security resilience through policies and programs that link immediate hunger relief interventions with a long-term strategy for sustainable growth.

- **Technology innovation:** Technology continues to create opportunities to improve the productivity and sustainability of the food system. Perhaps the most exciting and most controversial technological innovation is biotechnology, specifically genetically modified organisms (GMOs).

- **Sustainability:** The adoption of the Sustainable Development Goals (SDGs) by all nations will provide a powerful framework that will guide decision-making on policies and budgets by governments, private sector, and civil society to 2030. These goals hold the potential to set the global food system on a more sustainable path.

21

1. The degradation of natural resources

The productivity and sustainability of our global food system depends on the state of earth's natural resources: soil, water, climate, and biodiversity, both terrestrial and aquatic. Humans survive and prosper by manipulating these most fundamental resources to produce food through farming, animal husbandry and fisheries. But our food system is emerging as a major contributor to the breaching of our planetary boundaries that define "a safe operating space for humanity."[1]

Twelve thousand years ago, at the dawn of the Neolithic Era, the human population, comprising mainly hunters and gatherers, was probably no more than 10 million. In 2015, our planet struggles to nourish 7.3 billion people, with the daunting prospect of provisioning 9.5 to 13.3 billion inhabitants by the end of the century, according to recent UN estimates. The changes launched with the Industrial Revolution have brought unprecedented advances in science, technology and longevity. Agriculture now occupies 38% of the world's terrestrial surface. But the wider ecological consequences of human activity on our food system are becoming clearer and more troubling.

Agricultural land is being degraded through deforestation, soil erosion, nutrient depletion, salinization, waterlogging, overgrazing, desertification, and industrial pollution. Across Asia, Africa and Latin America, forests continue to make way for agriculture in response to population and income growth. Nutrients essential for plant growth are lost through erosion and extraction without replenishment. Seventy percent of freshwater extraction is allocated to agriculture. Water is being removed from the earth's surface and also from aquifers at an unsustainable rate. Our rivers, lakes and oceans are being overfished and polluted. Global biodiversity – the genetic foundation of our food system – is in retreat. Species and genotypes are becoming extinct at an alarming rate. And now, the earth's seemingly unique climate – which supports our agriculture, forests and fisheries – is threatened with catastrophic warming through the apparently inexorable increase in greenhouse gas (GHG) emissions.

Natural resource degradation adversely affects all four dimensions of food and nutritional security: availability, access, utilization, and stability. Reduced crop and animal productivity and depleted aquatic resources diminish local availability and access through higher prices. The poor are most affected, as a greater share of their income goes to buy food. They reduce consumption and shift to lower-cost products, often with adverse nutritional consequences. The inherent nutritional quality of food can be reduced by lower nutrient content and the accumulation of toxins. Reduced diversity of available and accessible food can also result in low-quality diets. Declining water quality, including fecal contamination, leads to diarrheal disease and the inability to utilize the nutrients from food. Climate change and variability affect the stability of food and nutrition security.

Halting and reversing natural resource degradation are essential for improving the world's nutrition. It is widely agreed that further expansion of the land frontier through deforestation must be avoided. Thus, sustainable intensification of *existing* agricultural land – producing more food, more efficiently, and with less damage to the environment – will be essential if we are to meet growing population demands for food and better nutrition.

Desertification, exacerbated by climate change, is threatening the livelihoods of pastoralist communities in northern Kenya and across Africa. Source: Jess Fanzo

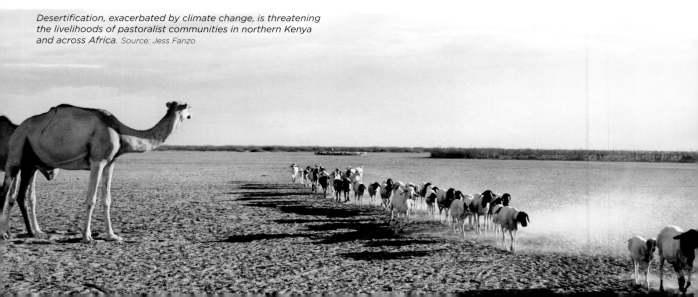

2. Climate change

The evidence is clear. Human activity, primarily through unrelenting fossil fuel consumption, ongoing clearing of forests, and food production, is changing the earth's climate. Increased GHG emissions from these actions are causing temperatures to increase, in turn, resulting in extreme and harmful conditions such as heat waves, typhoons, droughts, floods, and rises in the sea level. These conditions put populations at greater risk of food and nutritional insecurity. Broad consensus has been reached on the importance of a "2°C guardrail" to protect the planet from the most dire consequences. More recent analysis suggests this "guardrail" will not be enough to avoid catastrophic rises in the sea level.

Our climate is one of our natural resources. It makes the earth unique among all known planets. It is a fundamental building-block of the food system, providing temperatures and rainfall favorable to the management of farming systems that meet our nutritional requirements. Even with the more conservative estimates concerning climate change, we can expect disruptions of the food system, which will cause greater instability of food production and distribution and will result in shortages, price increases, periodic price spikes, unplanned migrations, and refugee emergencies. At the same time, agriculture, forestry and related land uses are major contributors to GHG emissions.

Climate change is also likely to exacerbate degradation of other natural resources, including our land, water and genetic resources. These trends will place unprecedented stress on the ability of the global food system to ensure a state of food security, defined by the World Food Summit in 1996 as: "when all people at all times have physical and economic access to sufficient, safe, and nutritious food to maintain an active and healthy life." Climate change threatens to undermine much of the progress achieved over the past 50 years. The world's poor, who are already most vulnerable to food insecurity and undernutrition, will be hardest hit.

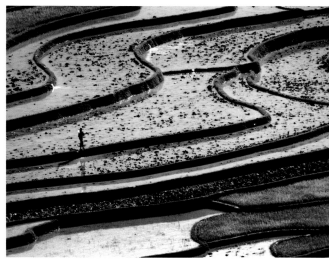

Rice terraces in northern Vietnam: worldwide, 70% of freshwater extraction is allocated to agriculture.
Source: International Rice Research Institute.

In response to the growing challenge of global climate change, there has been increasing attention to developing and promoting food systems that both reduce GHG emissions and decrease vulnerability to a changing, more variable climate. The World Bank, FAO and the CGIAR all highlight the need for "Climate-Smart Agriculture" (CSA) as an approach to managing landscapes to achieve increased productivity, enhanced resilience and reduced GHG emissions. This concept should extend to Climate Smart *Food Systems* by applying a value-chain approach which ensures that broader economic, social and environmental objectives are met in anticipation of climate change. This approach goes beyond CSA to incorporate dietary choices, food losses and waste, processing and packaging, and transport infrastructure. Thus, the design and deployment of Climate Smart Food Systems will require a multisector and multistakeholder approach.

3. Urbanization

Major economic and demographic transitions have had significant impacts on health outcomes of the global population, including fertility and mortality rates as well as disease patterns and health outcomes. Parallel to these transitions, diets, physical activity and body composition have also shifted. This phenomenon is also known as the nutrition transition. One of the main drivers of this nutrition transition is urbanization, which is an integral part of a broader structural transformation that has been long observed in Asia and Latin America and is rapidly emerging in Africa. People are leaving behind their rural livelihoods

and moving to urban centers. This expanded population growth within urban environments is putting increasing pressure not only on the planet and our global food system, but also on where people are able to get work, and how they live.

Globally, more people live in urban areas than in rural areas, with 54% of the world's population residing in urban areas as at 2014. In 1950, 30% of the world's population was urban, and by 2050, an estimated 66% will be urban. Africa and Asia remain rural, with 40% and 48% of their populations living in urban areas. This will change in the coming decades, with both regions urbanizing faster than other regions of the world. By

2050, 56% and 64% respectively will be urban. Just three countries together – India, China and Nigeria – are expected to account for 37% of the projected growth of the world's urban population between 2014 and 2050.

Urbanization is affecting food supply and demand in both positive and negative ways. While it is thought that increased urbanization displaces arable land needed for agriculture, the relationship between urban populations and rural producers is more complex. More and more people live in cities: they have relatively sedentary occupations and lifestyles, and often have higher disposable incomes. The lifestyles of urban consumers will increasingly dictate what food is grown by producers and how that food is traded, processed, distributed, and marketed. City dwellers will increasingly want access to a greater diversity of foods including meat, dairy products and convenient, ultra-processed foods. On the supply side, economic growth and global trade will change the way food is produced, processed and sold, creating new markets for rural producers. The rapid transformation of the food retail sector – the so-called supermarket revolution – is being observed in virtually all parts of the developing world.

Not all movement to urban centers has a positive influence on nutrition and wellbeing. Currently, a quarter of the world's inhabitants live in slums or poorly constructed shantytowns.[2] Limited access to social services, safe and nutritious food, and poor public health infrastructure leaves shantytown populations at high risk of both communicable and non-communicable diseases. These shifts will require delicate decisions as to how much quality food should be produced, what type, where, and how. Nutrition outcomes will surely be affected in the absence of proper planning, infrastructure, and health and social services, and many of the lower- and middle-income countries lack these. Our food system networks will have to change to ensure that food is accessed in an equitable way that crosses geopolitical boundaries.

4. Globalization

Globalization describes a historical and ongoing process of integration of economies across countries through the trade of goods and services, along with flows of labor, investment and technology across national borders. Globalization may include broader considerations of culture, politics and the environment. Indeed, the Millennium Development Goals and the recently agreed Sustainable Development Goals allow us to extend the concept further to include global solidarity and partnership to end poverty and achieve more inclusive and sustainable societies. This section will focus on just two important manifestations of globalization that directly affect the food system: agricultural trade and land acquisition.

Economists are well known to welcome trade without distortions as a means of improving the efficiency of markets in delivering agricultural commodities and food at the lowest cost. The Doha Round of international trade negotiations launched by the World Trade Organization in 2001 has sought to reduce distortions in global agricultural trade caused by high tariffs and other barriers, export subsidies, and other forms of domestic support, and to enable increased global trade. Also known as the Doha Development Round, the negotiations were additionally intended to improve the trading prospects of developing countries. Progress towards agreement remains slow, with most countries retaining entrenched positions designed to either protect or advance their own trade.

Notwithstanding the ongoing inefficiencies of global agricultural trade, food commodities are moving across international borders at unprecedented levels. The most obvious impacts are lower prices in importing countries of many internationally traded commodities (e.g., chicken exports from Brazil) and increased domestic prices of new, internationally traded commodities (e.g., quinoa produced in Peru). These trends are changing food consumption patterns all over the world, with mixed results.

The case of quinoa, an ancient, nutrient-rich grain, is illustrative of a new commodity on the international market. Peru was forecast to export 40,000 MT of quinoa (valued at US$180 million) in 2015 to become the world's leading exporter of this commodity. With growing demand from international markets, quinoa production more than doubled in Peru between 2011 and 2014, mainly through an increase in yield per hectare. While farmers have benefited from increased international demand, the impact of more expensive quinoa on domestic consumption and its dietary consequences remains a concern, although it is not yet fully understood.

Since the global food crisis of 2007–08, there has been rising interest in the transnational acquisition of agricultural land. Governments of some food-importing countries have sought to improve their food security by investing in land beyond their borders. Corporations and other private investors have seen the rising prices of agricultural commodities as an opportunity to invest in, and develop, agricultural land in land-rich regions such as Africa, Latin America and Central Asia. Advocacy groups, civil society organizations and academics have claimed that such investments have often resulted in the displacement and inadequate compensation of traditional owners, the corruption of proceeds from sale or lease of land, human rights violations, and environmental degradation. The Land Matrix Global Observatory, an independent global land monitoring initiative that promotes transparency and accountability in land investment, estimates that transnational acquisitions totaling 38 million hectares have been recorded in 1340 deals initiated since 2000. The impact of these transactions on food security, nutrition and poverty remains unclear.

5. Consumer behavior

Changing demographics, incomes, lifestyles, and preferences influence demand for specific foods. Overall, global diets are shifting towards higher-quality, nutrient-dense products such as meat, dairy products, and oils – but also towards more processed foods. This demand does not always equate to healthy decisions for people or the environment.

While consumers have come to exercise a more prominent role in the modern food system, they are not fully informed as to how it works, the foods it produces, and the environmental footprint it creates. They are also not sufficiently informed as to what constitutes a healthy diet.

There are exceptions. Many consumers are still poor and lack the resources to access higher-quality diets. Instead, they can only purchase what would be considered less healthy options – processed foods, high in sugar and fat, with high energy content for every dollar spent. In much of the world,

the cost of even basic diets which meet mainly caloric needs exceeds daily wages, on account of escalating food prices. Unfortunately daily consumption of this low-quality, high-energy diet increases the risk of obesity and of the chronic, non-communicable diseases associated with being overweight.

Consumers are increasingly articulating their preferences for foods they want to consume, and there is growing interest – especially in high-income settings – in consuming healthier diets. At the same time, however, many consumers are also becoming increasingly remote from the production of food, mainly on account of urbanization. The growing scientific complexity of food production and processing has placed greater burdens on consumers, who often lack the knowledge to understand nutritional or food sciences. Concomitantly, new information about diet and health is continually being released by the media for consumers to decipher. This often cryptic and contradictory information has left many consumers confused as to what comprises a healthy diet, and what foods they should eat. Yet consumers are increasingly being asked to make choices concerning complex issues regarding the nutritional content and health-giving properties of food.

Providing consumers with useful information and better skills that allow them to choose healthier foods can help influence consumer demand in a healthier direction. This

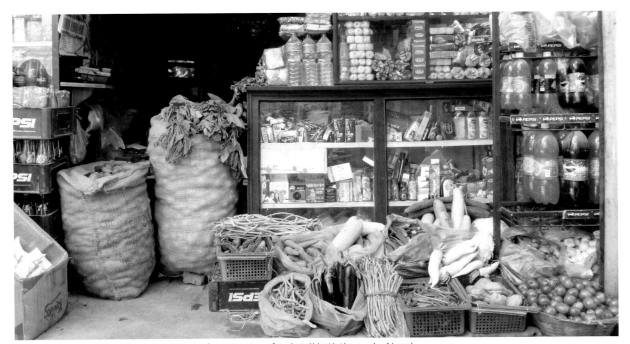

Processed and packaged foods compete for space at a food stall in Kathmandu, Nepal.
Source: Jess Fanzo

behavioral shift may affect what is in the food supply. Educating consumers about commercial agriculture and enhancing the public's understanding of food production methods may have long-term benefits in maintaining consumer confidence. Food labeling, informative health statistics on menus, nutrition literacy programs, cooking classes at school and work, and useful dietary guidelines can all help here. Furthermore, price incentives for healthy foods in underserved areas, health-related food taxes, and stricter regulation on advertising junk food to children can help consumers make healthier choices.

6. Culture and tradition

Culture is inherent in agri*culture*. Because food is the product of agriculture, food serves as a powerful expression of how we tie ourselves to the land and preserve our social traditions. The types of foods we consume, the preparation and cooking practices involved, and the way we eat those foods all articulate who we are and why we eat as we do. Food systems are consistently shaping our culture and traditions and vice versa.

Taste, health, social status, cost and resources all influence which foods we choose to eat, but culture and tradition are also key factors. Embedded in tradition and culture are

social events and gatherings, holiday traditions, special occasions, and religious or ritual observances that call for particular foods. This can be both positive and negative. On the positive side, food choice can be deeply personal and can often hinge on our ideals, sense of identity and habits. Food itself is central to our sense of identity, often showing the geography, diversity and hierarchy of a certain culture.

Food taboos can influence health and nutrition outcomes, and are practiced among most human societies. Some religions define certain food items as appropriate for human consumption and others less so. Dietary restrictions and rules may govern particular phases of the lifespan. Many of these taboos occur during pregnancy and lactation, including appropriate food intake, energy-expending activities, and food restrictions. Cultural perceptions of food behavior and activity can have significant impacts on women's lives and their food security and nutritional status.

The food environment around us is changing how we make food choices and how we access, prepare and consume food, including the ever growing influence of supermarkets but also of restaurants, vending machines, small kiosks, *bodegas*, and corner stores. Half a century ago, most food was grown for household consumption by smallholder farmers living in

Because food is the product of agriculture, food serves as a powerful expression of how we tie ourselves to the land and preserve our social traditions. Source: Mike Bloem

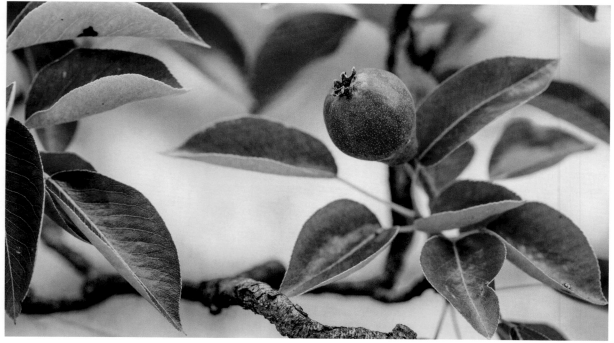

rural areas. Food was also purchased at small, local markets. With globalization, there is a growing trend whereby more and more food purchased by consumers has traveled longer distances and is purchased in supermarkets. These changing purchasing patterns have been influenced by rapid urbanization, income growth, and the expansion of modern retailers, processors and distributors. Additionally, more and more households are moving out of rural areas into urban centers, where they utilize modern supermarkets and are changing the cultures and traditions around food, sometimes both positively and negatively.

7. Government policies

Governments can affect the productivity and sustainability of food systems at all levels: local, national and global. Policies on regulations, subsidies, and taxes can shift the investment decisions of all participants along the food value chain, including producers, processors, traders, and consumers. Government policies and related budget allocations in infrastructure, procurement, research, and public information can similarly alter the priorities of these stakeholders.

In developing countries, governments have long been concerned with price stability and its impact on social stability. Rice economies in Asia have sought to buffer their domestic prices from price instability in the world market, although this has often come at a high cost and at a disadvantage to domestic producers. During the food crisis of 2007–08, some governments – with the intention of protecting their consumers – closed their borders, exacerbating fears and contributing to the price spike that plunged millions of people into food insecurity and poverty.

Many governments have advocated policies that support improvements in agricultural productivity. The Asian Green Revolution is viewed by many as a triumph of supportive government policies in the form of research and extension investments, rural credit, input subsidies, commodity price support, and infrastructure investments, mainly in irrigation and transport. For more than a decade, similar policies have been promoted by African governments, and their impact is now becoming apparent.

Whether in rich or poor countries, governments make policies and investment choices with a view to the consequences on their *own* sustainability. Democratically elected governments with vocal and influential rural constituents are reluctant to remove historical policy support, as seen with the case of agricultural subsidies in the United States, Europe and Japan. The US Government

Accountability Office estimates that agricultural subsidies and insurance cost its taxpayers some US$20 billion annually. Benefits accrued to politically influential agribusiness corporations and large-scale farmers have prevented any meaningful reform of these programs until recently. In Malawi, the government of President Bingu wa Mutharika boosted corn production in 2005 with a fertilizer subsidy, leading to national food security *and* a resounding re-election in 2009. Food can be a highly politicized commodity.

Governments and businesses must work in harmony to create synergies that bring benefits to producers and consumers alike. For example, the Alliance for a Green Revolution in Africa (AGRA) is creating value by building the governance and management capacity of small and medium-sized enterprises and farmer groups while at the same time building institutions that promote market efficiency and regional trade. To provide a more equitable food system, such policies must be coupled with social safety nets so as to ensure that the poorest consumers are food- and nutrition-secure.

Another area where governments influence the food system is through national dietary guidelines, which by their nature change over the course of time. The Dietary Guidelines for Americans provide the basis for federal food and nutrition policy and education initiatives, aiming to foster healthy eating habits and reduce the incidence of nutrition-related chronic diseases. First released in 1980, the Guidelines are updated and published every five years in a joint effort of the US Department of Health and Human Services and the US Department of Agriculture. Many countries have similarly established national guidelines that reflect the science on food and diets, while adapting to local culture and food availability. The establishment and dissemination of evidence-based dietary guidelines is an essential component of an effective national food and nutrition strategy which, in turn, influences the food supplied in schools, military institutions, hospitals, and government food assistance programs. It also affects the way the food industry formulates its food products.

It is evident that sound government policies are necessary, but not sufficient, for enabling a productive, sustainable and equitable food system. Governments operate within complex and context-specific political economies with a wide range of consequences. Professor Peter Timmer argues that "there is scope for more or less government involvement, depending on institutional capacity and the willingness of citizens to be taxed to pay for it, but 'none' has never been the right answer,"[3] He concludes that getting policies right is "a tricky balance that requires constant analysis, experimentation and learning."

8. Conflict and fragile states

The food system can serve as a lens through which to view the most important problems of society. One of these is conflict and violence and the many fragile states that are climbing out of war and genocide.

Countries and areas in protracted crisis are "environments in which a significant proportion of the population is acutely vulnerable to death, disease and disruption of livelihoods over a prolonged period of time."[4] Areas in protracted crisis and fragile states have some commonalities, including competition for natural resources, poor governance, inadequate access to nutrition, health and social services, dysfunctional institutions, loss of assets, food insecurity that impacts livelihoods, and persistent hunger.

The trigger for violent conflict or crisis may be natural, such as a prolonged drought, or economic, such as the change in price of a country's major staple or cash crop. Whatever the reason, these crises are both causes and effects of food insecurity and inadequate or inequitable access to assets. As well as being a consequence of conflict, food insecurity can of itself lead to conflict. Environmental scarcities and food insecurity do not always lead to conflict, but can escalate situations into violence. Most of the countries currently experiencing conflict are classified by FAO as "low-income food deficit," and have high burdens of undernourishment and high numbers of stunted children.

Conflict impacts global food security as well. Geopolitical conflicts cross the borders of different food systems. Fragile and failed nation-states are often suffering under the repression of extreme poverty and are touched by war and strife. These fragile states influence, and are in turn influenced by, global market forces, and food security is often one of the first factors to be affected.

Food systems that are repeatedly put under stress by conflict tend to move from predictable food value chains to instability and volatility. Violent, armed conflict can lead to the destruction of crops, livestock, land, and water systems, as well as disruptions in infrastructure such as roads and other transportation modalities, markets, and the human resources required for food production, processing, distribution, and safe consumption. Those participating or instigating war and conflict often use hunger as a weapon: "they use siege to cut off food supplies and productive capacities, starve opposing populations into submission, and hijack food aid intended for civilians."[5]

The response mechanisms adopted by the international community – such as the UN Committee on Food Security's Voluntary Guidelines on the Responsible Governance of Tenure of Land, Fisheries and Forests – are disparate and generally ineffective to address conflict, protracted crisis and fragile states. There is a critical need to enhance food security resilience through specific policies and programs that link immediate hunger relief interventions with a long-term strategy for sustainable growth. This would include rebuilding local institutions and support networks, building the capacity of farmers to adapt and reorganize, providing recovery measures for rural livelihoods, and supporting vulnerable groups. But challenges remain. Most actions are short-term, with narrow analysis and responses. There is a need to think about short and long-term approaches at the same time, with a major objective being resiliency.

9. Technology Innovation

Innovation in agriculture arguably began with the first attempts to domesticate food crops more than 12,000 years ago. More formal efforts to improve farming methods probably began at the Rothamsted Estate in the southeast of England in the 1840s, when John Bennet Lawes initiated research into the effects of fertilizers on crop growth. This research, coupled with the first manufacture of artificial fertilizers, also at Rothamsted, provided the foundation for modern scientific agriculture. Important discoveries were being made in parallel in Germany by Justus Freiherr von Liebig, a professor at the University of Giessen who is today considered the founder of organic chemistry. Yields were improved further in the early 20th century with the development of the Haber-Bosch process that used atmospheric nitrogen to produce ammonia (the core ingredient of nitrogen fertilizer) supplying the most important nutrient for food production.

Driven by advances in crop breeding, most notably the development and commercialization of hybrid corn in the United States, plus the rapid mechanization of many traditionally manual agricultural processes, global food production grew at an unprecedented rate. But while corn and wheat yields increased in the first half of the 20th century, mainly in temperate climates, there was little progress in tropical environments, where populations were most rapidly growing. It was only the advent of the Green Revolution, led by the efforts of Norman Borlaug and MS Swaminathan that, at the very least, postponed Thomas Malthus' 1798 predictions of "gigantic inevitable famine." Cereal production more than doubled in Asia between 1970 and 1995, while the population increased by 60% and agricultural land increased by only 4%. Agricultural

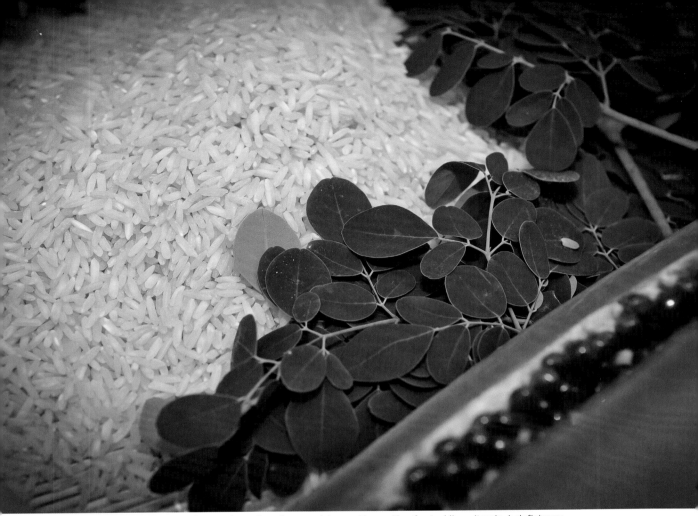

Golden Rice, produced through genetic engineering, provides another option for tackling vitamin A deficiency.
Source: International Rice Research Institute.

technology in the form of new seed varieties, fertilizer, and irrigation had provided breathing space for the planet.

Technology continues to create opportunities to improve the productivity and sustainability of the food system. Precision agriculture draws on progress in information technology, including GPS and the use of drones, to manage fields more efficiently through greater sensitivity to crop needs and field characteristics, for example enabling fertilizer and water to be applied at appropriate rates, reducing waste and environmental damage. While mainly applied in industrial agricultural settings, these new technologies are yet to realize their potential for improving agricultural efficiency for smallholders in low-income countries. In Africa, the Bill & Melinda Gates Foundation is supporting efforts to better understand soil and landscape resources and improve their management using the recent advances in soil spectroscopy, spatial-temporal statistics, geospatial mapping, aerial imaging, and cloud computing. These new approaches are being applied by the Africa Soil Information Service across several countries.

Perhaps the most exciting and most controversial technological innovation to shape the food system is biotechnology – specifically, genetically modified organisms (GMOs). Commercialized in the United States since 1996, GMOs have polarized communities within the global food system. For the most part, farmers have embraced genetically modified crops: a record 181.5 million hectares of biotech crops were grown across 28 countries in 2014, representing some 12% of global crop lands. Concerns about health and environmental risks appear to be waning as growing scientific evidence points to compelling economic, social and environmental benefits in most settings.

Research is showing potential for adaptation to climate change through genetic improvement to incorporate such traits as tolerance to heat, drought, submergence, and salinity. Biotechnology and other advanced breeding methods are also opening new frontiers for improvement in the nutritional quality of food e.g., Golden Rice to combat vitamin A deficiency, as well as vitamin A rich maize, high-zinc wheat, and high-iron pearl millet. These breeding methods complement important advances in the large-scale use of food fortification and micronutrient powders in combatting global malnutrition.

10. Sustainability

In 1972, the Club of Rome published "The Limits to Growth," outlining the need for a "great transition…from growth to global equilibrium."[6] This landmark document warned of the trends in population, industrialization, food production, and resource depletion. But the authors argued that these trends were not inevitable and that it was possible to establish a more sustainable global equilibrium "so that the basic material needs of each person on earth are satisfied and each person has an equal opportunity to realize his individual human potential."

The Brundtland Commission in 1987 defined sustainable development as "development that meets the needs of the present without compromising the ability of future generations to meet their own needs." This "intergenerational" concept was adopted by the Rio Earth Summit in 1992 and has remained a dominant conceptual framework for sustainability to this day.

More recently, beginning with the UN World Summit on Sustainable Development in Johannesburg in 2002, the term "sustainable development" was reformulated by the international community to comprise three interdependent and mutually reinforcing pillars: economic growth, social inclusion, and environmental protection. This vision of sustainable development was reinforced through the Rio+20 Summit and indeed has provided the foundation of a new set of global development goals: the Sustainable Development Goals (SDGs).

The SDGs embody an important principle of universality. We are now all accountable for an improved quality of life, one that can be shared by all and sustained over time. SDG2 commits UN member states to "End hunger, achieve food security and improved nutrition, and promote sustainable agriculture." Among SDG2's several targets are universally applicable commitments to end all forms of malnutrition by 2030, with an implication to address both undernutrition and overnutrition. SDG2 also calls on nations to fulfill the mandate of the Doha Development Round. Other SDGs address universally important needs to combat climate change, reduce food waste, and conserve terrestrial and marine resources.

International agreement on the SDGs will provide new impetus to rethink the way we produce, distribute and consume our food. From the outset, the SDGs have been criticized for their complexity and comprehensiveness. But a *sustainable* global food system will not be easy to achieve. There is no single sector or technology fix that provides a pathway to sustainability. Business as usual is not an option. And for the first time in history, there is a consensus that all of us will be held accountable for a shared development agenda and shared solutions that address food system issues in all countries and at all levels of income.

My personal view

Glenn Denning

Today's food systems are a complex, dynamic product of many interacting forces. In one sense, the food we consume is a remarkable feat of technical ingenuity and environmental adaptation against the forces of nature and population. Thanks to farmers, pastoralists and fisher folk, we have skillfully manipulated our land, water, and genetic resources to *more or less* feed the planet. Advances in science and technology, especially over the past century, have held at bay the "gigantic inevitable famine" predicted by Thomas Malthus in 1798.

This tells only part of the story, however. Almost 800 million people continue to go hungry. Micronutrient deficiencies affect perhaps 2 billion. At the same time, we are faced with an epidemic of overweight and obesity that is beginning to undermine past gains in longevity and quality of life. All of this is unfolding in a world that is rapidly urbanizing and globalizing, and in a bio-physical environment that is under stress from unrelenting population growth and the unsustainable exploitation of natural resources, while being at the same time increasingly subject to the effects of climate change.

There has never been a better time to think and act with sustainable development as our vision. The adoption of the SDGs by all nations in September 2015 provided us with a powerful yet challenging framework to guide decision-making on policies and budgets by governments, the private sector, and civil society to 2030. These goals hold the potential to set the global food system on a more sustainable path – one that meets the needs of present and future generations, while simultaneously ensuring that our food systems are economically viable, socially inclusive and environmentally sustainable.

Further reading

1. Degradation of natural resources

Rockström J, Steffen W, Noone K et al. A safe operating space for humanity. Nature 2009;461: 472–475.

Oliver MA, Gregory PJ. Soil, food security and human health: a review. European Journal of Soil Science 2015;66: 257–276.

Dobermann AR, Nelson D. Beever D et al. Solutions for Sustainable Agriculture and Food Systems. Technical report of the Thematic Group on Sustainable Agriculture and Food Systems. Paris, France and New York, USA: SDSN, 2013.

2. Climate change

Hansen J, Sato M, Hearty P et al. Ice melt, sea level rise and superstorms: evidence from paleoclimate data, climate modeling, and modern observations that 2°C global warming is highly dangerous. Atmospheric Chemistry and Physics Discussions 2015;15:20059–20179.

Pachauri RK., Allen MR, Barros VR et al. Climate Change 2014: Synthesis Report. Contribution of Working Groups I, II and III to the Fifth Assessment Report of the Intergovernmental Panel on Climate Change. 2014: 151.

Neufeldt H, Jahn M, Campbell BM et al. Beyond climate-smart agriculture: toward safe operating spaces for global food systems. Agric Food Secur 2013;2:10-1186.

3. Urbanization

Reardon T, Timmer CP. Five inter-linked transformations in the Asian agrifood economy: Food security implications. Global Food Security 2014;3:108–117.

Popkin BM., Adair LS, Ng SW. Global nutrition transition and the pandemic of obesity in developing countries. Nutrition Reviews 2012;70:3–21.

Satterthwaite D, McGranahan G, Tacoli C. Urbanization and its implications for food and farming. Philosophical Transactions of the Royal Society of London B: Biological Sciences, 2010;365(1554), 2809–2820.

United Nations, Department of Economic and Social Affairs, Population Division (2014). World Urbanization Prospects: The 2014 Revision, Highlights (ST/ESA/SER.A/352)

4. Globalization

World Trade Organization. The Doha Round. https://www.wto.org/english/tratop_e/dda_e/dda_e.htm USDA Foreign Agriculture Service. Quinoa Outlook. 12/23/2014.

The Land Matrix Global Observatory. http://www.landmatrix.org/en/

5. Consumer behavior

Aggarwal A, Monsivais P, Drewnowski A. (2012). Nutrient intakes linked to better health outcomes are associated with higher diet costs in the US. PLoS One, 7(5), e37533.

Hawkes C, Jewell J, Allen K. A food policy package for healthy diets and the prevention of obesity and diet-related non-communicable diseases: the NOURISHING framework. Obesity reviews, 2013;14(S2):

159–168.

Keats S, Wiggins S. Future diets: implications for agriculture and food prices. London England:ODI, 2014.

6. Culture and tradition

Counihan C, Van Esterik P. (2013). Food and culture: A reader. Routledge. Gómez MI, Ricketts KD. Food value chain transformations in developing countries: Selected hypotheses on nutritional implications. Food Policy 2013;42:139–150.

Pelto GH, Backstrand JR. (2003). Interrelationships between power-related and belief-related factors determine nutrition in populations. J Nutr 2003;133(1):297S–300S.

7. Government policies

Alliance for a Green Revolution in Africa (AGRA), 2015 Transformed livelihoods: AGRA's impact in Africa, Nairobi, Kenya Timmer CP. Food Security and Scarcity: Why Ending Hunger is So Hard. University of Pennsylvania Press, 2015.

8. Conflict and fragile states

FAO and IFAD Food insecurity in protracted crises – An overview 2012. High level expert Forum Rome Italy, 2012.

Pingali P, Alinovi L, Sutton, J. Food security in complex emergencies: enhancing food system resilience. Disasters 2005;29(s1):S5–S24.

Quinn J, Zeleny T, Bencko V. (2014) Food Is Security: The Nexus of Health Security in Fragile and Failed States. Food and Nutrition Sciences 2014;5(19):1828.

9. Technology innovation

DeFries R. The Big Ratchet: How Humanity Thrives in the Face of Natural Crisis. Basic Books, 2014.

Pingali PL. "Green Revolution: Impacts, limits, and the path ahead." Proceedings of the National Academy of Sciences 2012;109:12302–12308.

Barrows G, Sexton S, Zilberman D. Agricultural biotechnology: The promise and prospects of genetically modified crops. Journal of Economic Perspectives 2014:99–119.

Aldemita RR, Reaño IM, Solis RO et al. Trends in Global Approvals of Biotech Crops (1992–2014). GM crops & food just-accepted (2015): 00-00.

10. Sustainability

Meadows D et al, The Limits to Growth. 1972

http://collections.dartmouth.edu/published-derivatives/meadows/pdf/meadows_ltg-001.pdf

Brundtland Commission Report, Our Common Future, 1987

http://www.un-documents.net/our-common-future.pdf

Transforming Our World: The 2030 Agenda (including the SDGs), Aug 1, 2015.

https://sustainabledevelopment.un.org/content/documents/7891TRANSFORMING%20OUR%20WORLD.pdf

Sachs JD. The age of sustainable development. Columbia University Press, 2015.

References

1   Rockström J, Steffen W, Noone K et al. A safe operating space for humanity. Nature 2009;461:472-475.

2   http://unhabitat.org/wp-content/uploads/2014/07/WHD-2014-Background-Paper.pdf, accessed September 3, 2015.

3   Timmer CP. Food Security and Scarcity: Why Ending Hunger is So Hard. University of Pennsylvania Press, 2015.

4   FAO and IFAD (2012) Food insecurity in protracted crises – An overview 2012. High level expert Forum Rome Italy.

5   Messer E, Cohen MJ, Marchione T. Conflict: A cause and effect of hunger. Environmental Change and Security Project (ECSP) 7: 1–16. Washington DC: Woodrow Wilson Center for Scholars, 2001.

6   Meadows, Donella et al, The Limits to Growth. 1972. http://collections.dartmouth.edu/published-derivatives/meadows/pdf/meadows_ltg-001.pdf

Population Growth and Malnutrition

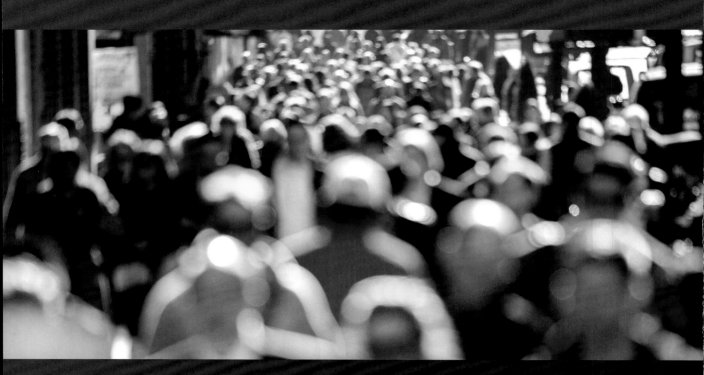

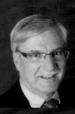

Michael J Klag
Dean, Johns Hopkins
Bloomberg School of Public
Health, Baltimore, MD, USA

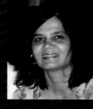

Parul Christian
Senior Program Officer,
Women's Nutrition, Bill &
Melinda Gates Foundation,
Seattle, WA, USA; Professor,
Department of International
Health, Johns Hopkins
Bloomberg School of Public
Health, Baltimore, MD, USA

"Population growth is an important driver of economic progress. Every stomach comes with two hands attached. Every mouth is backed by a creative human intelligence. We can solve the problems that are caused by our growing numbers. In fact, we have been doing so for many centuries now."

Steven W Mosher (born 1948), American social scientist and President of the Population Research Institute

Key messages

- The speed at which the world's population is increasing is without precedent and poses a wide range of complex challenges for nutritionists, agriculturalists and public health professionals alike.

- Life expectancy has also increased rapidly, especially in the developed world.

- At the same time as the world's population has been rapidly growing, childhood mortality rates have seen a dramatic decline.

- There will be a third more mouths to feed by 2050. Food production will have to rise considerably to meet this demand, and Sub-Saharan Africa will require special attention.

- Overall population growth will fuel the growth of urban areas, and the rise of urban populations will have wide-ranging health implications.

"The scale, severity and duration of the world food problem are so great that a massive, long-range, innovative effort unprecedented in human history will be required to master it."

US PRESIDENT'S SCIENCE ADVISORY COMMITTEE, 1967

The magnitude of global population growth

The world's population reached 7 billion on October 31, 2011 according to the United Nations Population Fund; according to the United States Census Bureau, this milestone was attained on March 12, 2012.[1] In the 1970s, it had been at approximately half this figure. The speed at which the world's population is increasing is entirely without precedent (**Figure 1**). It places enormous strain on the planet's resources, and poses a wide range of complex challenges for nutritionists, agriculturalists and public health professionals alike.

A little over two centuries ago, the world's population was 1 billion (**Table 1**). It was to grow sevenfold in the ensuing two centuries. It took just 123 years to double, under the influence of the Industrial Revolution and the accompanying advances in science and medicine. It took 46 years to double from 2 to 4 billion, but only 39 years to double from 3 to 6 million; and an additional 1 billion was added 12 years later.

In part, this dramatic increase occurred due to a phenomenon called the "population momentum," as a larger percent of the population was in its reproductive years during the period in question. The World Bank defines population momentum as: "The tendency for population growth to continue beyond the time that replacement-level fertility has been achieved because of a relatively high concentration of people in the childbearing years."[2] Even as fertility rates began to decline around the 1970–80s due to the effect of family planning programs, the previously high fertility rates resulted in continuing accelerated population growth. The rate of change in the world population was the highest during the 50-year period from 1925 to 1975, at 100 to 200 percent (**Table 1**).

Assuming a medium fertility variant or at replacement levels, by 2050 the world population will be 9 billion and by 2100, 10 billion (**Figure 2**). Much of this increase will occur in developing countries, with the population of high-income countries remaining relatively constant (**Figure 3**).

Figure 1 | **World population since 10,000 BCE**

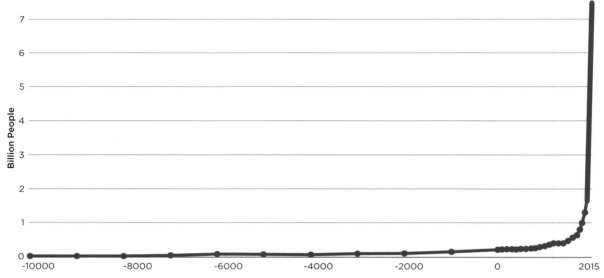

Source: https://ourworldindata.org/world-population-growth/, accessed July 8, 2016

Figure 2 | **Estimated and projected world population, billions, 1950–2100**

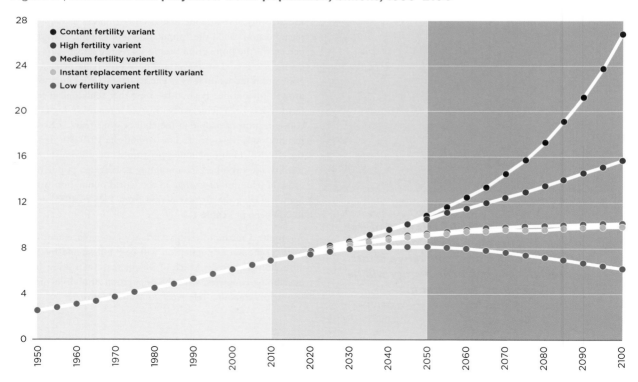

Source: United Nations, Department of Economic and Social Affairs, Population Division (2011): World Population Prospects: The 2010 Revision. New York. (Updated: April 15, 2011)

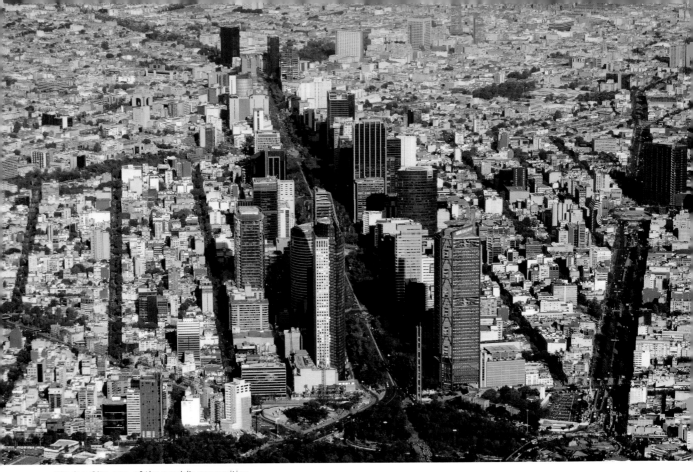

Mexico City, one of the world's megacities

Table 1 | **World population milestones**

Year	World Population	Interval
1804	1 billion	
1927	2 billion	123 years later
1960	3 billion	33 years later
1974	4 billion	14 years later
1987	5 billion	13 years later
1999	6 billion	12 years later
2011	7 billion	12 years later

Change in population profiles over time

In many European countries, the total fertility rate – the average number of children a woman will have during her lifetime if she experienced the current age-specific fertility rates and if she survived through the end of her childbearing years – is below the level of 2.0 which is required to replace the population without increasing it. In Germany, for instance, it is only 1.4. In the USA, it stands at just above this figure, at 2.1. China, with its policy of one child per family, had a total fertility rate of 1.7 in 2014, according to the World Bank, whereas India scored a higher than replacement level at 2.5. Countries in Africa, by contrast, demonstrate a very high total fertility rate, with Niger scoring highest of all at 7.2. With certain exceptions, most

countries in Africa and Asia have a high total fertility rate. Family planning strategies are urgently needed in these countries, both to limit the number of children born and to ensure appropriate intervals between births.

Meanwhile, life expectancy has grown rapidly, especially in the developed world. In the USA, for example, it increased by 56% for males and 63% for females between 1900 and 2000. The proportion of the population aged over 65 is projected to more than treble from 7% (111 million people) to 23% (450 million) by 2050. By 2050, the Western Pacific Region will have the second oldest population of all WHO regions – just below Europe where 25% of the population will be aged over 65. With a projected population of 450 million older people by 2050 globally, the Western Pacific Region will have far more older people than any other world region. At the same time as the population growth has been occurring and fertility rates have been declining, childhood mortality has been dramatically declining globally. It is projected to continue to do so across different regions, although the decline has slowed somewhat in recent years in Sub-Saharan Africa.

Overall population growth will fuel the growth of urban areas, which may become home to 50% of the world's population by 2050. The number of megacities is expected to grow to 36 by 2025, from a baseline of two in 1970 (Tokyo [Japan] and New York-Newark [USA]). These two cities are predicted to be accompanied in the top ten by Delhi (India,

32.9 million), Shanghai (China, 28.4 million), Mumbai (India, 26.6 million), Ciudad de México (Mexico, 24.6), São Paulo (Brazil, 23.2 million), Dhaka (Bangladesh, 22.9 million), Beijing (China, 22.6 million) and Karachi (Pakistan, 20.2 million). Tokyo's population will grow from its 1970 figure of 23.3 to 38.7 million, and New York-Newark's from 16.2 to 23.6. London, the first great metropolis of the Industrial Revolution, will occupy only 36th place, with a population of 10.3 million. Despite the massive increase in the size of existing megacities, more and more of the population will be residing in smaller urban areas, as these get built in response to overall population growth (**Figure 4**). After 2050, rural populations are predicted to remain stable, while the urban population of the planet will continue to grow.

Figure 3 | **Growth in developing v. developed countries 1965–2050**

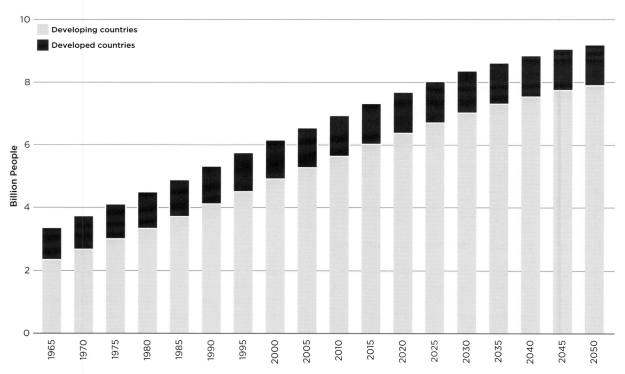

Source: Population Division of the Department of Economic and Social Affairs of the United Nations Secretariat (2007)

Figure 4 | **Urban and rural populations by development area, 1950–2050**

Billion People

- ● More developed regions urban populations
- ● More developed regions rural population
- ● Less developed regions urban populations
- ● Less developed regions rural population

(Y-axis: 0, 1, 2, 3, 4, 5, 6)

(X-axis: 1950, 1960, 1970, 1980, 1990, 2000, 2010, 2020, 2030, 2040, 2050)

Source: UN, World Urbanization Prospects: The 2011 Revision

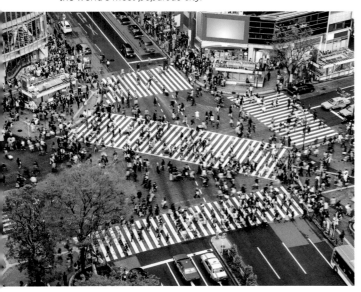

Aerial view of Shibuya in Tokyo, Japan – the world's most populous city.

Sub-Saharan Africa

Sub-Saharan Africa in particular will require special attention. Although the rate of population growth in this region is declining rapidly, it will continue to increase from 770 million in 2005 to 2 billion by 2050. Chronic hunger and malnutrition are already high in Sub-Saharan Africa, and so this region will face a special challenge in the years to come. Vulnerability to climate and dependence on rainwater for irrigation makes the agricultural economy of Sub-Saharan Africa as a whole extremely fragile, and this tendency has been accentuated by lack of appropriate investment in agriculture in recent decades. The development of smallholder farming may be key to the region's success in the future. There is cause for hope, however, when one reflects that Asia had only two staple crops during the "Green Revolution" masterminded by Norman Borlaug in the 1960s and '70s: Africa has no fewer than eight. Borlaug, who developed high-yielding, disease-resistant, semi-dwarf varieties of wheat, was credited at the time with saving a billion lives.

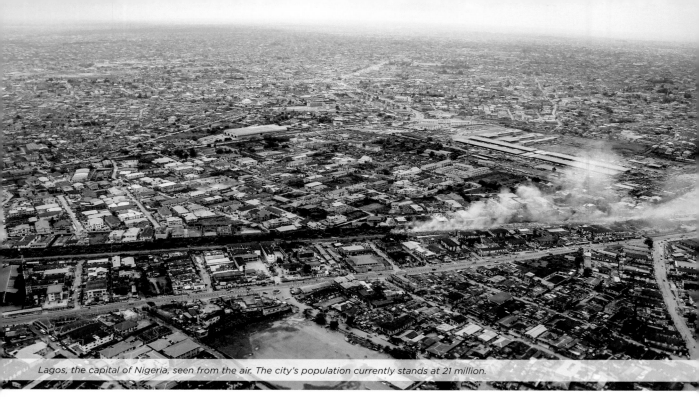

Lagos, the capital of Nigeria, seen from the air. The city's population currently stands at 21 million.

Figure 5 | **Total fertility by country, 2005–2010**

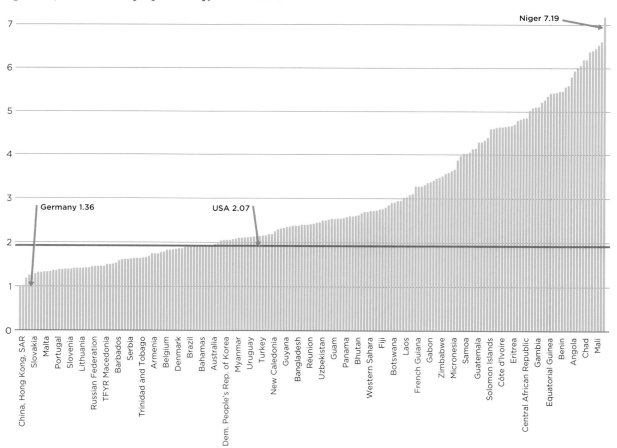

Germany 1.36

USA 2.07

Niger 7.19

Source: UN Department of Economic and Social Affairs – Population Division.

Figure 6 | **Gains in US life expectancy: 1900–2050**

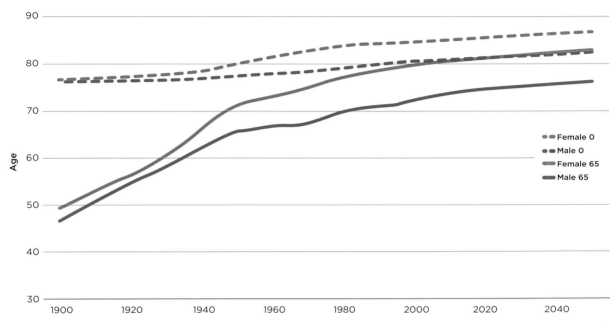

Source: Courtesy of Agree, 2011.

Figure 7 | **Childhood mortality, 1950–2050**

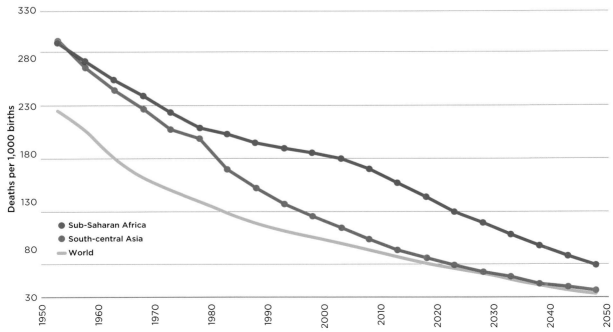

Source: WHO World Population Prospects: The 2004 Revision.

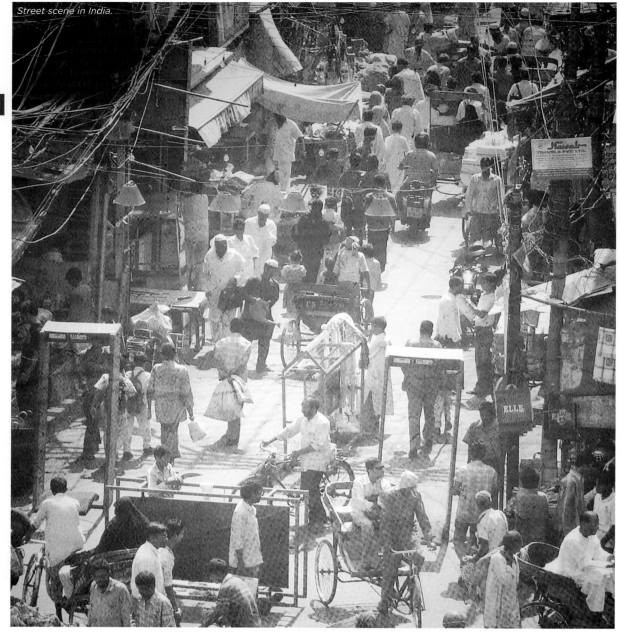

Street scene in India.

Urbanization and health

The growth of populations living in urban environments has wide-ranging health implications. One in three urban dwellers lives in slums, where nutrition, sanitation, and air and water quality are usually very poor. This amounts to 1 billion people worldwide. Urban air pollution kills approximately 1.2 million people each year around the world, mainly due to cardiovascular and respiratory diseases. Much of this pollution, although not all of it, is attributable to emissions from motor vehicles. The incidence of tuberculosis is also much higher in big cities. In the Democratic Republic of Congo, for example, 83% of people with tuberculosis live in cities.

Urban environments also tend to discourage physical activity and promote consumption of unhealthy, calorie-dense diets that are high in refined carbohydrates such as white flour and white rice. The process of refining a food not only removes the fiber; it also removes much of the food's nutritional value, including B-complex vitamins, healthy oils and fat-soluble vitamins. The consumption of the many processed foods that characterize the modern Western diet results in higher prevalence of obesity, diabetes and related non-communicable diseases, which account for 63% of deaths worldwide. Countering these factors, the provision of health services is more efficient in cities; but the growth of urban populations will create a host of practical, logistical and financial challenges, placing huge burdens on public health systems in general and healthcare budgets in particular (**Table 2**).

Global poverty has declined in the past two decades, and the global poverty ratio is predicted to fall from its 2005 figure of 21% to 2.5% in 2050.[3] Economic growth has occurred, but is highly variable within countries, and over time will even lead to higher income inequality within individual countries. In India, for example, the top 20% of earners in rural settings can only match the incomes made by middle and upper middle earners in cities. The lowest earners in urban settings are far ahead of the rural poor, who account for 80% of rural populations, and the urban top 20% of earners far outstrip all other categories.[4] Disturbingly, the GINI Index – a measurement of the income distribution of a country's residents that helps define the gap between the rich and the poor – is increasing in countries with high economic growth and high populations,

with greater disparities observable in urban than in rural areas. In absolute terms, however, large swathes of the world's population will still rise out of extreme poverty.

A recent USDA report predicts an improvement in the global food insecurity situation, projecting that only 6% of the world population will have inadequate access to food by 2026, compared to 17% at present. Decreased food prices and increasing incomes, especially in Asia, may be linked to this decline.[5]

Population growth is contributing to climate change, which is putting pressure on food systems and will impact agricultural yields. Food systems themselves contribute 19–29% of greenhouse gas emissions, and agricultural production accounts for 80–85% of total food systems emissions, although significant variation by country exists. The relationship between climate change and nutrition is discussed in detail elsewhere in this book.

An escalator in a crowded shopping mall. Economic growth is likely to lead to higher income inequality not just between nations but also within individual countries.

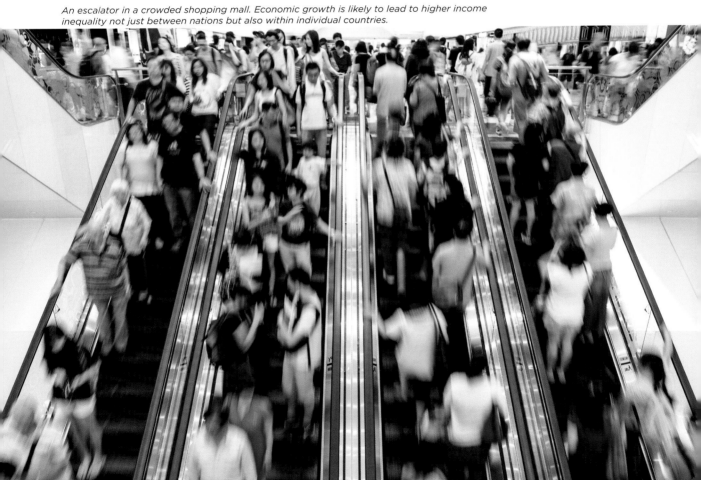

Table 2 | Implications of change for global health

Health effect	Confidence level
Increase in malnutrition and consequent disorders, including child growth and development.	High
Increase in death, disease, and injury from heat waves, floods, storms, fire and drought.	High
Mixed effects on malaria, with some contractions balanced by expanded geographic range and change in seasonality.	Very high
Change in the range of some vectors of infectious diseases.	High
Increase in diarrheal diseases.	Moderate
Increase in number of people exposed to dengue fever.	Low
Decrease in cereal crop productivity in low latitudes for even small temperature increases.	Moderate

Source: IPCC Fourth Assessment Report Climate, 2007.

The nutrition transition

Modernization, urbanization, economic development and increased wealth are also leading to predictable shifts in diet referred to as the "nutrition transition". This is broadly classified into five patterns (**Table 3**).

Most low-and middle-income countries are currently moving from pattern 3 (end of famine) to pattern 4 (consuming more energy-dense diets). This shift from traditional diets to Western-style diets has been a key contributor to the obesity epidemic in low- and middle-income countries. Meanwhile, childhood stunting (low height for a given age), an indicator of undernutrition in the earliest years of life, and which results in increased mortality and cognitive deficits, is still at unacceptably high levels. Although declines in stunting are observed worldwide, and the MDG target of halving the incidence of stunting worldwide by 2015 was nearly achieved, 162 million children were stunted in 2012, with particularly high levels of

Table 3 | The five patterns of the nutrition transition

Pattern	Description	Commentary
1	Hunter-gatherer	Individuals live highly active lifestyles, hunting and foraging for food. Diets typically are rich in fibrous plants and high in protein from lean wild animals.
2	Early agriculture	Famine is common, slowing individuals' growth and decreasing their body fat.
3	End of famine	Famine recedes as income rises and nutrition improves.
4	Overeating, obesity-related diseases	As income continues to rise, individuals have access to an abundance of high-calorie foods, and they become less active, leading to increases in obesity and obesity-related chronic diseases, such as diabetes and heart disease.
5	Behavior change	In response to increasing rates of obesity and obesity-related chronic diseases, individuals change their behavior – and communities promote behavior changes – to prevent these conditions.

Source: IPCC Fourth Assessment Report Climate, Behavior change

prevalence in south Asia, Sub-Saharan Africa, the Caribbean, and Oceania. Appropriate breastfeeding and complementary feeding practices are key to the prevention of stunting, as are adequate levels of sanitation and hygiene.

Meat consumption, which is important for meeting requirements for intake of animal protein as well as the micronutrients iron, zinc and vitamin A, is growing worldwide. There are, however, vast regional discrepancies in levels of meat consumption, with citizens of Bangladesh, Nigeria, Ethiopia, the Democratic Republic of Congo and Burma consuming an average of just 0–10 g meat per day and those of the USA, France and The Netherlands consuming 70–80 g daily. If the consumption of milk is included, over 70% of the world's population consumes less than 30 g of animal protein per day.[6] Nevertheless the consumption of meat, vegetable oils, sugar and pulses is projected to increase in developing countries, many of which are undergoing a

nutrition transition. This will place considerable demands on the world's food production systems, and alternative sources of food, such as fisheries and aquaculture, should be explored.

Outlook

According to the FAO, there will be a third more mouths to feed by 2050, despite an anticipated decline in fertility rates across the globe.[7] Food production will have to rise by 70% to meet this need, which will place huge demands both on the environment and on the world's agricultural systems. According to the best-case scenario, 4.5% of the world's population will be malnourished in 2050 (as opposed to 12.4% in 2005); the worst-case scenario puts this figure at 5.9% (**Tables 4 and 5**). Approaches to making agriculture more innovative, efficient and sustainable, and to ensuring that it delivers not just more calories but also improved nutritional content, are discussed in chapters 3 and 4 of this book.

Table 4 | **World food supply and demand projections: best-case scenario**

WORLD FOOD SUPPLY AND DEMAND IN MARKET FIRST SCENARIO

	World crop production (million metric tons)	Crop land (million hectares)	Yield (tonnes/hectare)	Crop loss ratio (percent)
2005	4,190	1,544	2.71	30.3%
2050	6,584	1,617	4.07	22.3%
percentage change	57.1%	4.7%	50.0%	
avg ann. percentage change	1.0%	0.1%	0.9%	

CALORIES AVAILABLE PER PERSON

	World	OECD	Non-OCED	Sub-Saharan Africa
2005	2,800	3,421	2,662	2,256
2050	3,207	3,635	3,135	2,588
percentage change	14.5%	6.3%	17.8%	14.7%
avg ann. percentage change	0.3%	0.1%	0.4%	0.3%

PERCENTAGE OF POPULATION MALNOURISHED

	World	OECD	Non-OCED	Sub-Saharan Africa
2005	12.4%	1.9%	14.8%	30.7%
2050	4.5%	0.0%	5.3%	18.5%

Source: Hillebrand E, White Paper, Expert Meeting on how to feed the world in 2050, FAO 2010.

Table 5 | **World food supply and demand projections: conservative estimates**

WORLD FOOD SUPPLY AND DEMAND IN TREND SCENARIO

	World crop production (million metric tons)	Crop land (million hectares)	Yield (tonnes/hectare)	Crop loss ratio (percent)
2005	4,190	1,544	271	30.3%
2050	6,150	1,620	3.8	24.1%
percentage change	46.8%	4.9%	39.9%	
avg ann. percentage change	0.9%	0.1%	0.1%	

CALORIES AVAILABLE PER PERSON

	World	OECD	Non-OCED	Sub-Saharan Africa
2005	2,800	3,421	2,662	2,256
2050	3,099	3,648	3,013	2,507
percentage change	10.7%	6.6%	13.2%	11.1%
avg ann. percentage change	0.2%	0.1%	0.3%	0.2%

PERCENTAGE OF POPULATION MALNOURISHED

	World	OECD	Non-OCED	Sub-Saharan Africa
2005	12.4%	1.9%	14.8%	30.7%
2050	5.9%	0.0%	6.8%	21.4%

Source: Hillebrand E, White Paper, Expert Meeting on how to feed the world in 2050, FAO 2010.

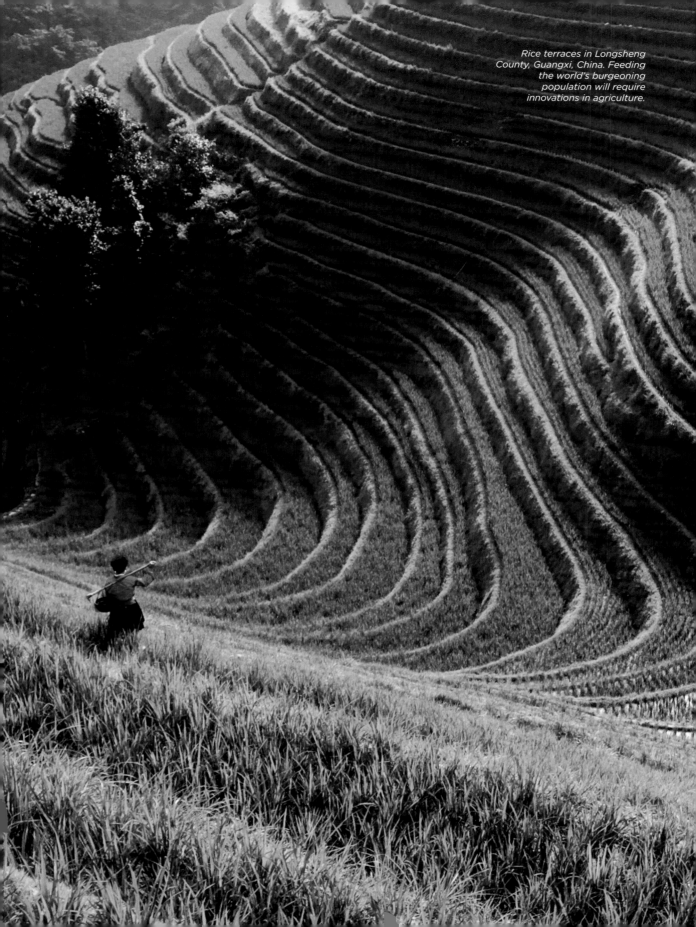

Rice terraces in Longsheng County, Guangxi, China. Feeding the world's burgeoning population will require innovations in agriculture.

My personal view

Michael J Klag

Population growth underlies many of the most important challenges facing the world today. In the future, the world will be more populous, especially in low- and middle-income countries, more urban, and with an older and more obese population which will be characterized by even greater economic disparities than is the case today. All these trends will impact poor countries more severely than wealthy ones.

Family planning is essential to curb population growth, and Family Planning 2020 (FP2020) has a key role to play here. FP2020 is a global partnership that supports the rights of women and girls to decide, freely, and for themselves, whether, when, and how many children they want to have. FP2020 works with governments, civil society, multilateral organizations, donors, the private sector, and the research and development community to enable 120 million more women and girls to use contraceptives by 2020. FP2020 is an outcome of the 2012 London Summit on Family Planning where more than 20 governments made commitments to address the policy, financing, delivery and sociocultural barriers to women accessing contraceptive information, services and supplies. Donors also pledged an additional US$2.6 billion in funding. It is very important that this goal be achieved.

Further reading

Rosen S, Thome K, Meade B. *International Food Security Assessment, 2016–2026. A report summary from the Economic Research Service.* USDA June 2016. *http://www.ers.usda.gov/media/2109786/gfa27.pdf*, accessed July 22, 2016.

Vermeulen SJ, Bruce M, Campbell BM. *Climate Change and Food Systems. Annu. Rev. Environ. Resour. 2012. 37:195–222. http://www.annualreviews.org/doi/abs/10.1146/annurev-environ-020411-130608*, accessed July 22, 2016.

The special challenge for sub-Saharan Africa. High Level Expert Forum – How to Feed the World in 2050. Rome: FAO, October 2013. *http://www.fao.org/wsfs/forum2050/wsfs-background-documents/issues-briefs/en/*, accessed July 22, 2016.

World agriculture: towards 2015/2030 Summary report. FAO, 2002. http://www.fao.org/docrep/004/y3557e/y3557e00.HTM, accessed July 22, 2016.

Cleland J, Bernstein S, Ezeh A et al. *Sexual and Reproductive Health 3. Family planning: the unfinished agenda. Lancet 2006; 368: 1810–27. http://www.thelancet.com/pdfs/journals/lancet/PIIS0140-6736(06)69480-4.pdf*, accessed July 22, 2016.

References

1   *http://www.worldometers.info/world-population/*, accessed December 14, 2015.

2   *http://www.worldbank.org/depweb/english/modules/glossary.html#momentum*, accessed July 8, 2016.

3   Hillebrand, E. *Poverty, growth and inequality over the next 50 years.* FAO, 2010.

4   Sen, A *(mimeo, 2004)* based on NSS data.

5   Rosen S, Thome K, Meade B. *International Food Security Assessment, 2016–2026. A report summary from the Economic Research Service.* USDA June 2016. *http://www.ers.usda.gov/media/2109786/gfa27.pdf*

6   FAOSTAT 2001.

7   FAO Expert Meeting, 2009.

Managing Value Chains for Improved Nutrition

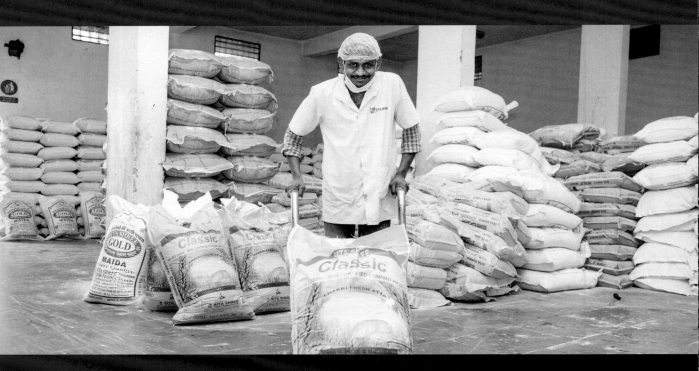

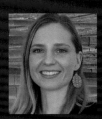

Shauna Downs
Postdoctoral Research Fellow, Institute of Human Nutrition and The Earth Institute, Columbia University, New York, NY USA

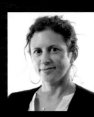

Jess Fanzo
Bloomberg Distinguished Associate Professor of Ethics and Global Food and Agriculture Policy in the Berman Institute of Bioethics and the School of Advanced International Studies at Johns Hopkins University, Baltimore, MD, USA

"The cost of a thing is the amount of what I will call life which is required to be exchanged for it, immediately or in the long run."

Henry David Thoreau (1817–62), *American, author, poet and philosopher, Walden (1854).*

Key messages

- Value chains involve many actors that influence the way in which food is produced, processed, distributed, marketed and consumed.

- The nutrition community needs to begin thinking in terms of "adding value" to improve the quality of the food supply.

- Making value chains more nutrition-sensitive can help improve the quality of the foods that are available, affordable and acceptable.

- Value chain analysis can be used in the context of both undernutrition and overweight & obesity and in low-, middle- and high-income country contexts.

- Value chain analysis can be used to examine the incentives and disincentives for the production and consumption of nutritious foods, and can help to inform interventions aimed at improving access to these.

Food value chains

The term "food value chains" describes the full range of activities required to bring a food product from conception, through the various phases of production, to delivery to end-consumers and eventually disposal following use. Production means the growing, raising or creation of the product. Sometimes production involves processing, which refers to the refining or altering of the original product with a view to adding value to it. Sometimes production involves manufacturing, which refers to the process whereby the product is produced on an industrial scale.

Food value chains in the developing world have undergone a rapid transformation in recent years. Only a few decades ago, most food in these regions was grown by family farms located in rural areas, and was intended for local domestic consumption. Food was also purchased at small, local markets. This has changed. Now, most food purchased by consumers in middle- and high-income countries has traveled longer distances and has touched several different actors across a food value chain. This has been influenced by changes in food consumption patterns that have been prompted by rapid urbanization, income growth, and expansion on the part of modern retailers, processors and distributors. Furthermore, increasing numbers of households are moving out of rural areas into urban centers, where they make use of modern supermarkets and are diversifying their diets, sometimes with both positive and negative consequences. The demand for more highly valued, nutrient-rich products such as meats, dairy, fruits and vegetables is growing. In addition, the markets for packaged, processed and ready-to-eat foods are expanding. This category includes breakfast cereals, confectionary, ready-to-eat meals, and carbonated soft drinks. Rural populations also depend on food value chains for their food purchases because most of them, including the very poor, are net-food buyers and are employed in the food sector or in industries supporting farming.

Gomez and Ricketts (2013)[1] developed a typology that divides food value chains that focus on providing nutritious foods into four broad categories to reflect different transformations. A simplified version of the four typologies is shown in **Table 1**, and includes traditional, modern, modern-to-traditional and traditional-to-modern food value chains.

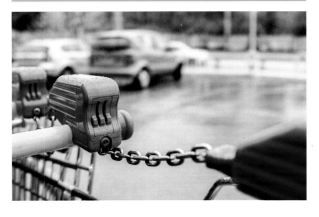

Cheap, energy-dense foods of low nutritional value are readily available in most countries worldwide.

Table 1 | **Typology of food value chains for nutrition**

Type	Description
Traditional	Traditional traders buy primarily from smallholder farmers and sell to consumers and traditional retailers in wet (mostly local) markets
Modern	Domestic and multinational food manufacturers procure primarily from commercial farms and sell through modern supermarket outlets
Modern-to-traditional	Domestic and multinational food manufacturers sell through the network of traditional traders and retailers (e.g., mom and pop shops)
Traditional-to-modern	Supermarkets and food manufacturers source food from smallholder farmers and traders

Consumers purchasing food through *traditional food value chains* most often purchase food directly from smallholder farmers and traders in local or regional wet markets, or from traditional retailers such as "mom and pop" shops, street vendors or roadside stalls. Traditional food value chains are mainly informal, and are common in small rural markets situated relatively close to production regions. Produce may, however, also travel greater distances to reach urban consumers, primarily in lower-income neighborhoods. Traditional markets may help increase access to affordable, nutritious foods such as fruits and vegetables, with the potential to improve micronutrient intakes; however, given the lack of post-harvest and distribution infrastructure, the availability of diverse foods that can enhance diet quality may be extremely limited.

Modern food value chains are largely driven by the expansion of modern retailers in developing countries, chiefly in urban areas. They involve both domestic and multinational food manufacturers and wholesalers, as well as commercial agribusinesses and farms. These value chains are often more streamlined, and have greater economies of scale, than traditional value chains. They are able to offer a wide assortment of fresh, as well as processed and packaged, food products all the year round, but they are unlikely to reach all consumers. Although the traditional food value chains often still predominate in low- and middle-income countries, modern value chains have grown considerably. They can influence nutrition outcomes both positively and negatively by facilitating the year-round availability of a wide variety of foods. These are aimed first and foremost at high- and middle-income households in urban areas. They exert a positive influence in that they provide nutritious food products all the year round, but they also contribute to overnutrition by increasing the availability of inexpensive, processed and packaged foods which are often high in sugar, salt and unhealthy fat.

Modern food value chains are the predominant typology in most high-income countries. There are fewer farmers operating in these systems, and many of their decisions in terms of what they grow are dependent on retailers and food manufacturers. In these food value chains, much of the power in the chain has shifted from the farm to retailers.

Modern-to-traditional food value chains often involve the distribution of processed and packaged foods made by food manufacturers and sold through traditional retailers. They allow for year-round distribution of processed and packaged foods, targeting lower-income consumers in urban areas as well as remote markets in rural areas. Increasing access to processed and packaged foods through modern-to-traditional food value chains has the potential to counteract undernourishment in rural areas while at the same time potentially increasing obesity in urban areas. Nevertheless, these food value chains provide an opportunity for implementing processed and packaged food fortification initiatives designed to combat micronutrient deficiencies.

Traditional-to-modern food value chains consist of smallholder farmers and traders selling primarily high-value crop and livestock products to supermarkets and food manufacturers. The participation of smallholder farmers and traders in these food value chains may increase incomes and thus help reduce undernutrition, particularly by indirect means such as increased opportunities for off-farm employment on commercial farms and in post-harvest businesses. However, smallholders often struggle to achieve the product quality standards demanded by modern retailers.

Actors across the food value chain

Food value chains involve many actors – farmers, agribusinesses, processors, wholesalers, distributors, retailers, and consumers. These influence what food is grown and the manner in which it is produced, processed, distributed, marketed and consumed, and whether or not nutritious foods are available, affordable and acceptable. The decisions made by one group of actors have implications for the others along the value chain. The private sector – from large multinational companies to small, local agribusiness enterprises – plays a key role in linking one end of the chain to the other.

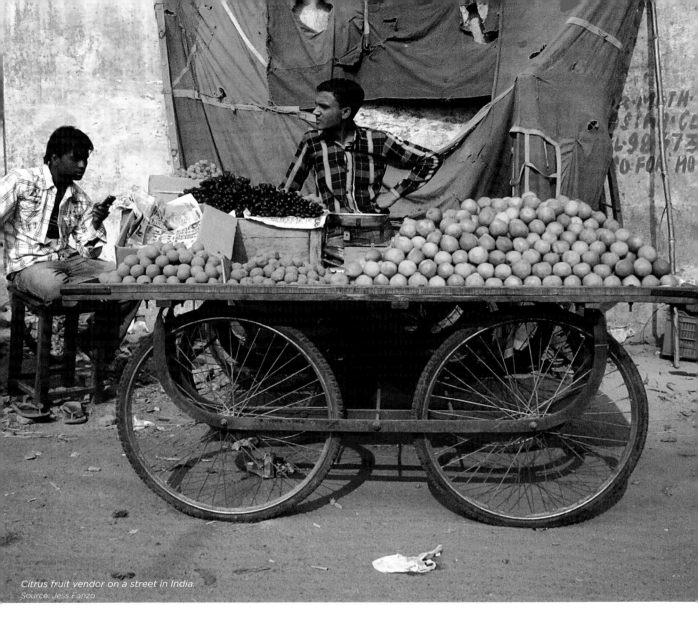

Citrus fruit vendor on a street in India.
Source: Jess Fanzo

Value for nutrition

Food value chain approaches are being closely examined with the objective of improving the livelihoods of food producers along with strengthening the supply side, but the nutritional value of diets is rarely considered in this connection. Food value chain approaches are also used in high-income contexts – mainly by the private sector – to streamline supply chains and maximize profits. In recent years there has also been a push to use value chains to identify ways of reducing carbon footprints and improving the quality of products being produced by some companies.

In low- and middle-income countries, the food value chain approach has mainly been considered with a view to improving the economic outcomes of cash cropping systems. More can be done within the value chain model, however, including ensuring that better partnerships with discrete sets of players can add value by introducing more nutrition into

the value chain. By including nutrition as an outcome of value chains, the supply and demand "ends" of the chain can be linked with a view to ensuring that the nutritional needs of the population are met.

The ultimate goal of *supply-side* initiatives is to improve the availability of food at the household level and to increase household income (in order to enhance access to food). However, evidence has shown that improvements in food supply and household income are not sufficient in themselves to improve nutritional status. To look at food value chains via a nutrition "lens," therefore, the demand side of the equation and the overall linkages of value chains to the food environment must also be taken into account.

The *demand side* relates to household decisions about the purchase of food, the allocation of resources to individual household members, and the knowledge of safe and nutritious food practices in the preparation of food and the feeding of children. Demand-side interventions focus on awareness, behavioral change, willingness to pay, knowledge transfer, and empowerment so as to increase demand for nutritious foods and thereby improve dietary intake. In this connection, "value" is defined not only in terms of economic impact (e.g., income earned) but also in terms of social impact as expressed by improved nutritional status and better health.

The links between what is produced on the farm, the consumer who buys that food, and the income received by the producer involves not just what the producer supplies or the consumer demands. The middle of the chain is also important. Food is stored, distributed, processed, retailed, prepared and consumed in a variety of ways that affect the access, acceptability and nutritional quality of what the consumer eats. Demand for healthier products can be stimulated when consumers value these higher quality products, and retail, packaging and marketing all have a role to play here. Food preferences are influenced by exposure to the eating behaviors of parents, caregivers, peers and role models; to the availability of foods inside and outside the home; and to cultural and social norms, as well as to new information and marketing. Demand for more nutritious foods can be encouraged by targeting food preferences through social marketing, nudges, modeling of healthy eating behaviors, and other means.

Adopting value chain approaches can be an effective way of identifying the causes of insufficient food availability, affordability and acceptability, and also of implementing effective solutions and creating long-term, sustainable benefits. Perhaps much of this effort can be realized by the agriculture sector. **Figure 1** depicts some of the ways in which nutrition interventions can leverage agriculture-focused value chain activities to address the double burden of malnutrition at both the market and the consumer level.

Nutrition-focused food value chains

Michael Porter first described value chains in the 1980s as a way of identifying how and where value can be increased along an internal business chain. Porter defines the value chain as comprising primary activities and support activities. **Figure 2** transforms this original definition of the value chain into a more nutrition-focused concept. The primary activities encompass the food value chain all the way from inputs into agricultural production right through to food labeling, marketing and retailing. The secondary activities relate to the supportive factors that increase the probability of adding nutrition value along the chain. Throughout the nutrition-focused food value chain, opportunities exist for creating shared value in terms of both economic and nutritional goals. **Table 2** provides an overview of potential indicators that can be used to conduct nutrition-focused value chain analysis.

Figure 1 | **Nutrition interventions can leverage agriculture-focused value chains for undernutrition and overweight/obesity**

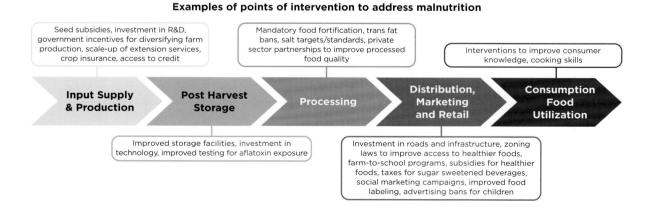

Examples of points of intervention to address malnutrition

Seed subsidies, investment in R&D, government incentives for diversifying farm production, scale-up of extension services, crop insurance, access to credit

Mandatory food fortification, trans fat bans, salt targets/standards, private sector partnerships to improve processed food quality

Interventions to improve consumer knowledge, cooking skills

Input Supply & Production → **Post Harvest Storage** → **Processing** → **Distribution, Marketing and Retail** → **Consumption Food Utilization**

Improved storage facilities, investment in technology, improved testing for aflatoxin exposure

Investment in roads and infrastructure, zoning laws to improve access to healthier foods, farm-to-school programs, subsidies for healthier foods, taxes for sugar sweetened beverages, social marketing campaigns, improved food labeling, advertising bans for children

Figure 2 | **A nutrition-focused food value chain framework**

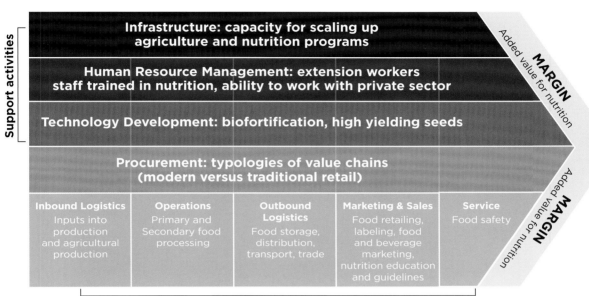

Source: Adapted from Porter and Miller, 1985

Table 2 | **Examples of indicators for conducting nutrition-focused value chain analysis**

Value chain step	Examples of potential indicators	
Input supply & production	• Yields • Production diversity • Access to inputs • Cost of inputs	• Use of inputs (irrigation, improved seed, fertilizer, etc.) • Time use • Farmer profit/incomes
Post-harvest storage	• Post-harvest losses	• Use of storage facilities
Distribution, marketing and retail	• Distance/access to markets • Transaction costs • Import/export flows • Availability and price of foods in markets (market analyses)	• Percentage of sales • Percentage spent on advertising • Food miles • Food waste
Consumption, food utilization	• Knowledge, attitudes and behaviors • Dietary intake and diet quality/diversity	• Intake of specific nutrients • Biomarkers of specific micronutrients • Food waste

Adapted from: Value chains and nutrition: A framework to support the identification, design, and evaluation of interventions.
IFPRI Discussion Paper 01413, January 2015.

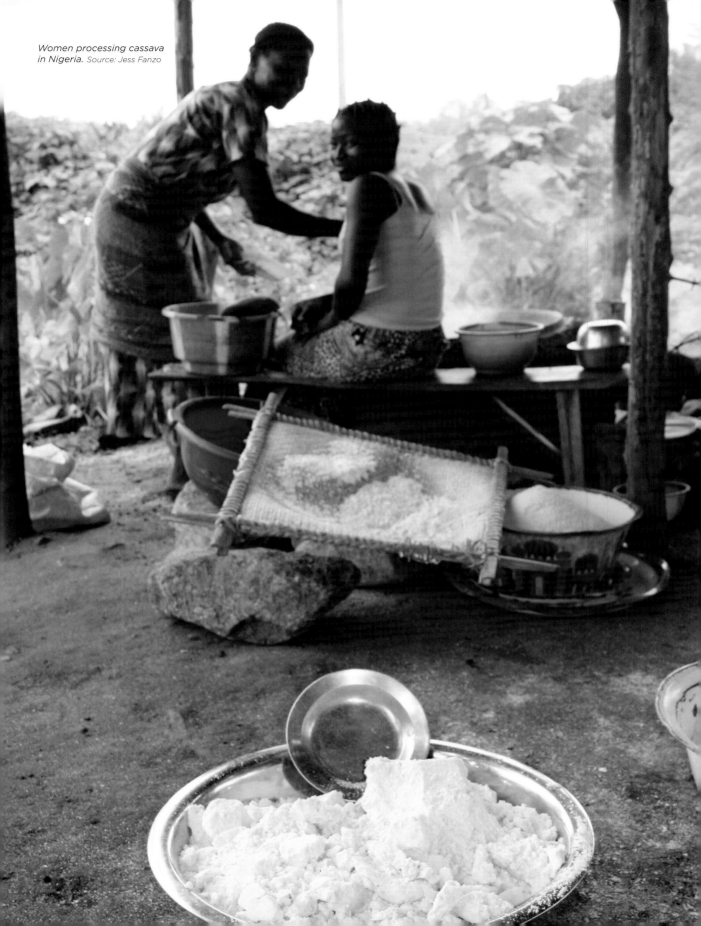

Women processing cassava in Nigeria. Source: Jess Fanzo

Primary activities of food value chains

Inbound Logistics: Inbound logistics encompass inputs into production as well as agricultural production itself. The actors involved in these processes include seed, irrigation and farming equipment companies, plus plant breeders, farmers and laborers, among others. Nutrition value can be added at this stage of the chain by producing nutrient-rich crops and maximizing the yields of those crops. For example, HarvestPlus has developed specific crop and nutrient combinations (e.g., rice biofortified with zinc in Bangladesh and India, and maize biofortified with provitamin A in Nigeria and Zambia) to deliver specific micronutrients to populations at risk of micronutrient deficiency mainly in Sub-Saharan Africa and South Asia. In the United States, Dow Chemicals launched canola and sunflower seeds to produce cooking oils that had a longer shelf life and were suitable for frying in order to enable product reformulation to facilitate the removal of trans fat from foods.

Operations: Operations include both primary and secondary food processing as well as the actors (mainly the food industry) involved in these processes. Nutrition value can be added at this point in the chain both by fortifying processed foods with micronutrients, fermenting foods, and by ensuring that processed foods are based on healthier inputs (for example, reductions in the levels of salt and trans fats). The private sector has a critical role to play at this point in the food value chain.

Outbound Logistics: Outbound logistics include food storage, distribution, transport and trade. Outbound logistics can occur directly after food production (also known as inbound logistics) or after food processing (also known as operations), depending on the type of product involved. Nutritional values can be improved at this stage of the food value chain by increasing access to nutrient-rich foods. Measures to achieve this include ensuring proper storage of foods so as to reduce wastage, distributing food more efficiently, and ensuring that infrastructure is in place to facilitate the transport of foods. For example, a dairy farming development assistance project in Zambia – which aimed to reduce household food insecurity among vulnerable groups by increasing incomes generated from the sale of milk and other dairy products – improved storage and transportation by means of technologies designed for milk aggregation and cooling. This increased the availability of safe, high-quality, cooled milk at milk collection centers and increased farmer profits, diet diversity and food security.

Marketing and sales: This is a very important step in the food value chain, whose function is to improve the acceptability, as well as the availability and affordability, of nutritious foods. Food retailers play a pivotal role by increasing access to foods that have a higher content of essential nutrients, such as vitamins and minerals, without having a higher energy density compared to similar foods. In urban populations, supermarkets are critically important in coordinating markets and determining prices. In rural populations, local markets, smallholder farms and "mom and pop" shops are important in that they provide access to nutritious foods such as fruits and vegetables and health products. In France, Intermarché (the country's third largest supermarket) launched an "inglorious fruits and vegetables" campaign aimed at getting consumers to purchase produce that would normally be tossed away for not meeting uniformity standards. The produce is sold at a 30% discount, potentially increasing access to low-income consumers while simultaneously reducing food waste. Similar initiatives have begun in Portugal, California and elsewhere worldwide.

Secondary activities of food value chains

The secondary activities of food value chains consist of infrastructure creation and management, human resource management, technology development, and procurement. In terms of adding nutrition value, these activities aim to support the primary activities in the chain and to increase the uptake of activities that are likely to improve the availability, affordability and acceptability of nutritious foods. For example, ensuring the presence of an adequate infrastructure increases the likelihood of being able to successfully scale up nutrition-sensitive agricultural programs and initiatives. In addition to improving infrastructure and human resource management, ensuring the development and uptake of appropriate technology by actors in the chain can help increase access to nutritious foods. So can streamlining the value chain by improving procurement. For example, reducing post-harvest losses is an important point for intervention along value chains, particularly in low- and middle-income countries, where a substantial proportion of food is lost before it ever leaves the farm gate.

Entry and exit points for nutrition across food value chains

Typically, extremely poor households in low-income countries subsist on monotonous staple-based diets; they lack access to nutritious foods, such as fruits, vegetables, animal-source foods (fish, meat, eggs, and dairy produce), fortified foods, and wild foods of high nutrient content. Lack of dietary diversity is closely associated with inadequate

53

intake of essential micronutrients and concomitant risks of a range of dietary deficiency diseases. In poor households around the globe, many rely on cheap foods that are caloric-dense, nutrient-poor, and high in sugar, salt and fat. The resulting deficiencies have far-reaching health and nutrition consequences, in both the short and the long term.

Targeting leverage points along the value chain can reduce the likelihood that nutrients will be lost from the value chain and also enhance the nutritional value of specific nutrient-rich foods. Exit points are caused by ineffective or inefficient harvesting, storage, processing, or handling, thereby reducing the availability, and raising the price, of nutrient-rich foods. The poor are at great risk of exposure to unsafe food, and since malnourished and micronutrient-deficient children are

most susceptible to the health risks associated with unsafe food or water, they have the most to gain from improvements in the nutritional value and safety of foods.

It is also important to understand potential entry points, and whether these are conceived to enhance (or prevent losses in) the nutritional value of foods during processing or to fortify (or restore the nutrient content of) foods. Entry points to educate and raise awareness among the different actors in the value chain are also important, as they stimulate demand for the target products. Economic constraints, lack of knowledge and information, and related lack of demand for nutritious foods are critical factors that limit the access of poor populations to such foods. **Figure 3** shows ways in which more nutrition could enter or exit food value chains.

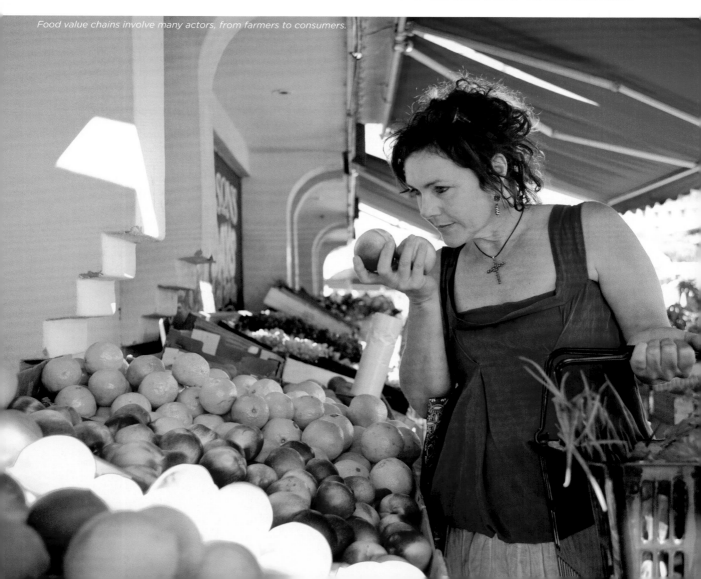
Food value chains involve many actors, from farmers to consumers.

Figure 3 | **Exit and Entry points along the value chain for nutrition**

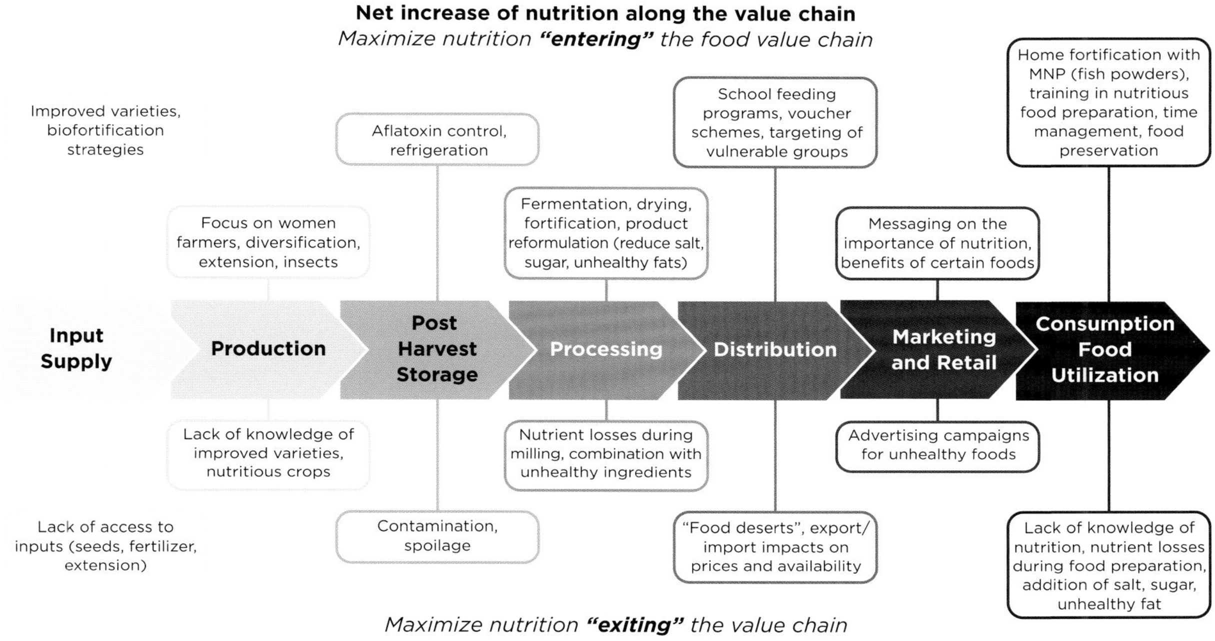

Net increase of nutrition along the value chain
Maximize nutrition "entering" the food value chain

Improved varieties, biofortification strategies

Aflatoxin control, refrigeration

School feeding programs, voucher schemes, targeting of vulnerable groups

Home fortification with MNP (fish powders), training in nutritious food preparation, time management, food preservation

Focus on women farmers, diversification, extension, insects

Fermentation, drying, fortification, product reformulation (reduce salt, sugar, unhealthy fats)

Messaging on the importance of nutrition, benefits of certain foods

Input Supply → **Production** → **Post Harvest Storage** → **Processing** → **Distribution** → **Marketing and Retail** → **Consumption Food Utilization**

Lack of knowledge of improved varieties, nutritious crops

Nutrient losses during milling, combination with unhealthy ingredients

Advertising campaigns for unhealthy foods

Lack of access to inputs (seeds, fertilizer, extension)

Contamination, spoilage

"Food deserts", export/ import impacts on prices and availability

Lack of knowledge of nutrition, nutrient losses during food preparation, addition of salt, sugar, unhealthy fat

Maximize nutrition "exiting" the value chain

Case Study 1

Identifying interventions to improve the quality of fat in India using a modified value chain analysis

Non-communicable diseases (NCDs), especially cardiovascular disease, are the leading cause of death in India. A serious dietary risk factor for NCDs is the consumption of industrially produced trans fat. The World Health Organization has called for its removal from the global food supply and has suggested it should be replaced by oils high in polyunsaturated (rather than saturated) fat for better health.

In India, trans fat consumption is probably high. The main source is a vegetable ghee called *vanaspati*, which is a partially hydrogenated vegetable oil that can contain upwards of 50% trans fat. *Vanaspati* is mainly used in fried snacks, bakery products and foods prepared by street vendors; however, it is also employed as cooking oil in the northern Indian states. The national Government of India has identified trans fat as a major contributor to the country's rising rates of NCDs, and in response has taken steps to begin regulating it. Although there has been success in removing trans fat from the food supply of high-income countries, low- and middle-income countries such as India may face

additional challenges such as large informal food sector, low enforcement capacity and low consumer awareness.

In order to examine the potential points for policy intervention and private-sector innovation to improve the quality of fats that are available, affordable and acceptable in India, a modified value chain analysis was conducted. A combination of interviews with key value chain actors, document analysis and analysis of existing data sources were used to: 1) examine the bottlenecks in the value chain for improving the availability, affordability and acceptability of healthier oils and 2) examine points for intervening to increase nutrition "entering" and reduce nutrition "exiting" the fats supply chain. Overall, key bottlenecks were: the low production of healthier oils in India; the low availability and use of healthier oils for product reformulation; wastage due to inefficiencies in the supply chain; use of *vanaspati* by street vendors; lack of consumer awareness regarding trans and saturated fat, and; the promotion of foods containing unhealthy fats (**Figure 4**).

Case Study 1 (continued)

Figure 4 | **Value chain analysis of oil chain in India**

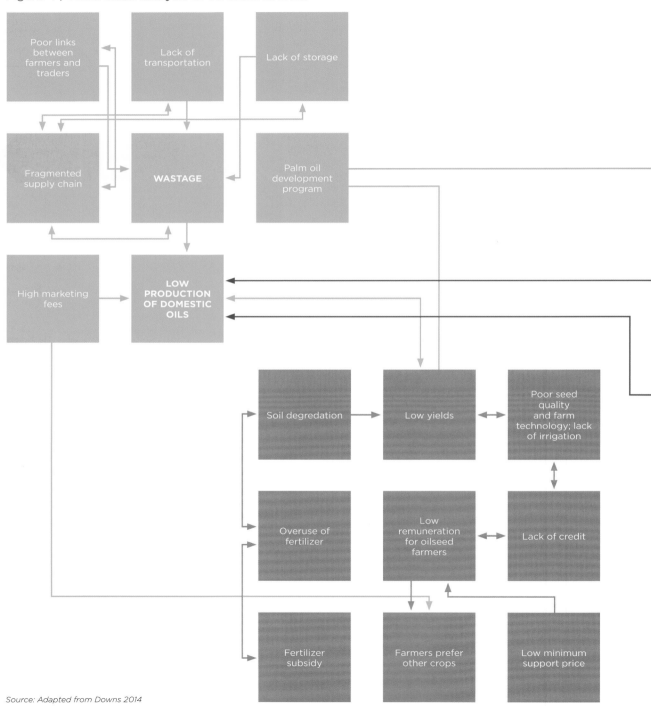

Source: Adapted from Downs 2014

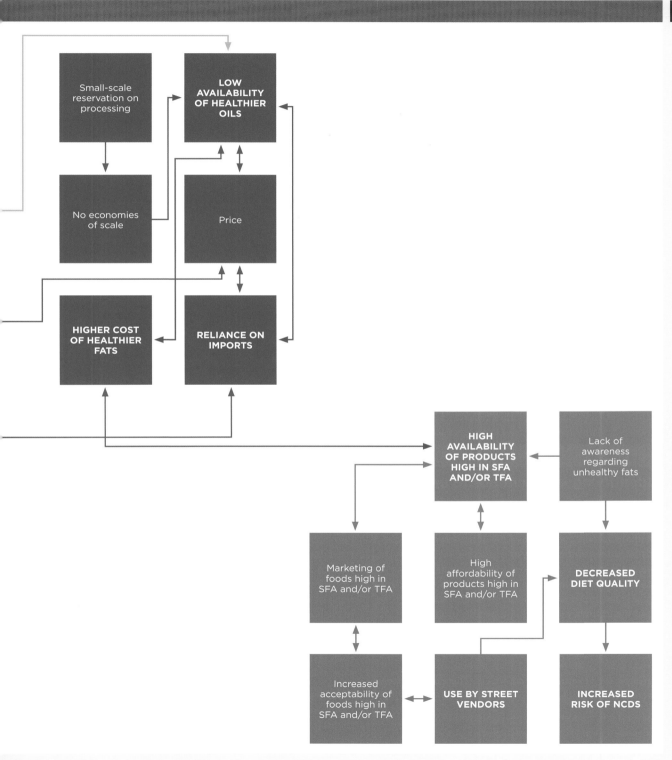

Case Study 1 (continued)

Figure 5 provides a summary of the potential levers to address these bottlenecks in order to improve the quality of fat that is available, affordable and acceptable in India. This value chain analysis highlighted the power of upstream determinants of the quality of fat and potential policy interventions at each step of the supply chain that would improve health. This systems-based approach helped to provide insight into what policies might work best in India.

It is clear from this work that a multisectoral whole-of-government approach to improving access to healthier oils

is required in India. Improving policy coherence among upstream determinants of the quality of the food supply (such as agricultural production) and downstream consumer-facing policies (such as trans fat limits and labeling) is necessary to ensure that product reformulation is done in such a way as to maximize health gains. Taking a value-chain approach to identifying innovative food policies is crucial in ensuring coherence between public health nutrition goals and the supply of foods that are available, affordable and acceptable.

Figure 5 | **Indian Case study: policy levers to improve the quality of the fat supply**

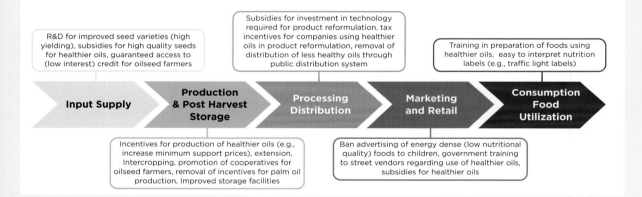

Net increase of nutrition along the fats value chain

Case Study 2

Identifying interventions to improve the vegetable value chains in Sierra Leone

The Koindagu district of Sierra Leone is known for its vegetable production, which is chiefly carried out by women and can account for much as 50% of household incomes. A detailed intervention analysis of small-scale commercial vegetable value-chain factors and opportunities was conducted in the district in order to identify the key entry points for improving nutrition for smallholder producers and their families involved in vegetable production.[3]

The main actors in this region involved in small-scale commercial vegetable production are female farmers, local traders, wholesalers, village loaning and sales groups, the government, and NGOs. There are challenges across the value chain.

Several entry points for improved nutrition were identified along the vegetable value chain:

Production component: First, on the production side, continuous cropping and burning of land has depleted the nutritional content of the soil and led to a reduction in vegetable yields. Second, during the dry season there is not enough water available, since adequate irrigation systems are lacking, which also results in low yields during certain times of the year. The government has begun offering workshops to increase farmers' understanding of the preparation of various crops for improved nutritional status, but no large-scale investments in irrigation have been made. Such investments would be key to growing nutrient-dense vegetables that can be sold at market.

Processing/packaging component: Processing and packaging are important tools to add value along the chain. Improved processing and packaging can increase

Case Study 2 (continued)

income and boost the availability of food by extending shelf-life, which would also allow for more household consumption, while a range of preservation techniques can make vegetables and fruits available all year. Currently, almost no processing of vegetables takes place. Small minorities practice some forms of processing by drying their vegetables and by making tomato paste. However, since processing is often not carried out correctly, or else done using unhygienic equipment, spoilage rates are still high. Introducing processed traditional vegetables into urban markets should be considered in areas that are closer to urban centers.

Transportation and storage component: Cold chain transport and storage pose major challenges to all key actors in Koinadugu due to a lack of infrastructure in the area. Because of the lack of built capital, most of the vegetables produced are sold immediately at the local markets, leaving little or nothing for home consumption. There is some investment by the private sector and NGOs for cold-room storage facilities in market places.

Marketing component: The main challenges faced when selling at the market are poor infrastructure and volatile prices. Improved infrastructure, access to transport and closer markets, as well as storage facilities, could all help improve nutrition by increasing household incomes. Access to transport and storage facilities, as well as markets situated within easy reach, would also reduce the spoilage rates of transported vegetables. Because Koinadugu is known for its vegetable production, urban traders come straight to the district, which offers a favorable context for opening new markets. The government is currently offering farmers training in bargaining and negotiating techniques.

Case Study 3

Initiatives to improve access to fruits and vegetables in low-income populations in New York City

Bottlenecks in value chains are not just a problem of the developing world. In many low-income neighborhoods in cities of the developed world, consumers experience 'food deserts' characterized by low availability and high cost of fresh fruits and vegetables. This creates a barrier to consumption for low-income populations, many of which are battling overweight and obesity, diabetes and other diet-related NCDs.

In an effort to increase fruit and vegetable consumption among lower socioeconomic groups in New York City, the city has implemented several initiatives aimed at improving both the supply and demand for fruits and vegetables. These initiatives are aimed at improving the availability and affordability of fresh produce.

In order to improve the availability of fruits and vegetables in low-income neighborhoods, New York City provided vendor licenses for Green Carts that sell fresh fruits and vegetables in low-income neighborhoods. An evaluation of this program found that the Green Cart Program was reaching low-income populations, some of which reported increasing their fruit and vegetable consumption since shopping at the Green Cart.[4] The city has also adopted other measures to improve the availability of fresh produce, including the Healthy Bodega Initiative, which aims to increase the availability, quality and variety of healthy foods in bodegas and the Food Retail Expansion to Support Health (FRESH) program, which provides zoning and financial incentives to promote the establishment and retention of grocery stores in underserved neighborhoods.

At the consumer level, the city has begun providing Farmers Market Health Bucks Coupons (worth US$2) to consumers who spend five dollars of their food stamps at farmer markets and for those who participate in nutrition and cooking classes sponsored by the Health Department. In addition, some hospitals serving low-income families have begun providing "prescriptions" for fruits and vegetables for children who are overweight or obese in an effort to increase their fruit and vegetable intakes. Patients exchange their prescriptions for Health Bucks to purchase a Fresh Food Box, or they can use them at farmers markets throughout the city.

These initiatives have the potential to address bottlenecks in the value chain and enable low-income consumers to access fresh fruits and vegetables with the potential to improve nutrition and health outcomes among the city's vulnerable.

Source: *New York City Department of Health: http://www. nyc.gov/html/doh/html/living/eating-well2.shtml.*

Conclusion

Value chains are not a new concept, and many working in agriculture and business have been not only utilizing this concept, but also putting value chains into practical use. Yet very little has been done to ensure that nutrition is included in the chain. This is probably a reflection of the cross-disciplinary nature of food value chains.

Analysis of food value chains requires an understanding of nutrition, agriculture, food technology, economics, and marketing, among other things. However, the training received by nutritionists in these other areas is often inadequate for this task. For this reason, many unanswered questions exist that require further research. Nevertheless, food value chains for nutrition have a role to play in terms of identifying innovative ways of improving the availability, affordability and acceptability of nutritious foods both in the context of undernutrition and in the context of overweight/obesity, and there is currently a push for conducting food value chain analyses in an integrated manner with various stakeholders. This will require buy-in from various actors in the value chain and will need to target both supply-side and demand-side dynamics.

There is probably a role for policy in terms of supporting actions along the food value chain that can contribute to healthier consumption patterns; however, there is also a role for the private sector. Applying a "business lens" to nutrition may help identify opportunities for integrating nutrition into food value chains with the goal of increasing the availability, affordability and acceptability of nutritious foods.

Further reading

Value chains and nutrition: A framework to support the identification, design, and evaluation of interventions: http://ebrary.ifpri.org/utils/getfile/collection/ p15738coll2/id/128951/filename/129162.pdf

Value Chains for Nutrition: http://cdm15738. contentdm.oclc.org/utils/getfile/collection/p15738coll2/ id/124837/filename/124838.pdf

Improving Nutrition through Agriculture. Viewing agriculture-nutrition linkages along the smallholder value chain: http://edepot.wur.nl/173655

Food value chain transformations in developing countries. Selected hypotheses on nutritional implications: http://www.fao.org/fileadmin/templates/ esa/Papers_and_documents/WP_13_05_Gomez_ Ricketts.pdf. Accessed March 14, 2015.

My personal view
Shauna Downs

Our current food system is flawed. Cheap, energy-dense foods of low nutritional value are readily available in most countries worldwide, while consumers often struggle to access nutritious foods at an affordable price. Moreover, what we eat is making us sick. There are over two billion people worldwide who are overweight or obese while at the same time undernutrition persists, sometimes within the same country, city or household.

Many countries now face the challenge of simultaneously tackling undernutrition and the growing burden of diet-related non-communicable diseases. In order to ensure that the food supply delivers the diverse, high-quality range of foods needed to promote good nutrition and health, changes are needed. The incentives in our current food system are misaligned: there is a disconnect between what is produced and what is recommended for good nutrition.

Policy is an important tool to address this disconnect and to reorient the incentives in the food system toward the production and consumption of nutritious foods. Value chain analysis is a useful tool to help map out where those incentives lie and to identify potential levers for policy interventions or for private sector innovation.

I believe that the more the nutrition and public health community think in terms of identifying – economically viable – opportunities for "adding value," the more we shall be able to achieve in terms of improving the quality of the food supply. Applying a "business lens" to tackle food system problems has the potential to lead to real change for the better.

References

1   Gómez MI, Ricketts KD. Food value chain transformations in developing countries: Selected hypotheses on nutritional implications. Food Policy 2013;42:139–150.

2   Downs SM. Reducing trans fat in the Indian food supply: A food systems approach. University of Sydney. Sydney, Australia. http://ses.library.usyd. edu.au/handle/2123/11646.

3   Njoro J, Nyahabeh A, de Hoogh I et al. An Analysis of the Food System Landscape and Agricultural Value Chains for Nutrition: A Case Study from Sierra Leone, ICN2 Second International Congress on Nutrition. FAO and WHO, 2013.

4   https://sipa.columbia.edu/system/files/GreenCarts_Final_June16.pdf.

Towards a Balanced "Healthy Diet" for the 21ˢᵗ Century

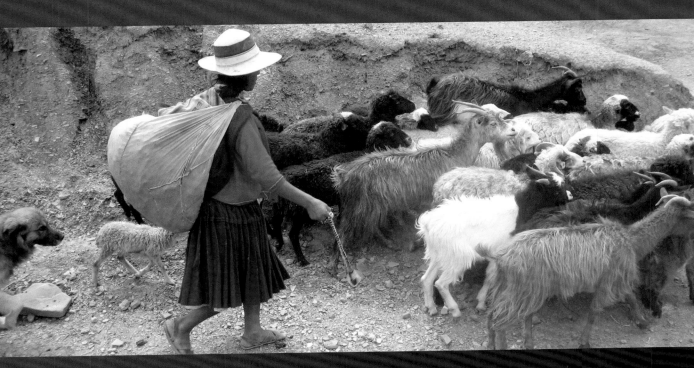

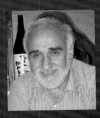

Ricardo Uauy
Professor of Public Health Nutrition, London School of Hygiene and Tropical Medicine, University of London, UK, and Department of Pediatrics, Catholic University of Chile

"Let food be thy medicine and medicine be thy food."

Hippocrates, *(c. 460 – c. 370 BC), known as "the Father of Western Medicine."*

Key messages

- Changes in diet and physical activity levels are chiefly responsible for the recent increase in nutrition-related chronic diseases.

- The problems of diet-related diseases cannot be addressed by the traditional model of single-nutrient deficiency or excess.

- Consumers will make healthier dietary choices if they have a practical option to do so.

- Diets must return to ones based predominantly on plant foods, with limited processing and a limited proportion of refined carbohydrates (need to limit intake of sugar[s])

- An adequate diet may be obtained from many different combinations of foods, but no individual combination has universal applicability.

Writing from the perspective of 1957, the British nutritionist Anne Wilbraham reflected on the precariousness of the concept of the "balanced diet." She observed: "Much was accomplished during the Second World War when, owing to rationing and control, it was difficult to obtain an ill-balanced diet [in the United Kingdom]. In the doubts that at present assail us as to the subtle dangers to health of too much of the wrong kinds of foods the lessons of wartime nutrition should not be forgotten. For it remains true that the foundations of good health are laid in the early years of life and that if boys and girls are properly nourished until maturity is reached they will be the better fitted to withstand hardship and privation in later life. It remains for us to be certain as to the nature of 'proper nourishment', a necessity which points to the need for more research on the problems of human nutrition."[1]

Almost 60 years later, and on the other side of the Atlantic, the sustxainable food systems activist Ellen Gustafson meditated on the process of collective amnesia that has led to a crisis in public health around the world since Wilbraham penned the above lines. She commented: "Roughly 30 years ago (about the time I was born), a series of shifts – some well-intentioned – led to the current global food system and modern American diet. During the 1950s, farming and food production, patterns of food delivery and consumption, even the way we *thought* about food careered off the tracks. The food systems we live with today were formed by innovation, technology and abundance. But they were also formed by food science that forgot what food is, and why we eat it. They were formed from farm subsidies and food aid that were intended to save farmers and save lives, but ended up destroying both. They were formed from farm consolidation that resulted from well-intentioned, misunderstood legislation. They were formed by the genetics of hunger – and the genetics of profit. The system operated confidently under this principle: By producing cheaper, more shelf-stable food, it meant we could feed "more" hungry people. That sounded like a solution. In fact, it sounded like the perfect solution. Yet it was a misguided measure that created an even bigger problem that has been three decades in the making. As a result, today America's largest exports aren't civilian aircraft and semiconductors, intellectual property or even corn. America's largest exports are bad food, bad food policy, crippling hunger, and escalating obesity."[2]

To assess the requirements of a balanced diet that will meet the needs of a rapidly expanding global population in the 21st century, it is first necessary to consider the evolution of human eating habits, in order to outline the drivers which, in today's global village, still inform so many of our eating choices.

Human nutritional needs and foods available to meet them

The foods produced since the advent of agriculture have evolved depending on prevailing environmental conditions that affect the climate, solar radiation, soil characteristics and water resources. These conditions, fundamental for the development of agriculture in prehistoric times, continue to play an important role in defining modern agriculture. Human diets have similarly changed from ones based on a predominantly gatherer-hunter or scavenger mode of existence to the present agriculture-based model.

Humans in pre-agricultural times depended on foraging for plant foods such as seeds, fruits and nuts, as well as hunting small animals; if they inhabited the land/water interface, they were able to collect mollusks and algae, and to catch fish. They were also likely to have been scavengers of meat and fat protected by bone (such as brain and marrow) left over from the hunt by predators larger and stronger than humans. Agriculture evolved in very specific ecological settings that facilitated the domestication and selection of the four main crops upon which we still rely for our food supply: wheat, rice, corn and potatoes In these settings, these crops became the key foods to support the expansion of human populations to the current level of over 7 billion individuals.[3,4]

Traditional dietary patterns have changed with time, and have withstood the test of human evolution. Indeed, most naturally occurring dietary patterns meet or exceed the nutritional needs of populations, although this is not the case where social or economic conditions limit access to food (purchasing capacity) or where cultural practices restrict the choice of foods consumed. However, within the framework of our present understanding of food-health relationships, it seems likely that a large variety of foods can be combined in varying amounts to provide healthy diets. Thus, it is difficult to determine a precise indispensable intake of individual foods that can, when combined with other foods, provide nutritionally adequate diets under all conditions. Perhaps the exception that proves this rule is human milk, now accepted as a source of complete nutrition (with the exception of iron) for the first 6 months of life, provided enough sun exposure is allowed to prevent vitamin D deficiency (in urban settings within temperate regions of the globe, levels of sunlight may not be sufficient, however, necessitating supplementation of the diet with vitamin D).

The prevailing view is that a large set of food combinations is compatible with nutritional adequacy, but that no given set of foods can be extrapolated as absolutely required or sufficient across different ecological settings. Recent trends in the globalization of food supplies provide clear evidence that dietary patterns, and even traditionally local foods, can move across geographical niches.[4]

The modern approach in defining the nutritional adequacy of diets and dietary recommendations has progressed over the past two centuries in accordance with the scientific understanding of the biochemical and physiological basis of human nutritional requirements in health and disease. The definition of essential nutrients and nutrient requirements has provided the scientific underpinnings for nutrient-based dietary recommendations. However, there are obvious limitations to the reductionist nutrient-based approach, since people consume foods and not nutrients. Moreover, the effect of specific foods and dietary patterns on health goes well beyond the combination of essential nutrients the food may contain. For example, if we neglect to integrate bioavailability or nutrient interactions in defining trace element recommendations, we will not be able to assess the true nutritional value of foods.[4,5]

In addition, factors unrelated to diet commonly exert a key influence on the health effect of diets; for example, parasitic infections rather than iron deficiency may be the cause of anemia in many parts of the world. Similarly, if we continue to ignore or undervalue the essential role of physical activity in achieving energy balance, dietary recommendations will fail to meet the goal of preventing obesity and other nutrition-related chronic diseases.

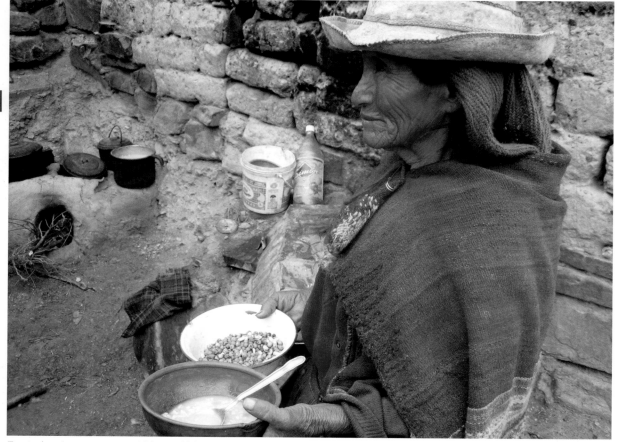

Toasted grains serve as a nutritious midday snack in the Bolivian Highlands (Altiplano).
Source: Ricardo Uauy

The nutrition transition

Many parts of the world are currently undergoing the so-called "nutrition transition." This is defined as changes in the food and nutrition profile of populations as a result of the interaction between economic, demographic, environmental, and cultural factors in society. Taking the Latin American region as an example, it can be seen that nutritional patterns have changed considerably, being now marked by an increase in the consumption of high-energy-density foods (high in fats and sugars) and a decrease in physical activity, with sedentary urban populations predominating.[7,8,9,10,11,12,13] Social and economic progress has improved environmental sanitation, contributing to a decline in infectious diseases. At the same time, higher income has fostered the consumption of high-energy-density foods and reduced the consumption of grains, legumes, and other sources of fiber. The result has been a gradual increase in life expectancy at birth and a greater proportion of obesity and other nutrition-related chronic diseases (type 2 diabetes, cardiovascular disease, certain types of cancer, and osteoporosis) in the total burden of disease.

Until recently, it was commonly thought that these non-communicable diseases were associated with excess – that is, with a wealthy environment. Another theory is that differences between countries are due to differences in genetic susceptibility, which would lead to the conclusion that this is a problem for individuals and almost a necessary evil or – even worse – a sign of social and economic progress. The reality in Latin American cities is that nutritional problems associated with nutritional imbalances, especially the imbalance between energy intake and energy expenditure, are most frequently observed in poor urban populations. Changes in diet and physical activity, as well as the wider food environment, can explain most of the increase in nutrition-related chronic diseases, which have reached epidemic proportions in many countries in recent decades. Clearly, this is the result of environmental changes, since genetic drift occurs over longer periods. What is certain is that our current genes were selected over the past six million years of our species' evolution in order to maximize the use of ingested energy and store as much of it as possible for when it would be needed. Today, in an environment that no longer demands physical labor to produce a little food, these same genes help to produce obesity, insulin resistance, and the associated metabolic consequences: diabetes, dyslipidemia, atherosclerosis, and hypertension.

Highly processed products

Highly processed products are made from processed substances extracted or refined from whole foods – e.g., oils, hydrogenated oils and fats, flours and starches, variants of sugar, and cheap parts or remnants of animal foods – with little or no whole foods. Products include burgers, frozen pizza and pasta dishes, nuggets and sticks, crisps, biscuits, confectionery, cereal bars, carbonated and other sugared drinks, and various snack products.

Most are made, advertised, and sold by large or transnational corporations and are very durable, palatable, and ready to consume, which is an enormous commercial advantage over fresh and perishable whole or minimally processed foods. Consequently, their production and consumption is rising quickly worldwide. In the global north – i.e., North America and Europe – highly processed products have largely replaced food systems and dietary patterns based on fresh and minimally processed food and culinary ingredients that have less fat, sugar, and salt. In the global south – i.e., Asia, Africa, and Latin America – highly processed products are displacing established dietary patterns, which are more suitable socially and environmentally.

Highly processed products are typically energy-dense; have a high glycemic load; are low in dietary fiber, micronutrients, and phytochemicals; and are high in unhealthy types of dietary fat, free sugars, and sodium. When consumed in small amounts and with other healthy sources of calories, highly processed products are harmless; however, intense palatability (achieved by high levels of fat, sugar, salt, and cosmetic and other additives), omnipresence, and sophisticated and aggressive marketing strategies (such as reduced price for super-size servings), all make modest consumption of highly processed products unlikely and displacement of fresh or minimally processed foods very likely. These factors also make highly processed products liable to harm endogenous satiety mechanisms and so promote energy overconsumption and thus obesity.

Source: *Profits and pandemics: prevention of harmful effects of tobacco, alcohol, and ultra-processed food and drink industries. Moodie R, Stuckler D, Monteiro C et al, on behalf of The Lancet NCD Action Group, The Lancet, published online February 12, 2013, http://dx.doi. org/10.1016/S0140-6736(12)62089-3 (modified).*

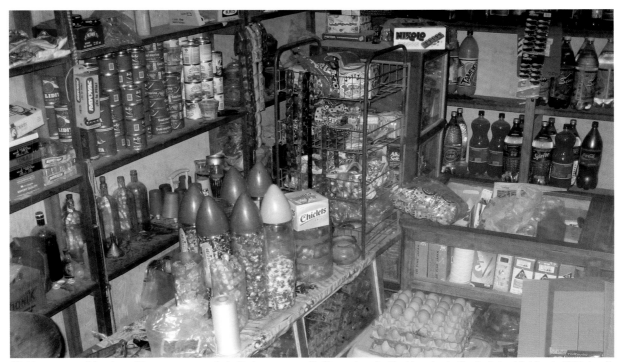

Highly processed foods and beverages on sale in Caripuyo, a small village close to Cochbamba in the Bolivian Highlands (Altiplano).
Source: Ricardo Uauy

What drives food choices?

It is normally believed that food choices depend essentially on the law of supply and demand. Thus, the consumer's preference is the basis of the demand and determines the supply. This model posits consumers as the principal driver of supply, with industry merely meeting their needs. In this case, the factors that usually determine food purchases and consumption patterns are the consumer's income, the prices, and the intrinsic and perceived quality of the products.

A more in-depth analysis of what drives consumption reveals that nowadays supply does not passively wait to respond to demand but has a life of its own and actively influences the choice of goods for purchase and consumption. That is, we buy and consume what is offered to us, not what we need to live a healthy life. What drives supply, and hence consumption, today is largely dominated by the factors that determine the productivity of the food-production chain. In this model, demand and consumption are determined by the ways we produce, process, distribute, trade, market, and advertise food. All these factors are beyond the consumer's control, and they operate mainly on the maximization of profit. The food production chain responds to the need to produce progressively cheaper food and to promote the highest possible consumption. As evidenced daily in the press, the eagerness to maximize profits creates both advantages and risks. The possibility of producing safe and less expensive food is no doubt the greatest advantage. However, the risk of ignoring concerns about a safe and healthy diet is also inherent in a model that puts commercial interests above consumer health. Some say that the responsibility for resolving this dilemma lies with the consumer, and that it is enough to provide information through nutritional labeling, public service announcements about healthy eating, or nutritional guidelines that promote healthy eating. What is certain is that the food production chain and the engines that drive the food supply are very powerful, and that they do not have a real counterpart in the efforts to educate, guide, and facilitate the selection and consumption of safe, wholesome food by the consumer.

Table 1 | **Annual growth rate (%) of volume consumption per person in low- and middle-income countries, and high-income countries**

	Low- and middle-income countries	High-income countries
Packaged food	1.9%	0.4%
Soft drinks	5.2%	2.4%
Processed food	2.0%	1.4%
Oil and fats	1.6%	−0.1%
Snacks and snack bars	2.4%	2.0%
Alcohol	2.8%	1.1%
Tobacco*	2.0%	0.1%

*Tobacco data are in retail sales per person.

Adapted with permission from Stuckler D, Nestlé M. Big food, food systems, and global health. PLoS Med 2012; 9: e1001242

In this battle the consumer is David, since the forces that drive supply are largely invisible and unidentifiable, and have powerful resources that motivate and determine consumer behavior. Thus, we enter a restaurant or eatery, attracted by an environment that for a few minutes makes us feel like members of the "first world" and as good as anybody else – an environment with a little luxury that sparkles like the stars, where each piece of furniture, container, and product is an icon that in some way symbolizes our aspirations for success, where our ancestral hunger for sweet, salty, and fatty foods is whetted with tempting offers of more food for less money, a double portion for a few cents more, buy two and get one free, buy an A + B + C combination meal for a moderate price and experience bliss in this paradise of consumption for the sake of fun and instant gratification. The dilemma is between personal responsibility coupled with an environment that encourages healthy eating and an active life versus an environment that can discourage healthy food choices and promote a sedentary life. Certainly, we can help our consumers in the uphill battle against environmental influences, but we will be much more successful if at the same time we can make the hill less steep by promoting changes in the environment that will make the healthy choice the easy one.

Table 2 | Potential supply- and demand-side interventions in the food production chain to modify food consumption – for example, in this case to reduce saturated fat intake

Link in the food production chain	Food policy instruments with nutritional impact	Examples of impact on fat consumption affecting quantity or quality of fat intake	Effectiveness in reducing intake of saturated fat
Food production	Subsidies or price supports	Subsidies for feed production	Very negative
		Support for dairy products; price guarantees for producers	Very negative
	Import and export quotas	Export incentives for vegetable oil	Uncertain
		Restrictions and/or tariffs on meat imports	Uncertain
Food processing	Quality grading	Definition of the level of quality (changes in the criteria for selecting quality, e.g., lean versus fatty)	Very positive
	"Identity standards"	Identity standards — switch to low-fat milk and yogurt	Positive
	Nutrition labeling	Descriptors in nutrition labeling (e.g., low-fat milk, ice cream)	Very positive
Distribution, marketing, and advertising of food	Advertising campaigns for dairy products	Changes in the demand of government programs for milk products (low-fat to replace full-fat milk)	Negative
	Nutrition labeling	Use % lean in the labeling of ground meat	Negative
		Labeling in restaurant menus to indicate the quantity and quality of fat, low in saturated fat	Positive
	Marketing standards	Need for standardization of the various sector descriptors: agricultural, health, trade	Uncertain
Food choices and consumption	Nutrition labeling	Label indicating the quantity and quality of fat	Very positive
	Public information campaigns to promote good nutrition	Nutritional guidelines for consumer orientation	Very positive
		Icon to orient food choices (pyramid)	Very positive
	Promotion groups for specific products	Promotion of cheese, milk, meat, ice cream, eggs	Very negative

Source: Haddad L. Redirecting the diet transition: What can food policy do? IFPRI World Bank Paper. Washington, DC: International Food Policy Research Institute, 2003. Quoted in Uauy R and Monteiro CA, Food and Nutrition Bulletin, vol. 25, no. 2 © 2004, The United Nations University.

Reintroducing the balanced diet

The first order of business is to bring foods back as the source of nutrients, avoiding the concept of nutrients in isolation; vitamin and mineral deficits are still relevant, but by now we have a good idea how to solve these. Food, food preparations and patterns of food consumption need to be returned to the top of the list. This should include consideration of how crops are cultivated and processed, and how animals are husbanded and fed.

The problems of obesity and diet-related chronic diseases cannot be addressed using the traditional single-nutrient model. Entire diets need to be considered within the framework of the overarching food environment, not just specific nutrients. Furthermore, energy intake and output must be brought into balance. This is easier said than done: human beings are programmed to over-consume food energy and accumulate fat for energy reserves.

In terms of energy provision, a balanced diet is a problem for both poor and rich in today's world, since the prices of sugars, refined carbohydrates and oils are relatively low at present; thus it is comparatively easy to consume more energy than what a normal sedentary person expends. However, vegetables and other "healthy" foods such as legumes and fruits, as well as healthy fats, have become relatively more expensive and also less available within urban settings. Thus urban low-income populations are left with diets high in refined carbohydrates and unhealthy fats. If we then consider the high sodium content of industrially processed foods, we have the ideal mix of energy, fat and sodium to promote unhealthy weight gain and hypertension, which lead to cardiovascular diseases and cancer. After tobacco, obesity is the most prevalent cause of preventable cancer in the world today.[14]

The only way to balance energy input and output is to expend energy and then eat according to what has already been expended. This is clearly hard to achieve, since appetite regulation in humans was established at a time when most individuals were on the verge of malnutrition. Our food-related behaviors and metabolic responses are therefore set to provide energy stores (mainly as fat) in preparation for leaner times. The foods we prefer to eat were defined at a time in our evolution when we needed to be active in order to get a meal. Over the past millennium, human beings have become progressively less active. Unless our existences become more physically active, we will always be on the side of excess intake. The attempt to curb the appetite is a lost battle – as has become all too clear over the past decades. We must change our diets and return to traditional diets based predominantly on plant foods, with minimal processing and a limited proportion of refined

carbohydrates. As pointed out by Michael Pollan, we must grow our food and hunt the animal we expect to get on our plate.[15] "To each according to his needs" is the law of thermodynamics that we must observe.

Fats and carbohydrates are perfectly healthy energy sources if we burn them off by being physically active. The residual adverse effects of fats, if consumed within the constraints of energy balance, are minimal and only observed in the case of trans-fats (which are produced by industrial processing in order to prevent rancidity); traditional human foods, except for dairy, are mostly cis-fats, and are thus generally healthy. Most cultures have based their diets on a mix of predominantly vegetable sources of foods, selecting a mixture of legumes and cereals that results in a balanced amino-acid mix very close to optimal in terms of human nutritional needs. Examples include beans and rice, corn and beans, wheat and lentils, and modern versions of these preparations; some additional small portions of meat or fish and dairy make these blends perfect for human requirements.

Most fats and carbohydrates are perfectly healthy as energy sources if we match our energy expenditure to our food intake; it is only when these sources exceed our expenditure that they become a potential health hazard. Thus if we are able to define our food intake as that necessary to match our energy expenditure, we will avoid most of the present diet/food-related health concerns.

What can public policies do?

Public policies can modify the way the supply of food influences consumption patterns and health. Possible interventions include:

- Optimizing the food production chain to offer healthier products at lower prices for poor consumers;
- Eliminating subsidies and economic incentives for the production of foods rich in saturated fats and facilitating the production of foods low in animal fat;
- Reviewing the regulations governing the international food trade from a nutritional and health perspective;
- Reviewing the regulations governing the institutional food offered in schools, public utilities, the armed forces, and the workplace;
- Facilitating the selection and consumption of healthful foods at lower prices; and
- Providing consumer information at the point of purchase (e.g., via improved labeling).

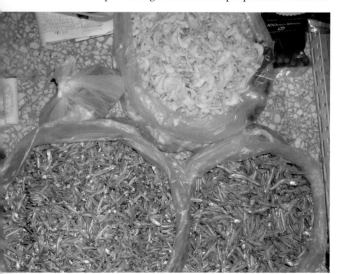

Dried seafood can be a valuable addition to the diet (market stall in Beijing). Source: Ricardo Uauy

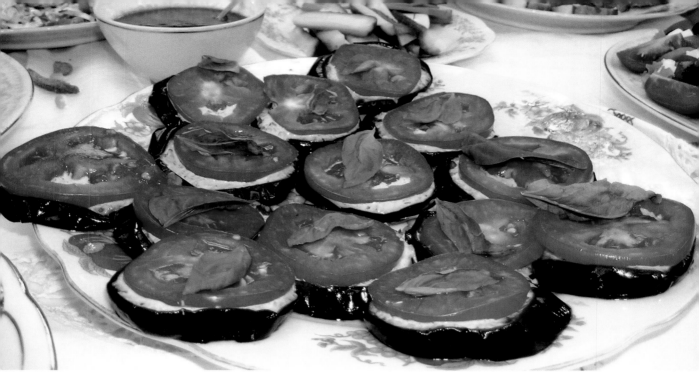

A healthy diet should contain high proportion of unprocessed fruits and vegetables. Source: Ricardo Uauy

Table 3 | **Food classification based on the extent and purpose of industrial processing**

Food group	Extent and purpose of processing	Examples*
Group 1: Unprocessed or minimally processed foods	No processing, or mostly physical processes used to make single whole foods more durable, accessible, convenient, palatable, or safe	Fresh, chilled, frozen, vacuum-packed fruits, vegetables, fungi, roots and tubers; grains (cereals) in general; fresh, frozen and dried beans and other pulses (legumes); dried fruits and 100% unsweetened fruit juices; unsalted nuts and seeds; fresh, dried, chilled, frozen meats, poultry and fish; fresh and pasteurized milk, fermented milk such as plain yoghurt; eggs; teas, coffee, herb infusions, tap water, bottled spring water
Group 2: Processed culinary or food industry ingredients	Extraction and purification of components of single whole foods, resulting in producing ingredients used in the preparation and cooking of dishes and meals made up from Group 1 foods in homes or traditional restaurants, or else in the formulation by manufacturers of Group 3 foods	Vegetable oils, margarine, butter, milk, cream, lard; sugar, sweeteners in general; salt; starches, flours, and "raw" pastas and noodles (made from flour with the addition only of water); and food industry ingredients usually not sold to consumers as such, including high fructose corn syrup, lactose, milk and soy proteins, gums, and preservatives and cosmetic additives
Group 3: Highly processed food products	Processing of a mix of Group 2 ingredients and Group 1 foodstuffs in order to create durable, accessible, convenient, and palatable ready-to-eat or to-heat food products liable to be consumed as snacks or desserts or to replace home-prepared dishes	Breads, biscuits (cookies), cakes and pastries; ice cream; jams (preserves); fruits canned in syrup; chocolates, confectionery (candies), cereal bars, breakfast cereals with added sugar; chips, crisps; sauces; savory and sweet snack products; cheeses; sugared fruit and milk drinks and sugared and "no-cal" cola, and other soft drinks; frozen pasta and pizza dishes; pre-prepared meat, poultry, fish, vegetable and other "recipe" dishes; processed meat including chicken nuggets, hot dogs, sausages, burgers, fish sticks; canned or dehydrated soups, stews and pot noodle, salted, pickled, smoked or cured meat and fish; vegetables bottled or canned in brine, fish canned in oil; infant formulas, follow-on milks, baby food

These listings do not include alcoholic drinks. The examples given are not meant to be complete. Many others can be added, especially to group 3, using the general principles specified in the text and as indicated in the second column.

Source: Monteiro CA, Levy RB, Color RM et al. A new classification of foods based on the extent and purpose of their processing. Cad. Saudi Publican, Rio de Janeiro, 26(11):2039–2049, November 2010.

My personal view

Ricardo Uauy

The world needs a food/nutrition-based perspective that examines the foods we need to preserve and augment our health and limits the production of foods that might compromise our health if consumed in excess. Thus food choices that support healthy consumption are promoted and choices that lead to unhealthy outcomes become less accessible as they exceed the "healthy limits." At present the lowest-priced foods are those are linked to adverse health outcomes, while healthier foods have become more expensive and less available.

Food processing as it stands today adds unhealthy components in order to preserve these foods and to promote their consumption; these additions are clearly linked to the chronic disease epidemic that we currently face. Returning to basic and minimally processed foods will improve our health and nutrition in multiple ways.

Further reading

Uauy R. *Defining and addressing the nutritional needs of populations. Instituto de Nutricion y Tecnología de Alimentos (INTA), University of Chile, Santiago, Chile, and London School of Hygiene and Tropical Medicine, London, UK. Public Health Nutr 2005;8(6A):773–780. DOI: 10.1079/PHN2005774.*

Uauy R *and Monteiro CA, Food and Nutrition Bulletin, vol. 25, no. 2 © 2004, The United Nations University.*

References

1 Drummond JC, Wilbraham A. *The Englishman's Food: Five Centuries of English Diet.* Jonathan Cape, London, 1939. New and revised edition published by Pimlico, London, 1991.

2 Gustafson E. *We the Eaters: If We Change Dinner, We Can Change the World.* New York: Rodale, 2014.

3 Food and Agriculture Organization of the United Nations (FAO). *Human Energy Requirements. Report of a Joint FAO/World Health Organization/ United Nations University Expert Consultation.* FAO Technical Report Series No. 1. Rome: FAO, 2004.

4 Food and Agriculture Organization of the United Nations (FAO)/World Health Organization (WHO). *Energy and Protein Requirements. Report of a Joint FAO/WHO Ad Hoc Expert Committee.* FAO Nutrition Meetings Report Series No. 52; WHO Technical Report Series No. 522. Rome/Geneva: FAO/WHO, 1973.

5 World Health Organization (WHO). *Energy and Protein Requirements. Report of a Joint Food and Agriculture Organization of the United Nations/ WHO/United Nations University Expert Consultation. Technical Report Series No. 724.* Geneva: WHO, 1985.

6 Popkin BM. *Nutritional patterns and transitions.* Popul Dev Rev 1993;19:138–57.

7 Albala C, Vio F, Kain J et al. *Nutrition transition in Chile: determinants and consequences.* Public Health Nutr 2002;5:123–8.

8 Monteiro CA, Conde WL, Popkin BM. *Is obesity replacing or adding to undernutrition? Evidence from different social classes in Brazil.* Public Health Nutr 2002;5:105–12.

9 Murray C, Lopez A, eds. *The global burden of disease.* Cambridge, Mass, USA: Harvard University Press, 1996.

10 Rivera JA, Barquera S, Campirano F et al. *Epidemiological and nutritional transition in Mexico: rapid increase of non-communicable chronic diseases and obesity.* Public Health Nutr 2002;5: 113–22.

11 Rodriguez-Ojea A, Jimenez S, Berdasco A et al. *The nutrition transition in Cuba in the nineties: an overview.* Public Health Nutr 2002;5:129–33.

12 James WPT, Smitasiri S, Ul Haq M et al. *Ending malnutrition by 2020: an agenda for change in the millennium.* ACC/ SCN Commission on Nutrition Challenges for the 21st Century. Food Nutr Bull 2000;21(Suppl):1–88.

13 Uauy R, Albala C, Kain J. *Obesity trends in Latin America: transiting from under- to overweight.* J Nutr 2001; 131:893S–899S.

14 World Cancer Research Fund International. http://www.wcrf.org/sites/ default/files/Breast-Cancer-Survivors-2014-Report.pdf.

15 Pollan M. *The Omnivore's Dilemma: A Natural History of Four Meals.* Penguin. 2007.

The Limits to Consumerism

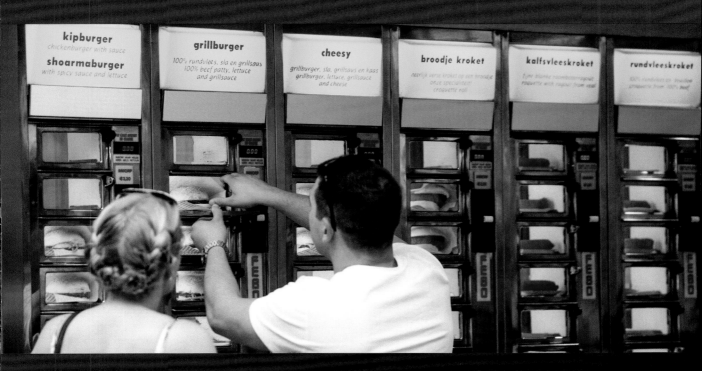

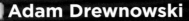

Adam Drewnowski
Center for Public Health Nutrition, University of Washington, Seattle, WA, USA

"Nature provides a free lunch, but only if we control our appetites."

William Ruckelshaus, *first head of the US Environmental Protection Agency (EPA).*

Key messages

- There are limits to free choice. Consumer food choices are driven by purchasing power and socioeconomic status.

- Calories have become cheap; nutrients remain expensive. Global diets are becoming energy-rich but nutrient-poor.

- Demographic shifts, urbanization, and climate change present additional problems for the global food supply.

- The agro-food industry needs to redress the global nutrition imbalance.

- Nourishing the world poses an immense public health challenge.

Consumerism and the drivers of food choice

Eat more stuff. Consumerism as a way of life encourages the purchase of goods and services in ever-growing amounts. Inherent to the consumerist ideology is the notion of choice. Faced with a variety of available foods, consumers can select those that are best suited to their wants and needs. Their collective food choices then influence different parts of the global food system: food production, distribution, and retail. In the consumerist view, the food industry is governed purely by consumer demand.

Choose more stuff. People are said to purchase foods for a whole variety of reasons. Their food choices are shaped by a complex mix of biology, economics, geography, and social interactions. An expression of cultural identity, consumer food choices are also influenced by personal preferences, attitudes, and beliefs. Understanding the underlying drivers of food choice requires an in-depth study of biological, psychological, economic, social, cultural, and geo-political variables. Such studies on consumer decision-making are vital, given that consumer food choice can determine both diet quality and population health.

Or so says conventional wisdom... In reality, there are limits to choice. What counts most is purchasing power: most people "choose" the foods that they can afford. The current hierarchy of global food prices is such that empty calories are cheap, whereas many nutrient-rich foods are much more expensive. As food purchases turn to low-cost refined grains, added sugars and added fats, the notion of consumer food choice becomes a well-nurtured illusion.

With the world hungry for better nutrition, there is a growing need to address the limits to choice and to correct the current nutritional imbalance. The price of healthier foods can help explain why the world's diets are becoming increasingly energy-rich but nutrient-poor. The price-driven economics of food choice behavior are not necessarily limited to low- and middle-income countries. Developed countries are affected as well. Malnutrition is one consequence seen across the socioeconomic spectrum: the dual burden of obesity and nutrient deficiencies shows how it is possible to be both undernourished and overfed.

The agro-food industry needs to ensure that the global food supply is nutrient-rich, affordable, sustainable, accessible, and appealing. Price supports, taxes, biofortification, food fortification, and enrichment are among the technological and policy options. Some of the relevant drivers of consumer food choice are described below.

Sustainable food and nutrition security

The Food and Agriculture Organization (FAO) of the United Nations has defined sustainable diets as nutritionally adequate, economically affordable, culturally acceptable, healthy, and safe. By the FAO definition, sustainable diets should be accessible, protective of both natural and human resources, and respectful of ecosystems and biodiversity.

Other than by price, how is the consumer to choose among different foods? These multisector criteria demand the creation of new metrics. Such metrics should include the foods' energy and nutrient density, affordability, acceptance, and impact on the environment, the latter expressed in terms of land and water use, and greenhouse gas emissions. Ideally, what is best for people should also be good for the planet.

However, no single diet or food pattern seems to fit all the desired criteria. First, studies showed that the most nutrient-rich diets were often the least affordable; it was empty calories that were cheap. Worse, some healthy yet affordable foods were not culturally acceptable and were rejected by lower-income groups. Second, studies showed that the most nutrient-rich foods were not environmentally friendly, whereas foods with low environmental impact were not necessarily nutrient-rich. On the one hand, animal products – meat and dairy – were rich in some key nutrients per calorie but also carried a heavier environmental cost.[1] On the other, some plant-based foods, including cereals, were more planet-friendly but could be nutrient-poor. Indeed, some studies identified a shocking paradox. By some reports, the plant food that was associated with lowest greenhouse gas emissions and low water use was sugar.

Can foods and diets be simultaneously low-cost, low-calorie, and nutrient-rich, environmentally friendly, good tasting and culturally acceptable? The answer is likely to be no. Some compromises will need to be made and consumer choices will likely be curtailed. In predicting consumer food choices, multiple factors will have to be taken into account.

An appetizing display of fruit and vegetables at the Mercat de Sant Josep de la Boqueria, a large public market in the Ciutat Vella district of Barcelona, Catalonia, Spain. Source: Adam Drewnowski

73

Energy density and nutrient density of foods

The energy density of foods is measured in terms of calories per gram (kcal/g) (**Figure 1**). The main determinant of this energy density is water, which provides bulk and volume but has no calories and no nutrients. Thus, the extremes of the scale are represented by plain water (0 kcal/g) at one end and oil (9 kcal/g) at the other. Carbohydrates, including sugar, and protein are in the mid-range of energy density, providing about 4 kcal/g. Dry refined grains, cereals, and fats, oils and sweets contain more calories per gram than do foods with higher water content, such as sugar-sweetened beverages (0.4 kcal/g) or fresh produce (<1 kcal/g).

The technique of ranking foods based on their nutrient content relative to calories has become known as nutrient profiling. Nutrient profile models distinguish between nutrients of public health concern and beneficial nutrients such as fiber, vitamins and minerals. For example, the typical American diet is too in high saturated fats and added sugars, whereas the consumption of fiber, potassium, calcium and vitamins D and E falls short of the recommended values. The goal of nutrient profiling is to correct this imbalance by identifying the chief dietary sources of empty calories. Accordingly, saturated fats, added sugars, and sodium were the nutrients to limit in nutrient profile models developed for

the US and for France. By contrast, fiber, potassium, calcium and vitamin D turned up among the nutrients to encourage.

Developing a nutrient profiling model can be a challenge, since most foods provide a variety of nutrients in addition to calories. The choice of index nutrients can depend on the nutritional concerns of a particular population and can be adapted to low- and middle-income countries. One function of nutrient profiling is to serve as a public policy tool.

Nutrient density of foods can be measured in terms of nutrients per calorie, nutrients per serving, or nutrients per unit weight (100 g) (**Figure 2**). Models have been based on nutrients to limit, nutrients to encourage, or on some combination of both. In some models, the presence of fat, sugar, and salt in excessive amounts was enough to disqualify a food from having a favorable nutrient profile, no matter what other nutrients it contained. Those were the noncompensatory models. An alternative approach was to balance multiple nutrients, allowing fat, sugar, or salt to be offset by the presence of protein, fiber, vitamins and minerals. Ideally, a nutrient profiling model should capture the overall nutrient quality of food and convey it to the consumer at a glance.

Figure 1 | **Relation between energy density of foods in the US food supply (kcal per 100g) and energy cost, measured in kcal per dollar.**

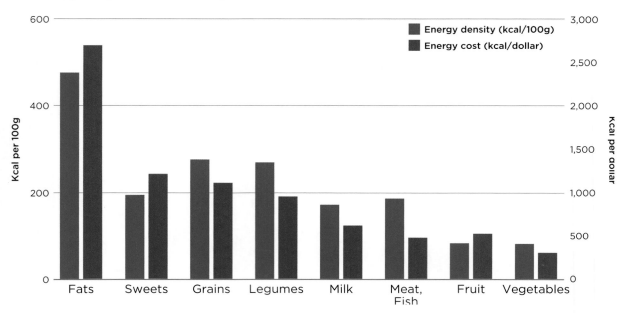

The Nutrient-Rich Foods (NRF) score

The Nutrient-Rich Foods (NRF) family of scores was based on a variable number of nutrients to encourage and on three fixed nutrients to limit: saturated fat, added sugar and sodium. The NRF9.3 variant of the score was based on protein, fiber, calcium, iron, potassium, and magnesium, vitamin A, vitamin C and vitamin E. These were the shortfall nutrients previously identified by expert committees and dietary guidelines. NRF versions have also used total and free sugars, as defined by the World Health Organization.

The final NRF9.3 algorithm was based on the sum of percent daily values (%DVs) for nine nutrients to encourage minus the sum of %DVs for the three nutrients to limit. Nutrient density calculations based on 100 kcal or on serving sizes performed better than those based on 100 g. Generally, weight-based scores cannot deal with the fact that foods are consumed in very different amounts. Higher NRF scores were associated with food patterns of lower energy density and higher nutrient content.

Importantly, the NRF profile made no formal distinctions between "good" or "bad" foods. Rather, foods and beverages fell along the nutrient density continuum. Fats and sweets, including sweetened beverages, were awarded low nutrient density scores, whereas low energy density salad greens, vegetables and fruit and low fat dairy were awarded higher nutrient density scores. The continuum of nutrient densities ran from sugar (low) to spinach (high). Since nutrient densities based on nutrient-to-calorie ratios, foods with low energy density tended to have higher nutrient density scores, when calculated per calorie.

The same nutrient profiling methods can be applied to complex meals, restaurant menus, or the total diet. Nutrient profiling methods can also be adapted to screen the food supply of low- and middle-income countries for nutritional value. There are some caveats. First, the selection of shortfall nutrients will need to be guided by population-specific nutrient needs. Bioavailability may be another concern, given wide disparities in local eating habits. Populations with vegetarian diets may be at risk for low intakes of bioavailable calcium, iron, zinc, vitamin B_{12} and vitamin D. In low income countries, Dietary Diversity Scores serve as proxies for dietary adequacy. Consuming a variety of foods, in addition to staple cereal crops, improves the likelihood that the diet does contain the required nutrients, vitamins and minerals.

Figure 2 | **Relation between nutrient density of foods in the US food supply (NRF 9.3 score) and energy cost, measured in kcal per dollar. NRF 9.3 is the Nutrient-Rich Food score**

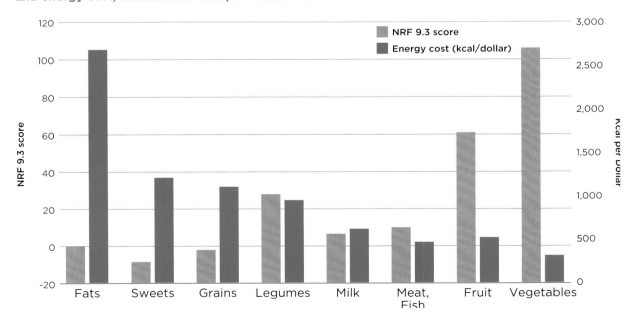

Food affordability metrics

Many consumer choices, if not most, are driven by food price. Whereas food nutrient density is calculated in terms of nutrients per calorie, food affordability is calculated in terms of calories or nutrients per unit cost. For example, studies have estimated the relative cost of calories, calcium, or potassium per penny, as provided by different food groups in the US food supply. As described below, milk and fermented milk products provided dietary calcium at the lowest monetary cost, as did some calcium-rich cheeses. Potatoes and beans were the lowest-cost sources of dietary potassium. Food affordability metrics have implications for public policy, since they can help health professionals and consumers alike to identify the most affordable items within each food group.

Based on USDA national prices for 98 vegetables, fresh, frozen, and canned, we calculated nutrient costs per 100 g, per 100 kcal, and per edible cup. Nutrient density was based on a nutrient profiling model that included fiber, vitamins A, C, and K, potassium and magnesium. Nutrient affordability was the cost associated with the provision of 10% daily value of each nutrient per cup equivalent.

Beans and starchy vegetables, including white potatoes, were cheaper per 100 calories than were dark-green and deep-yellow vegetables. Fresh, frozen, and canned vegetables had similar nutrient profiles and provided comparable nutritional value. However, not all vegetables were equally appealing. More than half of the vegetables listed by the USDA were never or rarely eaten by school-age children in the 2003–04 National Health and Nutrition Examination Survey (NHANES) database. For vegetables listed >5 times, potatoes and beans were the lowest-cost sources of potassium and fiber. Also providing high nutrient value per penny were carrots, orange-fleshed sweet potatoes, red and green peppers, spinach and broccoli.

A similar approach, applied to calcium content of milks and dairy products in France, showed that fluid milks, hard cheeses, and low-fat yogurts delivered calcium at relatively low monetary cost and without excessive amounts of calories or nutrients to limit. Comparable value metrics are being developed for whole fruits and juices, dairy protein sources and whole grains.

A social gradient in diet quality

Attaching retail food prices to dietary intake data has permitted the estimation of individual-level diet costs. Previously, data on food costs and food expenditures in the US were collected not at the individual but at household level. That simple innovation has led to new studies in nutrition economics that explored associations between diet quality and diet cost across different socioeconomic strata.

A market trader selling fresh vegetable in Colombia.
Source: Mike Bloem

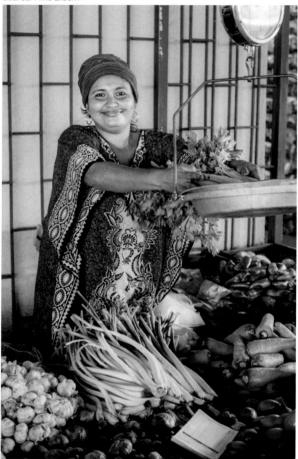

Merging dietary intake data from the National Health and Nutrition Examination Survey with the national food prices database allowed us to compute the cost associated with following the 2010 Dietary Guidelines for Americans (DGAs) (**Figure 3**). The monetary value of the diet was calculated by multiplying gram amounts of each food eaten by every NHANES participant by its mean national price per gram. The mean national food prices database was obtained from the USDA Center for Policy and Promotion. These values were then summed for each NHANES participant. To compare prices per calorie, the energy-adjusted diet cost was computed and expressed per 2,000 kcal/d diet. This type of standardization is also used by the World Bank to assess the cost of obtaining a 2,000 kcal/d daily ration, an indicator of food poverty.

The Healthy Eating Index (HEI) 2010, a measure of compliance with the 2010 DGAs, was the principal measure of diet quality. There was a strong positive association between quintiles of energy-adjusted diet costs and higher HEI 2010 scores (see **Figures 5** and **6** overleaf). As expected, those diets that were higher in green vegetables, whole fruits, whole grains, and seafood also cost more. By contrast, diets higher in refined grains, solid fats and added sugars cost less. As diet cost increased, the proportion of empty calories in the diet dropped. Not surprisingly, the more nutrient-dense and more costly diets were preferentially consumed by higher SES groups.

It is important to realize that these monetary costs reflected the intrinsic cost of the diet as opposed to actual food expenditures. The key assumption was that the foods were purchased at retail and prepared and consumed at home. However, the same assumptions go into the creation of the Thrifty Food Plan, the USDA-designed food pattern providing optimal nutrition at minimal cost.

These studies in nutrition economics suggest that, given our food supply, eating healthily generally costs more. Helping consumers identify foods that are nutrient-rich, affordable, and culturally acceptable would go a long way toward improving population diets and health.

Figure 3 | **Relation between energy density of foods in the US food supply and energy cost, measured in dollars per 1000 kcal and shown on a log scale. National food prices from the US Department of Agriculture.**

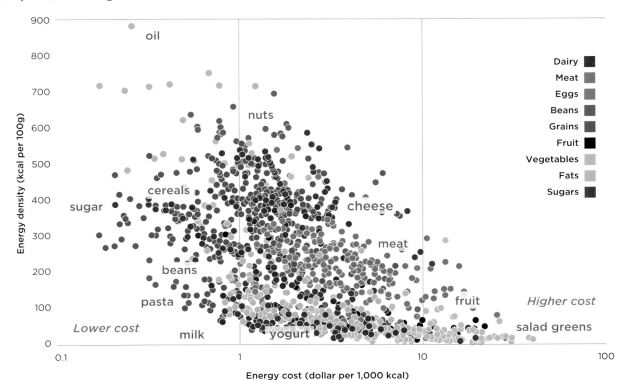

Figure 4 | **Relation between energy density of foods in Mexico and energy cost, measured in pesos per 100 kcal and shown on a log scale. National food prices from Mexico.**

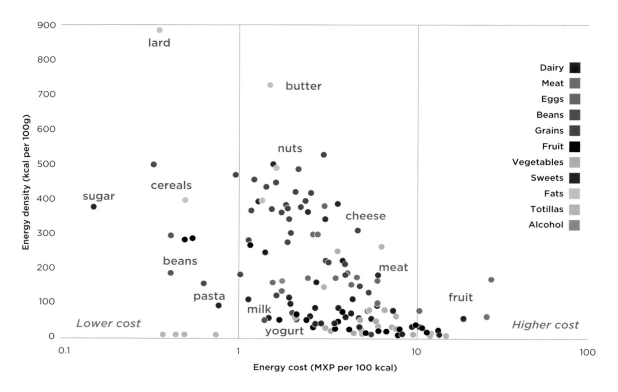

Nutrition resilience: eating better for less

The observed social disparities in diet quality cannot be wholly explained by differences in attitudes, beliefs, family, or culture. Food prices and diet cost also contribute to the observed social gradients in diet quality and health. However, within each population there are people who are able to construct higher quality diets at a lower than expected cost. For example, in a study based on NHANES data, Mexican-Americans were able to achieve Dietary Approaches to Stop Hypertension (DASH)-compliant diets at a lower cost than was estimated for some other groups (**Figure 4**).

The ability to promote healthier diets across diverse cultures and racial/ethnic groups has been referred to as cultural competence. Being able to create healthy food patterns, subject to economic constraints, is an example of economic competence that we call nutrition resilience.

Preliminary data analyses suggest that two factors may contribute to nutrition resilience. First, positive attitudes toward nutrition have been associated with higher-quality

diets, at every level of supermarket type, education and income. Offering nutrition education may be an integral component of dietary advice.

Second, frequent cooking at home was associated with higher HEI scores. This too has implications for public policy, since most likely to eat at home were large families, Mexican Americans, and groups of lower education and incomes. In past studies, frequency of home cooking was associated with better diets, improved family dynamics and lower childhood obesity rates. The phenomenon of nutrition resilience may therefore depend on family, culture, nutrition-related attitudes and cooking skills. Although food budgets still determine diet quality overall, it is possible to eat better for less.

In the absence of empirical data on the drivers of food choice, linear programming optimization models have been used to create nutritionally acceptable food patterns, subject to a variety of constraints. Here, the goal was to create food patterns that are simultaneously nutrient-rich, affordable, acceptable and appealing.

Figure 5 | Relation between quintiles of diet cost and diet quality for men in the US, as measured by the Healthy Eating Index 2010 (HEI 2010).

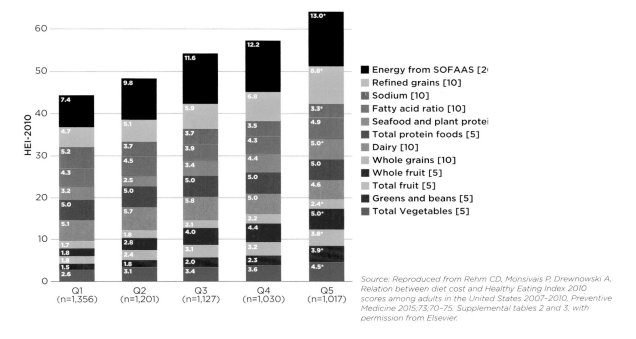

Source: Reproduced from Rehm CD, Monsivais P, Drewnowski A, Relation between diet cost and Healthy Eating Index 2010 scores among adults in the United States 2007–2010, Preventive Medicine 2015;73;70-75. Supplemental tables 2 and 3, with permission from Elsevier.

Figure 6 | HEI-2010 component scores by diet cost quintile among women in the US from NHANES 2007–2010.

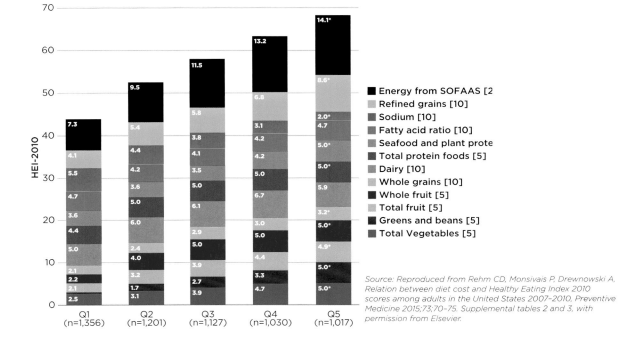

Source: Reproduced from Rehm CD, Monsivais P, Drewnowski A, Relation between diet cost and Healthy Eating Index 2010 scores among adults in the United States 2007–2010, Preventive Medicine 2015;73;70-75. Supplemental tables 2 and 3, with permission from Elsevier.

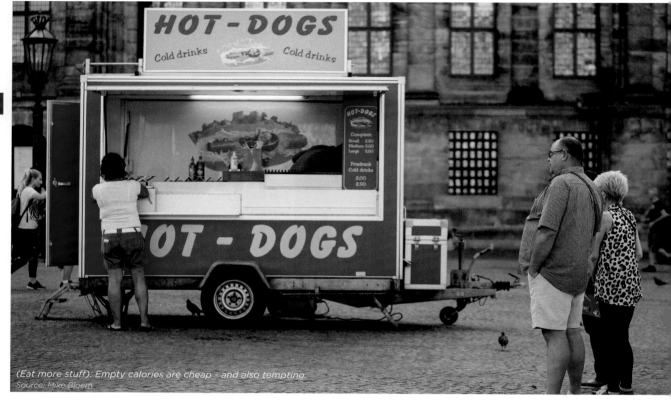

(Eat more stuff): Empty calories are cheap - and also tempting.
Source: Mike Bloem

More limits to consumer choice

The LMICs and the developed countries are beginning to share many of the same problems. First, the majority of the world's population will soon be living in emerging megacities, housing tens of millions of people, well away from farms, fields, and fisheries. As a result, short, local food supply chains will have to transition to urban or national systems of food processing, storage, distribution, and retail. Fresh local foods will give way to more processed foods.

Poverty in megacities will bring additional problems. Already, processed grains, fats, and sweets in the global marketplace cost less per calorie than do lean meats, seafood, low-fat dairy products, or fresh vegetables and fruit. As economies grow and incomes rise, many traditional foods give way to low-cost imported grains, added sugars and added fats. The dual burden of cheap ample calories and more scarce and more expensive nutrients is now a common feature of the food supply in both developed and developing countries.

Increasingly, poverty and obesity are becoming linked, a public health problem compounded by rampant urbanization. Supplying megacities with clean water and affordable nutrient-rich foods on a daily basis is a major logistic, environmental, and economic challenge. Cheap empty calories become the default option. Unless prevention systems are put in place, megacities — many of them both crowded and poor — are likely to become hotspots for rampant obesity and other non-communicable diseases.

Reducing disparities in nutrition and health

Developed and developing countries are beginning to share the same dietary burden – a food supply with increasingly cheap and ample calories that can readily become nutrient-poor. Some measures need to be put in place to assure a nutrient-rich food supply for all.

The argument that healthier diets cost more is politically charged. Some key objections were grounded in the core belief that all consumers exercise a significant degree of choice over what foods to buy. However, there is now an understanding that changing dietary behaviors may also require some economic incentives. Some of these interventions extend consumer choices. For example, some pricing interventions were intended to promote purchases of vegetables and fruit by lower-income consumers. By contrast, taxes on beverages and snacks were intended to restrict choice by limiting consumer access to the wrong foods by the same lower-income groups. However, not all food-based decisions stem from free choice. Regressive fiscal measures may also increase social inequalities in diet quality and so contribute to the already-widening gap between the rich and the poor when it comes to diet quality and health.

My personal view

Adam Drewnowski

Eating more calories once meant getting more nutrients. That was the long-standing principle of nutritional epidemiology. However, that relationship has been uncoupled in recent years by the low cost of energy-dense foods. Contrary to expectations, paying less for food easily translates into eating more. Cheap, energy-dense foods that pack ample calories into small volumes are easy to overeat. Processed foods built around refined grains, added sugars, and vegetable fats are energy-dense, inexpensive, and highly palatable, but can have minimal nutritional value. Consumer dietary "choices" are increasingly driven by the purchasing power of the individual household, especially among the world's poor. As empty calories sweep the globe, hidden hunger and obesity are no longer mutually exclusive: it is quite possible to be both undernourished and overweight. The food industry has an increased responsibility to ensure that the world food supply remains affordable, sustainable, and nutrient-rich.

The inclusion of food prices and diet cost in studies of diets and health allows for further insights into who is healthy and why. Food-focused studies have linked costly fresh produce, lean meat, and fish, nuts and berries with better health. By contrast, the consumption of low-cost fats and sweets has been linked to obesity and weight gain. Sociologists will argue that it is virtually impossible to separate the food from the consumer. In general, more costly diets are consumed by the rich, and cheaper diets by the poor. While this may not have been the intent, studies in nutritional epidemiology attest to the importance of socioeconomic determinants of health.

Further reading

Darmon N, Drewnowski A. Does social class predict diet quality? Am J Clin Nutr 2008; 87(5):1107–1117.

Darmon N, Drewnowski A. The contribution of food prices and diet costs to socioeconomic disparities in diet quality and health: A systematic review and analysis. Nutr Rev 2015;Oct, 73(10):643–60.

Darmon N, Vieux F, Maillot M et al. Nutrient profiles discriminate between foods according to their contribution to nutritionally adequate diets: A validation study using linear programming and the SAIN, LIM system. Am J Clin Nutr 2009; 89:1227–1236.

Drewnowski A, Kawachi I. Diets and health: How food decisions are shaped by biology, economics, geography, and social interactions. Big Data 2015;3(3):September 16, 2015. http://online.liebertpub.com/doi/abs/10.1089/big.2015.0014.

Drewnowski A, Specter SE. Poverty and obesity: The role of energy density and energy costs Am J Clin Nutr 2004;79:6–16.

Rehm CD, Monsivais P, Drewnowski A. Relation between diet cost and Healthy Eating Index 2010 scores among adults in the United States 2007-2010. Prev Med 2015;73:70–5.

References

1   *Environmental cost is typically defined in terms of energy, water and land use. While greenhouse gas emissions and the carbon footprint have captured popular imagination, the coming scarcity of water resources may turn out to be a more serious problem.*

The Economics of Poor Nutrition: Patterns, consequences and costs

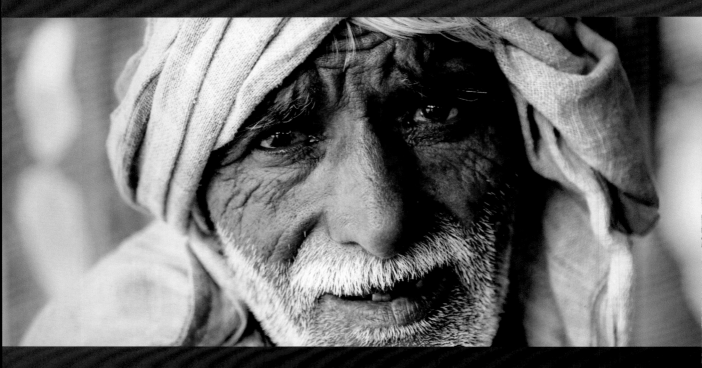

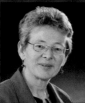

Source: Waterloo
Wellington Community
Care Access Centre

Susan Horton
CIGI Professor of Global Health Economics, Balsillie School of International
Affairs, University of Waterloo, Ontario, Canada

Acknowledgments:
The author would like to thank Daphne *Chen Nee Wu*
for her excellent research assistance in the development of this chapter.

"Once poverty is gone, we'll need to build museums to display its horrors to future generations. They'll wonder why poverty continued so long in human society – how a few people could live in luxury while billions dwelt in misery, deprivation and despair."

Muhammad Yunus, *co-recipient (together with the Grameen Bank) of the 2006 Nobel Peace Prize "for their efforts through microcredit to create economic and social development from below."*

Key messages

- Nutrition typically improves with higher income. In some cases, however, nutrition-related health states can worsen as income improves (obesity rates increase and breastfeeding rates decrease).

- Public policy is very important in improving nutrition – for example, it can drive investments in water and sanitation. Public policy is also important in providing education regarding healthy behaviors in the sourcing, preparation and consumption of food.

- The investments required to improve nutrition can be modest: micronutrients in particular are inexpensive.

- Investments in nutrition are good value for money, and in some cases provide returns several times the initial investment.

- Reducing stunting (chronic undernutrition), increasing breastfeeding and reducing anemia (all World Health Assembly targets) are key priorities both for health and for economic reasons.

The dimensions of nutrition

Good nutrition is essential for good health. The most important and obvious consequence of poor nutrition is poor health, and the extreme consequence is death. This holds true both for undernutrition and for overnutrition. But poor nutrition has more subtle consequences for human development. Children who are poorly nourished not only grow physically less well, but also develop cognitively less well. Poorer cognition is associated with lower educational achievement, and hence lower productivity in work, and ultimately lower national income. It is possible to estimate the economic losses associated with poor nutrition and even (for some conditions) the costs of preventing such losses. In this chapter, we summarize some of the economic evidence concerning poor nutrition.

An inappropriate quantity and quality of food in the diet is a key factor in poor nutrition; another important factor is the body's ability to absorb and utilize these nutrients, which depends on the health of the individual. These proximate factors in turn depend on underlying determinants – namely, food insecurity, inadequate care, unhealthy conditions, and lack of access to health services, according to the well-known UNICEF framework.[1]

Nutrition has a number of dimensions. The Millennium Development Goals (2000–2015) focused on underweight as the key nutrition indicator. More recently, the World Health Assembly identified six nutritional indicators with associated targets for 2025, namely stunting (the sign of chronically poor nutrition), breastfeeding, anemia, wasting (where children are thin for their height, due to recent nutritional inadequacy), low birth weight, and obesity. For reasons of space, we focus on the first three indicators here.

The next section examines the patterns and causes of stunting, inadequate breastfeeding, and anemia (focusing on iron-deficiency anemia). The third section examines the economic consequences of these three conditions, and provides some quantitative estimates. The final section provides some brief concluding remarks.

Patterns and causes of poor nutrition

Inadequate diets can have lifelong consequences, and there are critical periods during the first 1,000 days (pregnancy and the first two years of life) where this is particularly the case. Often, poor nutrition is associated with poverty. However, high-income countries are not exempt from nutritional problems. In this section, we examine the patterns of these nutritional problems using global maps, and discuss the causes. In the next major section, we will consider the effects on human functioning, which in turn have economic consequences.

Stunting

When visiting museums and viewing furniture and clothes from previous centuries, it comes as a surprise to see how much shorter people in high-income countries were in historical times. Similarly, when travelling in low-income countries, particularly in Asia, the height disparities among generations in the same country (and across countries) are striking. Achieved height is strongly influenced by nutrition over the early years of life. Child height-for-age is a sensitive indicator of long-term poor nutrition, and children who fall a specific distance below international growth standards are termed "stunted."

Stunting is highly correlated with income (**Figure 1**). The countries where over 30% of children are stunted are mainly low- and lower-middle income countries in Sub-Saharan Africa, South and Southeast Asia. As incomes rise, stunting levels decrease to lower levels (10–30%) in most of Latin America and some countries in Central Asia and North Africa, and they diminish below 10% in the OECD countries. We do not have up-to-date data on all OECD countries, since nutrition data often come from MICS (Multiple Indicator Cluster Surveys) or DHS (Demographic and Health Surveys), which are not undertaken in high-income countries. There are at least three important reasons why stunting and income are correlated.

Diets inadequate in quality and quantity are an important contributor to stunting. Deficiencies in specific micronutrients such as zinc are often associated with stunting. One reason that stunting and income are so strongly correlated is that low-income households often cannot afford more expensive foods such as animal-source foods and fruit and vegetables, which are higher than staples in various micronutrients.

Figure 1[2] | **Prevalence of stunting among children under five years**

Legend
< 9.9%
10-19.9%
20-29.9%
30-39.9%
> 40%
No data

Note: Data collected from WHO Global Health Observatory Data Repository for the most recent year available between 2007 and 2014.

Source: World Health Organization (WHO). Global Health Observatory (GHO) data. http://www.who.int.gho/health_equity/outcomes/stunting_children/en, accessed August 5 2015.

A second reason linking stunting and income is that in low-income households, children are also more likely to have health problems which limit their ability to absorb and use all the nutrients from their food. Poor families are less likely to have convenient access to clean water and sanitation, which directly affects nutritional status. Unsafe drinking water leads to a variety of infections (particularly diarrhea and dysentery) which inhibit the absorption of nutrients; inadequate sanitation leads to increased worm infestations, for example, and a variety of diseases proliferate where there is inadequate water for washing. Recent research suggests that diseases associated with unclean water and poor sanitation can have long-lasting effects and are associated with stunting.

Finally, household behavior in food preparation and personal hygiene is also strongly related to education, particularly of the mother. Education is, in turn, correlated with income.

Breastfeeding

Breast milk is the perfect food for babies, and exclusive breastfeeding to six months is recommended by the World Health Organization. Breast milk not only contains all the nutrients infants need, but also has a range of other health and cognitive benefits that we discuss below. WHO and UNICEF recommendations are that breastfeeding should be initiated early (preferably within one hour of birth), that infants should be exclusively breastfed to six months, and that breastfeeding should be continued to at least the age of two.

There are various ways to measure breastfeeding rates. We present the rates of "some" breastfeeding to six months (**Figure 2**), a measure that is available for around a hundred low-, middle- and high-income countries. Contrary to many other patterns of nutrition and income, it is the low-income countries in Sub-Saharan Africa and South and Southeast Asia

Figure 2[2] | **World rate of partial breastfeeding at 6 months**

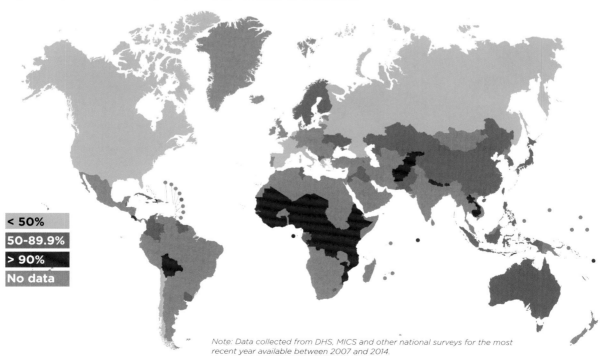

< 50%
50-89.9%
> 90%
No data

Note: Data collected from DHS, MICS and other national surveys for the most recent year available between 2007 and 2014.

Source: Victora C, Bahl R, Barros A et al. Breastfeeding in the 21st Century: Epidemiology, Mechanisms and Lifelong Impact. Lancet 2016;387:475-490.

which have the highest rates of breastfeeding. Middle-income countries in Latin America and in East and Central Asia have intermediate rates, while the lowest rates are in high-income countries in North America, Western Europe and Russia; however, some high-income countries (Australia, Japan and the Scandinavian nations) are in the intermediate group.

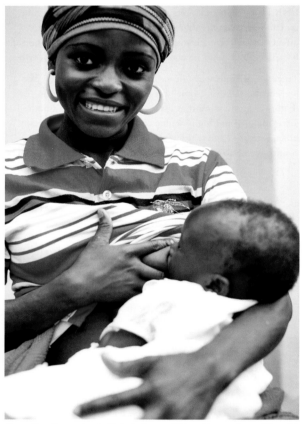

Breastfeeding rates in Sub-Saharan Africa (shown here, Nigeria) remain relatively high.
Source: Micronutrient Initiative

Breastfeeding rates and duration have tended to decrease as incomes increase, although more recently some upper-middle and high-income countries have intervened to try to reverse this trend. Many factors cause this tendency: urbanization and the increased rates of women's work outside the home are key, but strong marketing of formula, obstacles to breastfeeding in public places, and insufficient training of health personnel all contribute.[4] Data on the WHO-recommended breastfeeding rates (exclusive breastfeeding to six months, and continued breastfeeding to two years) are not even available for high-income countries, suggesting a lack of emphasis.

Reversing the declining trend towards breastfeeding is possible. Important factors include maternity leave of sufficient length (the ILO convention suggests 18 weeks) and workplace conditions that support breastfeeding. This should preferably be funded by social security, although this omits women who are self-employed or those in work not covered by social security. Passing domestic legislation to enforce the provisions of the International Code of Marketing of Breastmilk Substitutes can help to reduce harmful marketing practices. It is also important to train health professionals in the benefits of breast milk such that they can counsel and support new mothers.

Breastfeeding in the USA

The USA is one of the outlier countries in not requiring any paid maternity leave (as compared to the ILO recommendation for 14 weeks). Despite this, the breastfeeding rates in the US (although low) are higher than in Canada, and are increasing faster than in the UK (both Canada and the UK have a full year of paid maternity leave).

Some other measures in the US may help to explain the positive trends: the Surgeon General's Call to Action to Support Breastfeeding in 2011; legislation in most states protecting breastfeeding in public; mandatory insurance coverage (since 2012) for lactation counseling and breast milk pumps; and the requirement that employers provide time and space for the expression of breast milk.[4]

Anemia

Anemia is one of the most common nutritional deficiencies, affecting about 2 billion people worldwide. The WHO estimates that about half of these cases of anemia are associated with iron deficiency (hence approximately a billion people suffer from iron-deficiency anemia), while another billion are iron-deficient, but not anemic. That is, their body stores of iron are low, but not so low that the hemoglobin levels in their blood are below the level that is considered to be anemia. (It should be pointed out that anemia may have either nutritional or non-nutritional causes. The former is produced by a lack of essential nutrients, including vitamin A and the B-vitamins. The latter is induced by infections, inflammation and parasites.)

Anemia levels vary systematically by age and sex, being higher in adult women (who have higher iron requirements than men), and children. Pregnant and lactating women have particularly high needs due to the expansion of blood volume during pregnancy and the mechanisms by which the mother provides the iron stores for infants for the first six months of life. Children also have higher deficiency levels due to higher needs (associated with growth). We present information below on anemia in children aged 6–59 months – noting, however, that anemia rates in pregnant women are almost as high, and that those in women of reproductive age are relatively high.

Anemia is correlated with income (**Figure 3**). Anemia rates of 40% and above are observed in almost all countries in Sub-Saharan Africa, throughout South Asia, and in a few countries in Southeast Asia, Latin America and the Caribbean, primarily low- and lower-middle income countries. As countries move into the upper-middle income category, anemia rates become more moderate (20–39%), and rates are lower still in the high-income countries. However, anemia remains a problem even in high-income countries. There are two major reasons why anemia and income are correlated.

Firstly, some of the leading causes of anemia are micronutrient deficiencies (particularly of iron, but also of

B-vitamins and vitamin A). Secondly, infection is important. Infection with malaria, for example, increases anemia: since the malaria parasite utilizes iron from the bloodstream in the human host, one of the body's responses is to reduce iron availability in hemoglobin. Infection with hookworm is associated with anemia, since the parasite causes the human host to lose blood from the wall of the intestines.

Poor households consume fewer iron-rich foods: animal products are a good source of iron, in a form that is more readily assimilated by the body. Even a modest consumption of animal products also enhances the absorption of iron from non-animal sources. Absorption is also enhanced by vitamin C in the diet, obtained from fruit and vegetables, for example.

Poor households are also more likely to have inadequate sanitation, which increases the possibility of worm infections. They are less likely to possess and use insecticide-treated nets which help reduce malaria transmission. Malaria is more prevalent throughout Sub-Saharan Africa and South and Southeast Asia, and is also correlated with observed patterns of anemia.

Figure 3[5] | **Global estimates of the prevalence of anemia in infants and children 6–59 months, 2011**

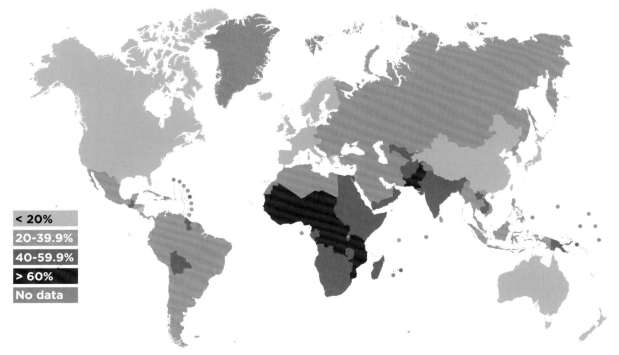

< 20%
20-39.9%
40-59.9%
> 60%
No data

Source: Reprinted from The global prevalence of anemia in 2011, World Health Organization (WHO), Geneva: World Health Organization, Page 19 of Annex, 2015.

Physiological and economic consequences of poor nutrition

Stunting

There are biological reasons why undernourished children are not only stunted, but also suffer cognitive deficits. Chronic undernutrition impacts brain development in ways that are manifested by attention deficits and poorer memory. It also harms the development of motor skills, which (along with greater lethargy and longer periods of illness) results in children interacting less with their environment, and limiting their learning. Stunted children are likely to enter school later than taller ones, are likely to achieve fewer grades in school, and are also likely to score less well in cognitive tests.

Economic studies find evidence that wages are associated with height. In low-income countries and in manual occupations, being taller is associated with greater physical strength and being able to work longer/harder, and hence to earn more. This relationship also holds true in high-income countries and non-manual occupations, because of the association with cognitive skills. One study[6] used the average effect of height on low- and middle-income countries, and in high-income countries, and estimated that undernutrtition (as measured by low adult height) accounted for a loss of 8% of world GDP in the twentieth century. Between a quarter and a third of this figure was due to lower achievements in school, and much of the rest probably due to lower cognitive skills (**Table 1**).

Table 1 | **Estimated costs of poor nutrition, and benefit:cost ratios for interventions, stunting, inadequate breastfeeding and anemia**

Intervention details	Loss as % GDP/GNI	Benefit:Cost ratio
STUNTING		
Study[6] uses data on adult height worldwide, combined with estimated effect of height on wages from 9 studies of high-income and 9 studies of low- and middle-income countries.[4]	8% of world GDP over 20th century	n/a
Study[5] uses data on stunting for 17 countries, combined with estimated effect of stunting on household income[7] and effectiveness of nutrition interventions.[7]	n/a	Median is 18:1; ranges from 3.6:1 to 48:1
BREASTFEEDING		
Study[2] uses worldwide data on some breastfeeding to six months, effect of some breastfeeding on IQ[6] and coefficient of effect of IQ on wages.[8]	0.49% of GNI (world average): range by country 0.01–0.80% GNI	n/a
Study[9] uses estimated losses due to inadequate breastfeeding for one country (Vietnam) compared to costs and effectiveness of a three-year subnational breastfeeding promotion program.		2.4:1
ANEMIA		
Study[10] uses effect of anemia on adult productivity from survey; effect of anemia on child cognitive skills from survey; and effect of adult cognitive skills on wages, for 10 countries with high anemia levels. Calculates present value of losses for current child population, and compares to cost of wheat flour fortification which can reduce anemia.	Median loss is 0.8% of GDP	Median benefit:cost ratio is 8.7:1

n/a means not applicable

Another estimate is based on a longitudinal study in Guatemala, which followed a cohort of children who had participated in a randomized controlled feeding trial at early ages, and found significant effects in adulthood.[9] Those who were stunted at age three scored one standard deviation lower in cognitive tests (for comparison, 15 IQ points is one standard deviation), while those who were not stunted achieved 3.6 more years of schooling, had higher

hourly earnings (20% more for men, 7.2% more for women), 20% higher household income, and (due to smaller household size and fewer children) 59% higher per capita income. Nutrition does not necessarily cause all these outcomes; stunting may also be a marker of multiple childhood deprivations, which in turn adversely affect the future life-course. These results were used in a second study[10] to make estimates of the rate of return to a package

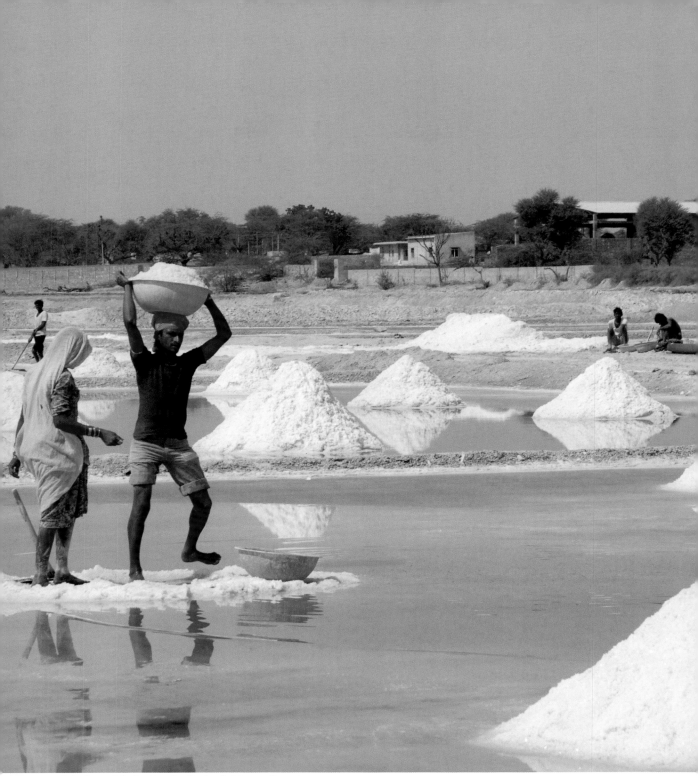

Bringing salt iodization the "last mile," to small producers.
Source: Micronutrient Initiative

of recommended nutrition investments. The authors estimated the returns for 17 different countries with high levels of stunting. The median benefit:cost ratio is 18:1 (being lower in countries with slower growth rates and/or lower stunting levels, and higher in countries with higher growth rates and/or higher stunting levels: Table 1). This indicates that improving nutrition can potentially be a very good investment.

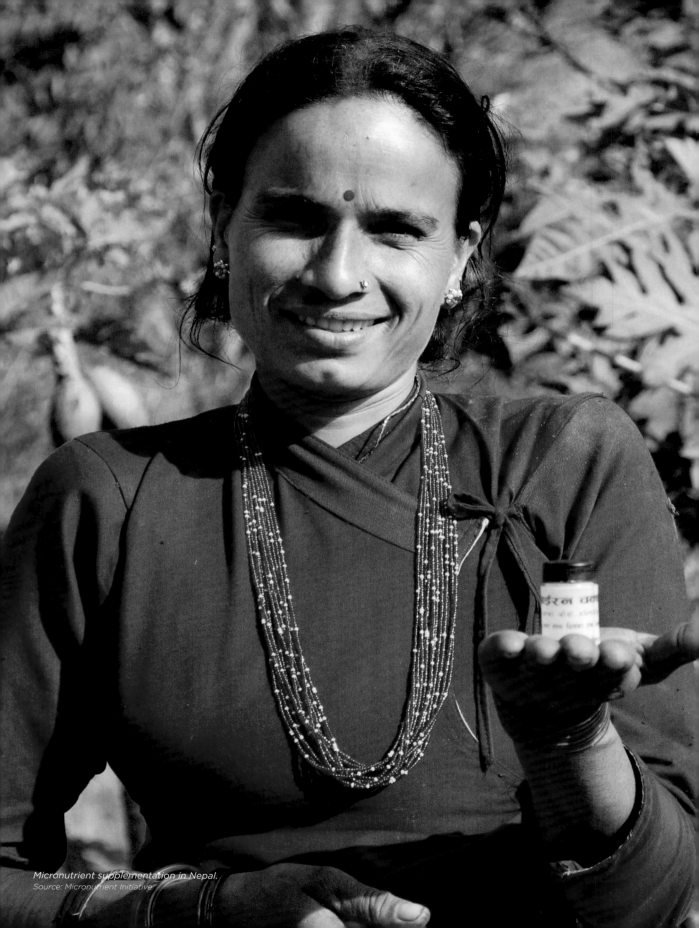

Micronutrient supplementation in Nepal.
Source: Micronutrient Initiative

Breastfeeding

Breastfeeding is a protective factor against child infection, both because the process of preparing breast milk substitutes can be unsanitary, and because the mother's milk confers immunities and antibodies to her baby. The relative risk of dying from common childhood infections is higher for non-breastfed infants. Breastfeeding also benefits the mother and reduces her risk of developing breast cancer. Recent research suggests that breast milk confers lifelong benefits by affecting the microbiome (in particular, the gut bacteria), and is "the most exquisite personalized medicine."[3] The composition of breast milk is also designed to promote brain development in ways that milk from animals such as cows is not. A recent survey[3] shows that "some" breastfeeding is associated with increased IQ, and the effect increases with the amount of breastfeeding.

One study[2] uses this relationship to estimate the global losses associated with inadequate breastfeeding (defined here as the proportion of infants under six months currently receiving some breast milk to six months, compared to all of them receiving it). The global losses are very large – averaging 0.49% of world Gross National Income (Table 1). In this case, it is the richest countries that lose the most economically: France, due to low breastfeeding rates but high income, loses 0.8% of its national income, whereas in Bhutan, where almost all infants are breastfed and income is low, the loss is only 0.01% of national income.

Another study[11] estimates the economic benefits of a comprehensive breastfeeding program in one large country, and compares these to the costs. The authors estimate that the returns are 2.4:1 (Table 1). Breastfeeding is one example of a nutrition intervention which is more pressing in the high-income countries, where the rates are the lowest but the economic costs are in the billions of dollars.

Anemia

We focus here on iron deficiency anemia, while noting that there are other causes of anemia (primarily infection), and that iron deficiency (without anemia) is also important. Iron plays an important role in many biological processes, and affects economic outcomes both through improved physical and improved mental capacity. Iron in hemoglobin in the blood is required to transport oxygen around the body, and people who are anemic cannot perform at maximum levels (e.g., run as fast), or for as long. This means that anemic adults undertaking manual work cannot work as hard, or as long, as adults without anemia, which in turn often

means that they earn less. More subtly, even workers in light manual work (e.g., in factories) also produce less if they are anemic.

Iron is also involved in brain development. Studies have shown that very young anemic children (below the age of two) are less outgoing and interact less with their environment, and that this therefore inhibits their ability to learn. Early limitations on cognitive development hinder subsequent performance in school, and this is compounded if the child remains anemic and is therefore less energetic and engaged while at school. One survey[10] estimates that anemia in early childhood is associated with a loss of about 8 IQ points.

Researchers have made estimates of the economic losses associated with iron deficiency. These losses are due to lower wages attributable to current levels of anemia (in adults), as well as owing to lower wages in adulthood on account of lower cognitive achievements in childhood. One study[12] makes estimates of the present value of lifetime economic losses if current levels of anemia persist, for ten countries with high levels of anemia. The median loss was 0.8% of GDP – a significant loss. The study further goes on to estimate the benefit:cost of iron fortification of staple foods, an inexpensive way to help reduce anemia levels. The authors estimate that the median benefit:cost ratio is 8.7:1.

Conclusions

The World Health Assembly has six nutrition targets for 2025. There are strong health reasons for these targets, and we have examined here the economic costs and benefits of the first three targets. In all three cases, the economic benefits of improving nutrition outweigh the intervention costs, and all three should be key public health priorities. Nutrition is a one world issue: While low-income countries may focus more on stunting and anemia, high-income countries need to focus on anemia (particularly in women of reproductive age, and children), and on increasing breastfeeding rates.

My personal view
Susan Horton

My first experience in a developing country came when I spent six months at the International Center for Diarrheal Disease Research in Bangladesh in 1979–80. During the 1970s, Bangladesh had been founded as a separate country and had undergone a major cyclone and a major famine. Undernutrition was all too evident a problem. This inspired me to work on nutrition in my economics research.

Thirty-five years later, Bangladesh – although still poor – has made substantial progress in improving nutrition. At the global level, progress on undernutrition has been made, with the Millennium Development Goals being one way of focusing attention on progress. Economics research has helped to show the benefits of nutrition as an investment, and that although the nutrition agenda is costly, it is affordable.

But more needs to be done. Even high-income countries face issues of "hidden hunger" – deficiencies of key micronutrients which harm child development. The growing rate of obesity is a "one world" issue facing rich and poor countries alike. Economics research will continue to play an important role in helping address these issues.

Further reading

Bhutta, ZA, Das JK, Rizvi A et al for Lancet Maternal and Child Nutrition & Interventions Review Groups Evidence based interventions for improving maternal and child nutrition: what can be done and at what cost? Lancet; 2013; 382 (9890); 452–477.

International Food Policy Research Institute. Global Nutrition Report 2014: actions and accountability to accelerate the world's progress on nutrition. Washington DC: IFPRI, 2014.

World Health Organization (WHO) Global nutrition targets 2025: policy brief series (undated). Available at https://www.who.int/nutrition/publications/globaltargets2025/en/. Accessed August 6, 2015.

References

1   UNICEF. A UNICEF policy review: strategy for improved nutrition of children and women in developing countries. New York: UNICEF, 1990.

2   World Health Organization (WHO). Global Health Observatory (GHO) data. http://www.who.int.gho/health_equity/outcomes/stunting_children/en, accessed August 5 2015.

3   Victora C, Bahl R, Barros A et al. Breastfeeding in the 21st Century: Epidemiology, Mechanisms and Lifelong Impact. The Lancet, 2016; 287: 475-490.

4   Rollins N, Bhandari N, Hajeebhoy N et al. Breastfeeding in the 21st century: Why invest, and what it will take to improve breastfeeding practices in less than a generation. Lancet Breastfeeding Series Paper 2. 2016; 287: 491-504.

5   World Health Organization (WHO). The global prevalence of anaemia in 2011. Geneva: World Health Organization, 2015.

6   Horton S, Steckel RH. Malnutrition: global economic losses attributable to malnutrition 1900–2000 and projections to 2050. In B. Lomborg (ed.) How much have global problems cost the world? Cambridge: Cambridge University Press, 2013.

7   Bhutta, ZA, Das JK, Rizvi A et al for Lancet Maternal and Child Nutrition & Interventions Review Groups Evidence based interventions for improving maternal and child nutrition: what can be done and at what cost? Lancet; 2013; 382 (9890); 452–477.

8   Hanushek, E, Woessmann L. The Role of Cognitive Skills in Economic Development. Journal of Economic Literature 2008; 46(3); 607–668.

9   Hoddinott J, Maluccio J, Behrman JR et al. The consequences of early childhood growth failure over the life course. 2011. Washington DC: International Food Policy Research Institute Discussion Paper 1073, 2011.

10 Hoddinott J, Alderman H, Behrman JR et al. The economic rationale for investing in stunting. Maternal and Child Nutrition 2013; 9(S2); 69–82.

11 Walters D, Horton S, Siregar AYM et al. The cost of not breastfeeding in Southeast Asia. Submitted, 2015.

12 Horton S, Ross J. The economics of iron deficiency. Food Policy 2003; 28(1); 51–75 Corrigendum Food Policy 2007; 32(1): 141–143.

The Economic Causes of Malnutrition

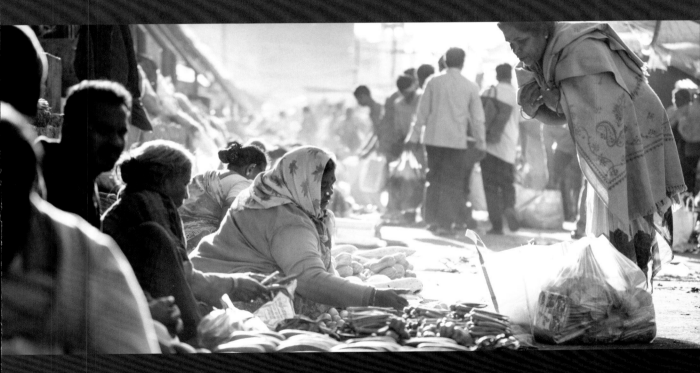

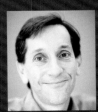

William A Masters
Professor, Friedman School of Nutrition Science & Policy,
Tufts University, Boston MA, USA

"*Life is better now than at almost any time in history. More people are richer and fewer people live in dire poverty. Lives are longer and parents no longer routinely watch a quarter of their children die. Yet millions still experience the horrors of destitution and of premature death. The world is hugely unequal.*"

Opening paragraph of The Great Escape *(2013) by Angus Deaton, winner of the 2015 Nobel Prize in economics for his work on the measurement of poverty and wellbeing.[1]*

Key messages

- For most people, nutritious foods are more widely available and affordable than ever before, yet malnutrition remains the world's leading cause of death and disability.

- Malnutrition is hard to eradicate, partly because it has different causes in different people.

- Economic analysis helps explain differences among people regarding both their food choices and the non-dietary factors that influence their nutritional status and health.

- By identifying the causes of malnutrition, economic analysis can help guide interventions and support changes that foster better nutrition.

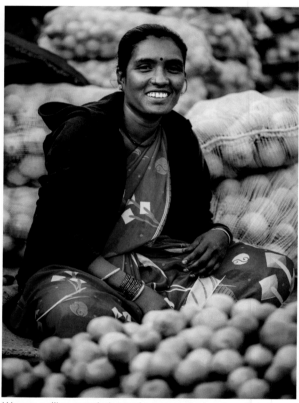

Woman selling mandarins and oranges at a local market at Karnataka State, India. Source: Mike Bloem

This chapter reviews the available evidence concerning differences among people, and changes over time, in four distinct dimensions:

1. The global, regional and national **availability** of nutrient-dense foods;

2. The **access** that individuals and households have to nutrient-dense foods;

3. The methods employed for food **use** that transforms foods into meals that people can consume; and

4. The non-dietary influences on people's nutrient **needs** that influence their nutritional status.

Malnutrition can be caused by a wide range of problems in each of these four dimensions. These causes can also be classified in a number of other ways, using a variety of conceptual frameworks. The approach taken in this particular chapter is complemented by Chapter 2.3, *The Economics of Poor Nutrition: Patterns, consequences and cost.*

Our approach takes a holistic or systems view and is concerned with aggregate outcomes at the population level, where all outcomes are interconnected: everything is caused by everything else. Individual social and biological pathways, from particular causes to specific effects, will be addressed in later chapters, drawing on research using biomedical and epidemiological methods. Here we are concerned with broad patterns, using economic methods to identify and explain society-wide outcomes.

Availability, Access, Utilization and Needs[4]

1. Availability: What makes a healthy diet more (or less) available to people, at prices they can afford?

Globally and regionally, nutrient-dense foods and fortificants are generally more available and affordable than ever in human history, but there are still large gaps of unmet need. Great opportunities therefore exist to improve the quality as well as the quantity of food supplies.

Market supplies of raw materials and foods can keep up with demand, but they do this at prices that fluctuate over time and space as well as in respect of food type. Affordability therefore depends on government policies and public investments.

Analysis of the most successful regions and time-periods allows us to conclude that meeting increased demand without raising prices requires research, education, infrastructure and institutions that are specific to the food sector. We can also see that, historically, periods of food crisis have led to surges in public investment and subsequent periods of abundance (and complacency).

2. Access: What makes a healthy diet more (or less) accessible to all people, at all times?

Within individual countries, there are consistent patterns of poor nutrition. Unfilled gaps are greatest for young women and children, as well as the poorest. Great opportunities therefore exist to improve distribution and food access.

Distribution of food access is closely tied to other entitlements such as education, healthcare, housing and transportation. Private markets to distribute nutrient-dense and fortified foods depend on government policies (e.g., trade, standards), institutions (e.g., quality assurance, enforcement) and infrastructure (e.g., rural electrification, roads and marketplaces). Nutrition interventions are cost-effective ways to fill any remaining gaps.

Analysis of the most successful regions and time-periods shows that market development goes a long way, but not the whole way, to facilitating universal access. It is also important to note that even the richest countries have ongoing nutrition interventions.

3. Utilization: What makes a healthy diet more (or less) user-friendly for the most vulnerable groups?

Food utilization is a major cause of poor nutrition. Storing, preparing, cooking and serving safe and nutritious food is surprisingly difficult, especially to support the nutrition requirements of healthy gestation and infancy. Great opportunities therefore exist to facilitate improved feeding practices.

Figure 1 | **Everything is connected: Availability, Access, Utilization and Needs**

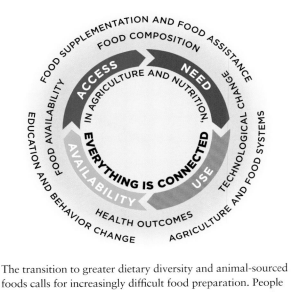

The transition to greater dietary diversity and animal-sourced foods calls for increasingly difficult food preparation. People shift quickly to packaged food and food consumed away from home, which exposes them both to nutritional and food-safety risks. Opportunities to improve begin with breastfeeding and complementary feeding, and they continue at every life stage.

Analysis of the most successful regions and eras indicates that availability and access are important factors, but that they are not sufficient in themselves to ensure a nutritious diet. Many kinds of labeling, norms and standards are needed to ensure a safe and healthy diet.

4. Needs: What changes in non-dietary factors alter dietary needs and nutritional status?

Dietary needs are not uniform or constant. Individual circumstances drive large differences in total energy and nutrient needs – for example, due to the effort of labor, the state of the individual's gut health, and the burden of various types of disease. Improving non-dietary factors strengthens the link between nutrition and health.

Dietary improvements reveal the role of other factors. Adjusting to changes in the effort of labor and physical exertion is difficult, while sanitation and environmental health pose major constraints.

From the most successful regions and time-periods, we can conclude that dietary intake is important but not sufficient to ensure health and wellbeing. The path towards good nutrition involves change at every step, and embraces all aspects of health.

Figure 2 | **Availability and access to food: Africa and South Asia still have far to go**

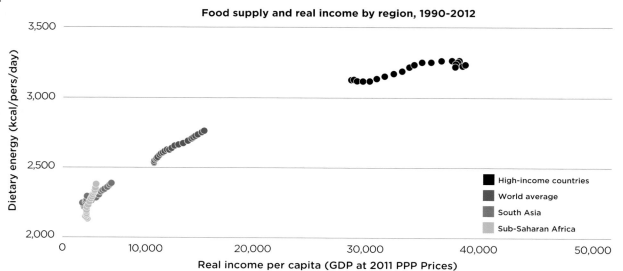

Food supply and real income by region, 1990-2012

Source: Author's calculations. Real income is from World Bank, World Development Indicators (April 2014), downloaded from http://data.worldbank.org. Food supply is from FAO, Food Security Indicators (December 2013), downloaded from http://www.fao.org/economic/ess/ess-fs. Each point is a 3-year average, from 1990-92 to 2010-12.

Figure 3 | **Utilization of food shifts to meet nutrient needs mostly from foods other than starchy staples**

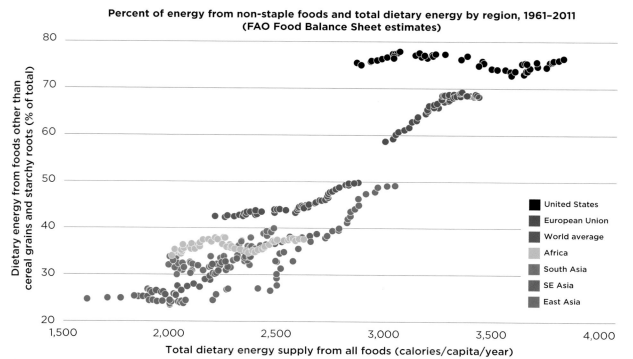

Percent of energy from non-staple foods and total dietary energy by region, 1961–2011 (FAO Food Balance Sheet estimates)

Source: Author's calculations from FAO Food Balance Sheets, http://faostat3.fao.org/download/FB/FBS/E (June 2015).

Using economics to explain malnutrition

The relationship between individual choices, separability, and population-level outcomes

The economics approach to studying malnutrition starts with individual choices, and the separability between production and consumption that arises when people sell or buy some of what they produce. This notion of separability is intrinsic to food production: even the most remote farmer, whatever their landholding and other resources, is rarely limited to consuming solely his or her own produce.

Separability in practice

Any one person's food consumption can be separated from their food production by their trade with other people. The Scottish philosopher Adam Smith, writing in 1776, focused *The Wealth of Nations* on the consequences of our human "propensity to truck, barter, and exchange one thing for another,"[2] thereby launching the modern economic approach to studying human societies.

Although access to markets may be heavily constrained by factors such as poor roads, inadequate transport, inclement weather, and many other obstacles, virtually everyone, in any part of the world, will be able to find attractive opportunities to sell certain things in order to be able to buy others. This is particularly true of foods, given the need for each person to consume various foods the whole year round, and the differences among farms that lead to specialized agricultural enterprises and diverse trading systems. Once each person can trade with many others, his or her production and consumption decisions become *separable*, with separate causes for one as opposed to the other.

At the individual level, separability ensures that the production – and hence the availability – of nutrient-dense foods is determined by agricultural conditions and prices, as farmers adjust their activities in response to the scarcity of each thing relative to their own farm's productivity. Similarly, dietary intake and nutritional outcomes among individuals is then determined by the relative scarcity of each thing, relative to people's household income and decisions regarding consumption. Different outcomes arise depending on individuals' access to nutrient-dense foods, which in turn follows from market opportunities (the real cost of what they buy, relative to the prices of all other things) relative to their livelihoods (the full income they earn from all sources).

The logic of separability is graphically illustrated in **Figure 2**, in which availability is shown by the curved blue set of production possibilities, from which people can access additional food by buying and selling along the dashed diagonal line showing real income. Dietary intake and health outcomes are determined by utilization along the red indifference curve, whose position indicates their need and level of wellbeing in terms of both nutrition and other aspects of living conditions.

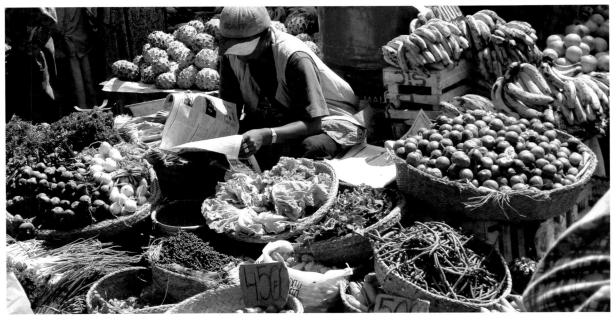

Stall on a fruit and vegetable market in Antananarivo, Madagascar. Source: Sight and Life

Individual choices

The logic of **Figure 4** is an abstract representation of ideas that are universally familiar in everyday life, but easily forgotten in the design of policies and programs to improve nutrition. Farmers almost never eat all they grow, or grow all they eat. Selling one thing so as to buy another is often the best way for farmers to meet their own nutritional needs, just as it is almost everyone's best way to acquire almost everything that can readily be bought and sold. Poor farmers usually try hard to limit what they must buy, but this is because they have so little to sell in exchange. Taking account of market behavior is often key both to predicting behavior and to designing interventions to improve farmers' circumstances.

Figure 4 | **Explaining individuals' choices**

Numerous studies have shown that production and consumption are separable when farm households have market access, and "non-separable" when they don't.

Most of the world's extreme undernutrition is among farm households as in the diagram to the right, with some buying and some selling of relatively nutritious foods, but many non-farm households also suffer from malnutrition as in the lower diagram.

- ● Consumption
- ● Production
- ● In self-sufficiency, production = consumption
- —— Production Possibilities Frontier
- —— Welfare of farm household in self-sufficiency
- – – – Welfare of farm household trading food
- ••••• Welfare of non-farm household
- – – – Income level of farm household
- ••••• Income level of non-farm household

Panel 1a. An individual farm household
(example shown is a *net seller* of this food)

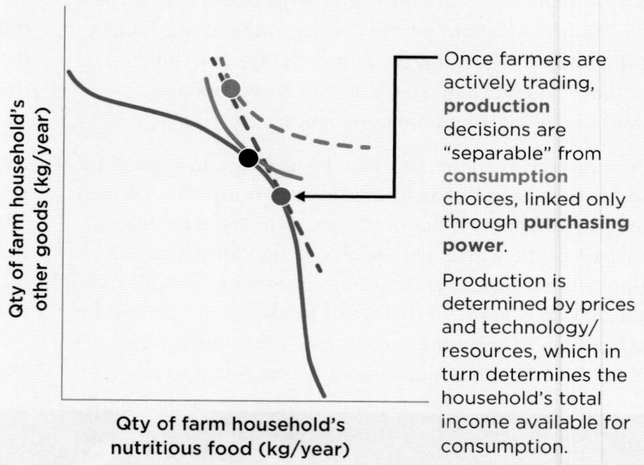

Qty of farm household's other goods (kg/year)

Qty of farm household's nutritious food (kg/year)

Once farmers are actively trading, **production** decisions are "separable" from **consumption** choices, linked only through **purchasing power**.

Production is determined by prices and technology/ resources, which in turn determines the household's total income available for consumption.

Panel 1b. An individual non-farm household
(non-farmers are *net buyers* of food)

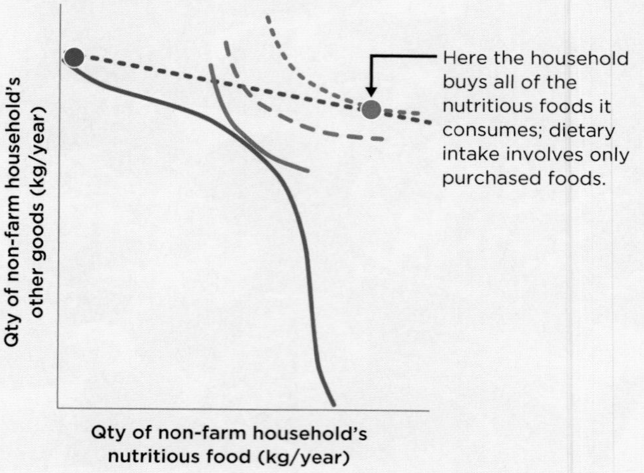

Qty of non-farm household's other goods (kg/year)

Qty of non-farm household's nutritious food (kg/year)

Here the household buys all of the nutritious foods it consumes; dietary intake involves only purchased foods.

Population-level outcomes

The economics approach to population-level outcomes focuses on the interactions among people, and the many kinds of exchange between them. **Figure 5** illustrates the economic interactions among individuals that generate observed outcomes at the level of a country or a subnational population.

The availability of a particular food is shown by the upward sloping blue "supply" line. Access depends on the dashed horizontal line showing the price at which this food can be bought or sold, while utilization and needs are illustrated by the downward sloping red "demand" line. These lines, and the resulting points, follow directly from adding up the choices of individuals illustrated in **Figure 4**, as they interact with each other at the population level.

Figure 5 | **Explaining population-scale outcomes**

Numerous studies have shown that countries and communities can improve nutrition outcomes by participating in markets, so that consumption becomes separable from production.

Some malnourished people are in communities whose situation is illustrated in the diagram to the right, as producers of a nutritious food which they sell to other people. They use the resulting income to buy other foods of varying nutritional quality. Many are in settings shown by the lower diagram, where their community produces some of a nutritious food, but can import more to a higher level of dietary intake.

Panel 2a. One community of households
(here, they *export* a particular nutritious food)

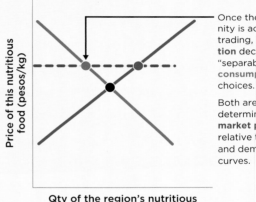

Once the community is actively trading, **production** decisions are "separable" from **consumption** choices.

Both are determined by **market prices**, relative to supply and demand curves.

- ● Consumption
- ● Production
- ● In self-sufficiency, production = consumption
- —— Supply curve
- —— Demand curve
- ▬ ▬ Price in trade with people elsewhere

Panel 2b. Another community of households
(here, they *import* this particular nutritious food)

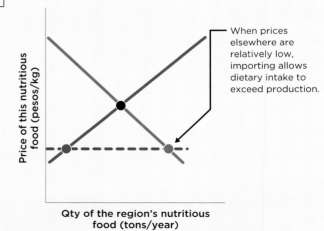

When prices elsewhere are relatively low, importing allows dietary intake to exceed production.

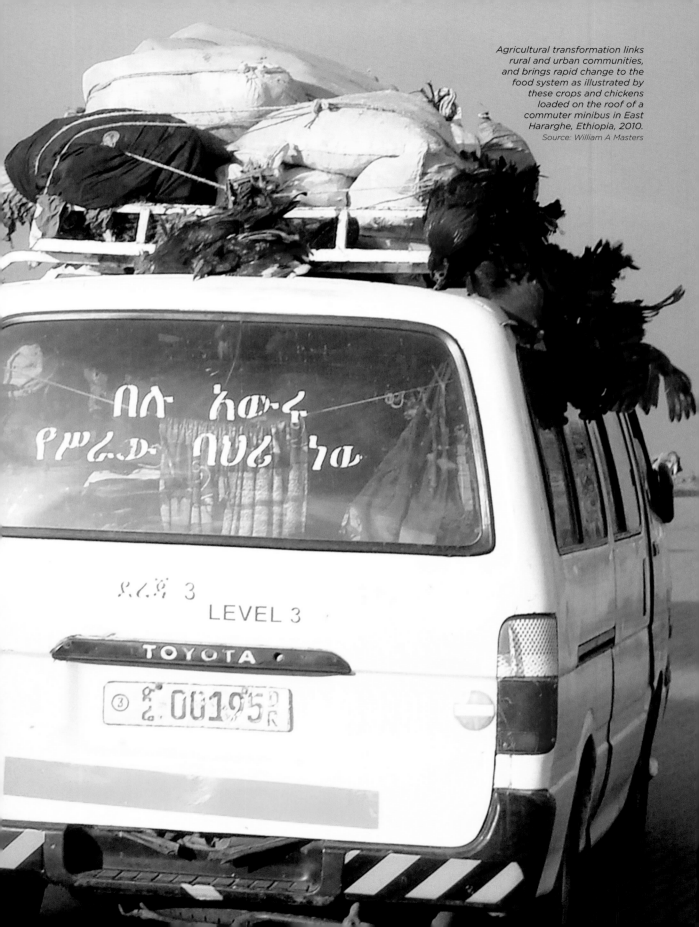

Agricultural transformation links rural and urban communities, and brings rapid change to the food system as illustrated by these crops and chickens loaded on the roof of a commuter minibus in East Hararghe, Ethiopia, 2010.
Source: William A Masters

Two structural changes associated with economic development:
Agricultural transformation and demographic transition

Agricultural transformation is a shift in employment and expenditure from food to other enterprises.

In the world's poorest societies, most people have no choice but to live in rural areas, relying on natural resources and household labor to obtain food, fuel and water. If opportunities arise to improve productivity, either within agriculture or in other activities, then people can save and invest, specialize and trade, ultimately moving into a wide array of services and manufacturing.

This transformation occurs within rural areas, and also allows migration to towns and cities, which sustains further economic development. The transformation out of agriculture as incomes rise explains why the poorest people and most malnourished children are typically found in the most agriculturallyoriented places, both across and within countries. Agricultural transformation creates the apparent paradox that people and places most heavily engaged in food production are the most likely to be malnourished, but that paradox can typically be resolved by controlling for real income.

Demographic transition is another kind of structural change with surprising implications for child nutrition.

This familiar shift towards longer life and then also lower fertility almost always starts with lower child mortality, often associated with an improvement in nutrition. That can quickly lead to a decline in birth rates, particularly if accompanied by opportunities for education, women's employment and access to contraception. In the meantime, however, there is a burst of population growth and a demographic burden of more children per household.

The rise in child dependency during the demographic transition helps explain why child malnutrition often worsens over time, before it improves. The demographic burden of child care falls disproportionately on young women, until declining fertility rates help the age structure swing back toward more working-age adults per child. The eventual rise in the workforce as a fraction of the population then offers a demographic gift that can fuel rapid economic development, particularly when combined with agricultural transformation and off-farm employment growth.

Demographic transition interacts with agricultural transformation in a way that often makes nutrition improvement harder in low-income countries, and then easier at higher-income levels. In poor countries, the non-agricultural sector is initially so small that even very rapid rates of off-farm employment growth cannot absorb all of the increasing number of working-age people. Despite successful year-to-year economic development and rapid urbanization, there will be a rising number of workers who have no choice but to farm, typically with less and less land and other natural resources per worker. That burden of declining land area per farmer in poor countries can be offset only by raising their crop yields, until the size of their country's non-agricultural sector has become large enough via its annual growth to absorb each year's increase in the adult workforce.

In summary, these two structural changes associated with economic development impose temporary burdens on child nutrition in low-income countries. By the arithmetic of year-to-year change, they serve to raise the number of children per adult and to lower the area of land per farmer in the early stages of structural change, making progress harder before it gets easier.

At later stages of economic development, child dependency rates and area per farmer can increase – both of which factors help the poorest and most malnourished escape more quickly from poverty. The development process may start earlier or later, varies widely in speed, and occasionally stalls altogether. But to the extent that economic development proceeds, it is characterized by remarkable similarities that help explain the patterns we see across countries and over time.

In that sense, successful societies are alike, even as their progress towards that shared destination involves a variety of diverse forces.

Adapted from: Masters WA. "Child Nutrition in Economic Development", in Duggan CP, Watkins JB, Koletzko B et al, eds., Nutrition in Pediatrics, 5th ed. Shelton, CT: PMPH-USA, 2016.

The separability between production and consumption:
Example of the fruit vendor from Makoni District, Zimbabwe

In 1986, as a young teacher in a rural school near Nyazura, Zimbabwe, I used to buy lemons and other fruit from a vendor named Amai Nickson, who would walk over the hill from a neighboring village to sell her wares. She was much poorer than the other villagers, and could rarely afford to eat the produce she sold. All her money went on more basic needs, including school fees for her children.

When I returned to Nyazura in 2010, I found Amai Nickson's[3] life much changed. She was now caring for grandchildren as well as her own youngest children (shown in the photo). She had saved up over the years and invested in her farm, including some backyard chickens. One consequence of these changes was that she could now buy fruit, instead of selling it. Amai Nickson's transition from seller to buyer of fruit is an example of how the relationships shown in Figure 4 can change over time and vary among neighbors, with differences explained by variation in income, market prices and the affordability of each food relative to farm production.

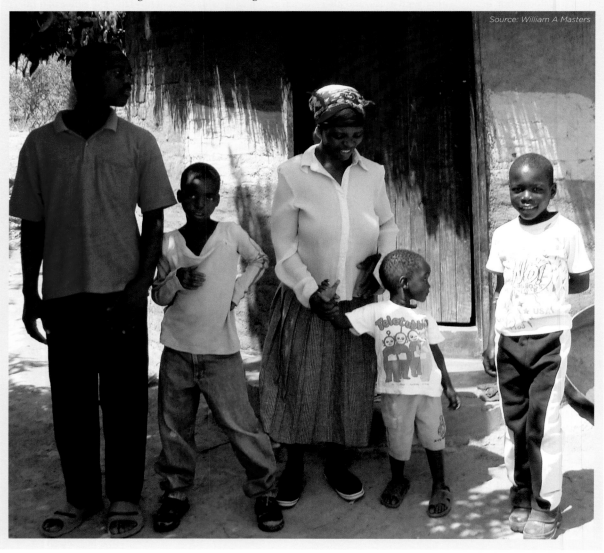

Source: William A Masters

Child nutrition and economic development

Individual choices and separability

Children's nutrition is both a cause and a consequence of broader health conditions, household income and living standards. Some of these changes are mediated by national or community-level policies and programs as well as medical interventions. Most of the patterns, however, occur autonomously as individuals respond to changing circumstances associated with economic development. These changes often occur slowly, without the conscious knowledge of those involved. They have only recently been documented, thanks to the accumulation of evidence from a wide range of social environments.

Leo Tolstoy's classic novel *Anna Karenina* begins: "All happy families are alike; each unhappy family is unhappy in its own way." This claim starts an epic, questioning search for whatever it might be that successes have in common. For economic development, an extensive social science literature documents wide variation in people's living conditions. These circumstances have often stagnated for centuries, with almost all people experiencing relatively poor health, low income and less preferred living standards, until new opportunities and forms of social organization trigger the onset of sustained improvement.

Rising income is eventually associated with large gains in adult height, weight, and many measures of health and even measureable increases in subjective wellbeing. It turns out that success in one dimension is typically accompanied by successes in other areas. Many different obstacles might slow development, but successful societies often move in similar directions as people gradually achieve similar objectives.

Many aspects of child nutrition are likely to change as children's families acquire more purchasing power. Surveys of several million children from more than a hundred countries over multiple decades allow us to look systematically at changes in child height, stunting and wasting, as well as various contributors to nutritional status. These include food availability and diet quality, sanitation and water supplies, breastfeeding behavior, treatment of childhood diarrhea, vaccination, and vitamin A supplementation. Each of these measures reflects a different aspect of child nutrition.

Many factors other than economic development clearly matter for child nutrition. Ethnographic studies describe in detail how children are raised, finding that social norms and beliefs can lead to a variety of choices regarding complementary feeding and other nutritional practices. These norms may eventually adjust to income changes, or may introduce variation that is unrelated to economic circumstances.

Adapted from: Masters WA. "Child Nutrition in Economic Development", in Duggan CP, Watkins JB, Koletzko B et al, eds., Nutrition in Pediatrics, 5th ed. Shelton, CT: PMPH-USA, 2016.

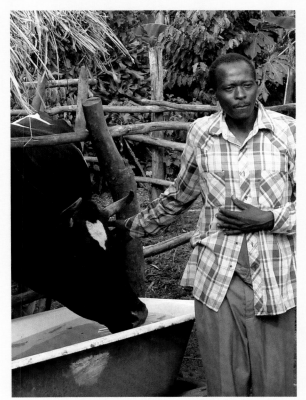

Recipient of Heifer International cow named Esther, Uganda.
Source: William A Masters

103

Agriculture and nutrition as a factor in health and development

Agriculture, nutrition, and health are interrelated through biological and behavioral pathways that tie these sectors to ecological and socioeconomic conditions.

Place-based factors constrain and influence people's nutrition and health outcomes at every scale and in every context. For example, rainfall, temperature, and soil nutrients interact with crop genetics to influence plant growth and food quality as well as farm incomes, which in turn influence food-purchasing and health-seeking behaviors, all of which combine to influence individuals' nutrition and health outcomes.

Ecological conditions also influence the growth and reproduction of pathogens, parasites, and disease vectors of all kinds, weighing heavily on the effectiveness of interventions aimed at meeting development goals.

Since the 2007–08 food-price crisis, increasing attention to agriculture and nutrition as a factor in health and development has led donors and governments to pursue more integrated national plans, with a view to capitalizing on potential synergies between sectors in each location. For example, countries as diverse as Nepal, Haiti, and Kenya all promote intersectoral coordination and interministerial collaboration to achieve common goals around enhanced nutrition, health, and food security. Indeed, the call for integrated action represents a new global agenda, as highlighted by the L'Aquila Joint Statement on Global Food Security, which argued that: "food security, nutrition and sustainable agriculture must remain a priority issue on the political agenda, to be addressed through a cross-cutting...approach."

The potential gains from integrated interventions call for enhanced research methods that explicitly account for biological and ecological relationships at their natural scale, to reveal regional-level effects that may be quite different from the sum of individual-level changes potentially observed in a limited-scale randomized control trial. However, the increasing focus of policies and programs on intersectoral integration to solve location-specific problems poses deep challenges for researchers, regarding how the value added from integration is most appropriately measured.

The challenge is illustrated by controversy and confusion regarding what constitutes appropriate evidence in relation to multisectoral programming at the village level or in economic development more generally. Programs that seek to link food, water, health, and nutrition at a regional scale are already being implemented around the globe, but few have been rigorously analyzed, and most remain focused on measuring siloed outcomes within sectors and then aggregating these as if their impact equaled the sum of their parts.

To measure synergies, we need a research agenda that explicitly addresses intersectoral linkages and the cost-effectiveness, replicability, and scalability of integrated processes.

Source: *Agriculture, nutrition, and health in global development: typology and metrics for integrated interventions and research, http://onlinelibrary.wiley.com/doi/10.1111/nyas.12352/full, accessed August 28, 2015 and lightly adapted.*

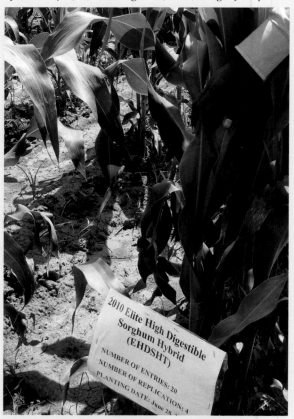

Testing new sorghum varieties at Melkasa Research Station, Ethiopia. Source: William A Masters

My personal view

William A Masters

When I was 20 years old, I took a semester off from school to live and travel in Haiti, where I saw widespread malnutrition in both rural and urban areas. I later worked in Colombia and Zimbabwe, before starting my PhD at Stanford. An especially inspiring teacher there was Reynaldo Martorell, whose research helped suggest new ways to overcome the many obstacles to good nutrition.

Prof. Martorell's teaching also opened the door to many new questions, and emphasized the need for each of us to use our own skills and perspectives to help solve problems collaboratively.

My own interests focused then, as now, on how people's behavior influences local agriculture, markets and nutritional outcomes. I like using economic methods in part because economics offers a platform for collaboration with natural scientists and health scientists, leading to the kind of fruitful partnerships discussed throughout this book.

Further reading

FAO. The State of Food Insecurity in the World Rome: FAO, 2015. http://www.fao.org/hunger/en.

IFPRI. Global Nutrition Report: Actions and Accountability to Accelerate the World's Progress on Nutrition. Washington, DC:IFPRI, 2014. http://globalnutritionreport.org.

Masters WA. Child Nutrition in Economic Development, in Duggan CP, Watkins JB, Koletzko B et al, eds., Nutrition in Pediatrics, 5th ed. Shelton, CT:PMPH-USA, 2016.

Masters WA, Webb P., Griffiths JK et al. Agriculture, nutrition, and health in global development: typology and metrics for integrated interventions and research. Ann N Y Acad Sci 2014;1331(1):258–269.

Masters WA. Economic Development, Government Policies and Food Consumption, chapter 14 in Jayson Lusk, Jutta Roosen and Jason Shogren, eds., Oxford Handbook on the Economics of Food Consumption and Policy. New York: Oxford University Press, 2011.

Norton G, Alwang J, Masters WA. Economics of Agricultural Development (3rd ed.). New York: Routledge2014.

Smith LC, Haddad L. Reducing Child Undernutrition: Past Drivers and Priorities for the Post-MDG Era. World Development 2015;68:180–204.

Vollmer S, Harttgen K, Subramanyam MA et al. Association between economic growth and early childhood undernutrition: evidence from 121 Demographic and Health Surveys from 36 low-income and middle-income countries. Lancet Global Health 2014;2(4):e225–e234.

References

1   Deaton, A. The Great Escape: Health, Wealth, and the Origins of Inequality. Princeton University Press, 2013.

2   Smith A. An Inquiry into the Nature and Causes of the Wealth of Nations, Book I Chapter 2, London, 1776. Penguin Classics, new edition 1982.

3   This phrase means "Mother of Nickson." In Shona society, both women and men are frequently called "Mother of" or "Father of" their firstborn child, even if they have other children.

4   The definitions employed here are the author's and are based on recent scientific insights and detailed economic analysis.

Diet and Non-Communicable Diseases: An urgent need for new paradigms

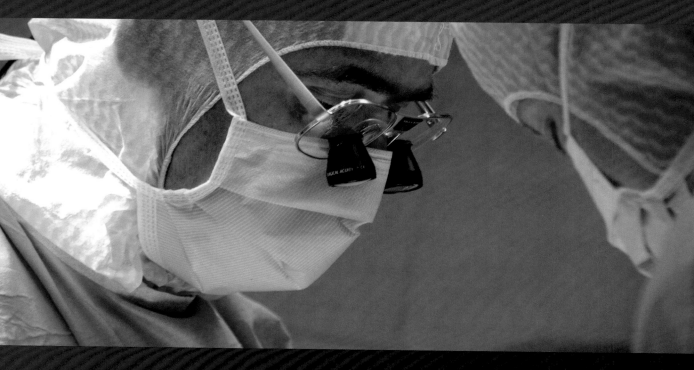

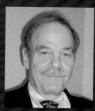

Henry Greenberg
Special Lecturer in
Epidemiology, Institute of
Human Nutrition, Mailman
School of Public Health,
Columbia University Medical
Center, New York, NY, USA

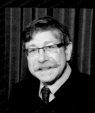

**Richard J
Deckelbaum**
Robert R Williams Professor of
Nutrition, Professor of Pediatrics
and Professor of Epidemiology;
Director, Institute of Human
Nutrition, and Department of
Pediatrics, College of Physicians
and Surgeons, Columbia
University Medical Center, New
York, NY, USA

"The voyage of discovery is not in seeking new landscapes but in having new eyes."

Marcel Proust (1871–1922), *French novelist, essayist and critic.*

Key messages

- Incidence and impact of non-communicable diseases (NCDs) will further increase, and will continue to do so at a younger age than we have been accustomed to in the US and Western Europe.

- NCDs have many risk factors, and lifestyle-altering interventions are necessary to mitigate them.

- Many countries worldwide are rapidly acquiring the characteristics that create a receptive milieu for NCDs.

- More people die annually from cardiovascular diseases (CVD) than from any other cause; approximately one third of these deaths occur in adults aged between 30 and 70.

- NCDs are very difficult to manage with traditional health measures, but innovative interventions do exist, and can be effectively implemented.

- To reduce the prevalence of NCDs, public health needs to engage more actively in the shaping of policies that influence health.

- The food industry should be encouraged to offer a portfolio of nutritious food products and food supplements to fill the nutrient gaps.

The spread of non-communicable diseases

Non-communicable diseases (NCDs) have emerged as the leading cause of human mortality and morbidity in low-, middle- and high-income countries. NCDs are not considered only as social burden; the economic costs of NCDs are also accelerating worldwide. By the year 2030, when the Sustainable Development Goals (SDGs) should have attained their targets, cardiovascular disease (CVD) will be the leading cause of death across the planet, exceeding mortality from HIV, TB, malaria, and maternal & child undernutrition combined. Despite these "costs," not to mention personal disabilities and social ailments, however, little progress has been made to date in limiting or diminishing the NCD epidemic.

The main NCDs include diabetes, cardiovascular disease (CVD), chronic respiratory disease, cancer, and mental health conditions. Obesity and overweight are frequently associated with the presence of one of more of these NCDs. In this chapter, the major emphasis will be on overweight and obesity and the root associations of these conditions with cardiovascular disease and diabetes. The text is presented as key themes that need to be considered in developing new paradigms to diminish the burden of NCDs. An overview of the basic epidemiology of these diseases will be considered, and this will be followed by recognized and underappreciated drivers for NCDs. The economic cost of NCDs will be considered, along with interventions and challenges to the new paradigms presented for successful control of this major burden to human health and productivity.

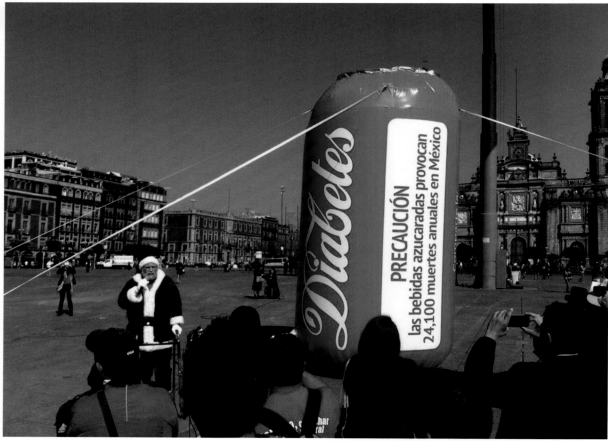

The global rise in the incidence of type 2 diabetes has been fueled, in part, by the consumption of carbonated beverages with a high sugar content. Source: Ricardo Uauy

1 Basic epidemiology of non-communicable disease risk factors related to diet

Aside from the role of genetics, the dominant risk factors for non-communicable diseases are behavioral; they relate to unhealthy diets, inadequate physical activity, exposure to tobacco smoke (and air pollutants), and excessive alcohol use. By and large they can be avoided, and if recognized at any time over the life course, they can be modified by changes in behavior and lifestyle, and/or with well-tolerated and inexpensive medications. However, because the risk factors are embedded in behavioral, cultural, and political realities, modifying the up-stream drivers is very difficult and requires the engagement of different sectors of government and other groups.

The major NCDs related to diet are cardiovascular diseases and diabetes mellitus (DM). There are also several others: respiratory diseases, mental health disorders, lower extremity arthritis secondary to obesity, several cancers, and dental caries. The key diet-related risk factors for CVD and DM include overweight/obesity, hyperglycemia, elevated blood lipids, and hypertension. (Here we do not focus on alcohol or tobacco, although the former could be included under the diet umbrella.) The leading risk factors for CVD (ranked by disability-adjusted life years, DALYs) in every region of the world are of dietary origin, and this excludes hypertension, which is categorized separately and is universally number two. (In Eastern Europe, hypertension is first and dietary second – see **Figure 1**). Hypertension, however, obviously has substantial contributory diet-related mechanisms.[1]

Figure 1 | Burden of disease attributable to 20 leading risk factors in 2010, expressed as a percentage of global disability-adjusted life years(DALYs). *SHS = second-hand smoke*

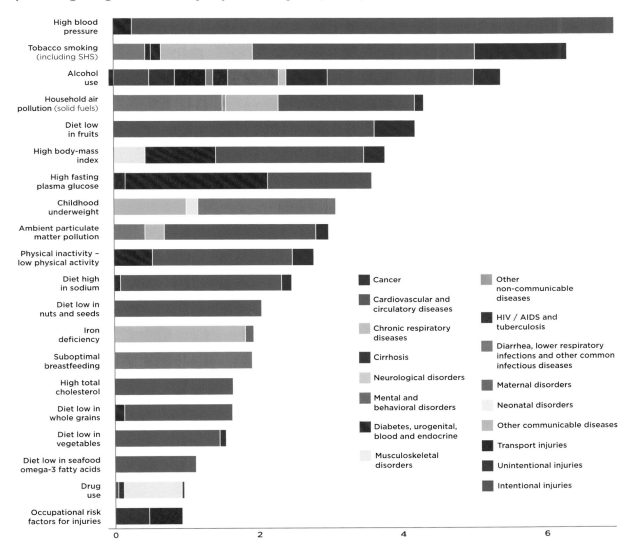

Source: Lim SS et al. A comparative risk assessment of burden of disease and injury attributable to 67 risk factors and risk factor clusters in 21 regions, 1990–2010: a systematic analysis for the Global Burden of Disease study, 2010. Lancet 2012;380:2224–2260.

Figure 2 | **Projected deaths by cause in high-, middle-, and low-income countries, 2004 to 2030**

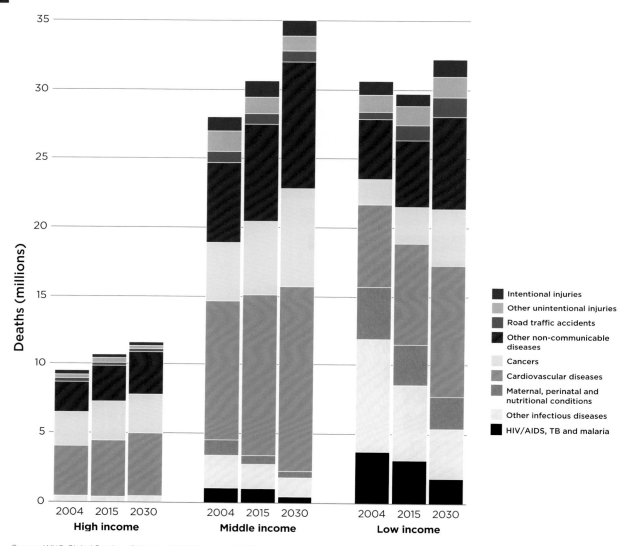

Source: WHO Global Burden of Disease 2004 Update, p. 24, "Projected deaths by cause in high, middle, and low income countries, 2004 to 2030." http://www.who.int/healthinfo/global_burden_disease/2004_report_update/en/. Accessed May 25, 2016.

Figure 2. illustrates how by 2030 CVD will cause the largest number of deaths not only in developed countries but also in low- and middle-income countries (LMICs), exceeding the mortality from HIV, TB, malaria, and maternal-child undernutrition combined.

From the Global Burden of Diseases (GBD) 2010[2] we learn that in the two decades between 1990 and 2010, the disease burden attributable to hypertension, alcohol consumption, high BMI, high fasting blood glucose, high sodium intake, and low fruit, vegetable, nut and whole grain consumption all increased significantly, while the disease burden attributable to childhood underweight, suboptimal breastfeeding and micronutrient deficiencies all decreased significantly (**Figure 3**). There is little likelihood that these trends will change in the near future in all regions of the world. The NCD expression will only increase, and will do so at a younger age than we have been accustomed to in the US and Western Europe.

Figure 3 | Global risk factor ranks for all ages and sexes combined in 1990 (left) and 2010 (right).
PM= particulate matter; UI= uncertainty interval; SHS= second-hand smoke

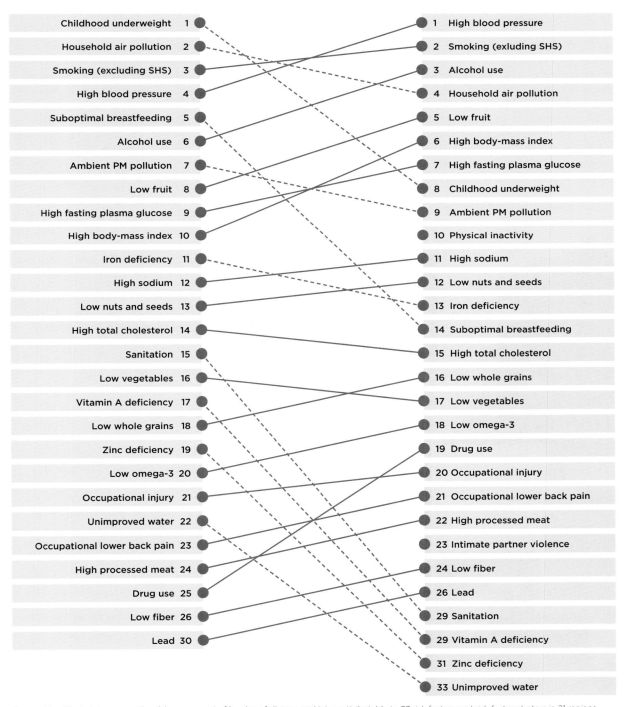

1990	2010
Childhood underweight 1	1 High blood pressure
Household air pollution 2	2 Smoking (exluding SHS)
Smoking (excluding SHS) 3	3 Alcohol use
High blood pressure 4	4 Household air pollution
Suboptimal breastfeeding 5	5 Low fruit
Alcohol use 6	6 High body-mass index
Ambient PM pollution 7	7 High fasting plasma glucose
Low fruit 8	8 Childhood underweight
High fasting plasma glucose 9	9 Ambient PM pollution
High body-mass index 10	10 Physical inactivity
Iron deficiency 11	11 High sodium
High sodium 12	12 Low nuts and seeds
Low nuts and seeds 13	13 Iron deficiency
High total cholesterol 14	14 Suboptimal breastfeeding
Sanitation 15	15 High total cholesterol
Low vegetables 16	16 Low whole grains
Vitamin A deficiency 17	17 Low vegetables
Low whole grains 18	18 Low omega-3
Zinc deficiency 19	19 Drug use
Low omega-3 20	20 Occupational injury
Occupational injury 21	21 Occupational lower back pain
Unimproved water 22	22 High processed meat
Occupational lower back pain 23	23 Intimate partner violence
High processed meat 24	24 Low fiber
Drug use 25	26 Lead
Low fiber 26	29 Sanitation
Lead 30	29 Vitamin A deficiency
	31 Zinc deficiency
	33 Unimproved water

Source: Lim SS et al. A comparative risk assessment of burden of disease and injury attributable to 67 risk factors and risk factor clusters in 21 regions, 1990–2010: a systematic analysis for the Global Burden of Disease study, 2010. Lancet 2012;380:2224-2260.

While the disease prevalence in most of Sub-Saharan Africa (SSA) seems relatively benign as far as expressed disease is concerned, the recent changes in the CVD risk factor profile tell a different story. In SSA between 1990 and 2010, hypertension has increased by 60%; dietary risk factors have increased by 45%; the prevalence of high plasma glucose has increased by nearly 30%; and, most impressively, the prevalence of a high BMI has tripled. In 2010, more than a third of the disability in SSA originated from non-communicable diseases, and CVD accounted for 6.8% of the total. While ischemic heart disease remains uncommon in SSA, stroke rates approach those in the developed world, probably related to a rapid increase in

Increasing wealth and urbanization are key drivers of NCDs.
Source: Donated by Jo Wilson.

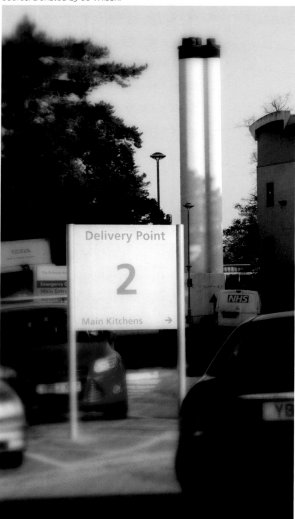

hypertension and inadequate methods to control it. No CVD risk factor has decreased over the past 20 years (2013 data). We have seen this scenario before; we know how it will end if no altering interventions are introduced. We know from the INTERHEART study[3] that "a risk factor is a risk factor is a risk factor." So the present trajectory of SSA will take this region to a NCD health picture much like Latin America or South East Asia in the next generation. And the speed with which these countries will travel to those destinations will be rapid. The drivers that accelerate this transition were discussed in Section 2.2.

Lack of access to integrated healthcare services for people who suffer from CVD and other NCDs is also an issue. Processed foods high in trans fats, saturated fats, sugar and salt, plus sugar-sweetened beverages, are associated with increased risk of hypertension, diabetes, elevated cholesterol and CVD. Increased urbanization and use of motorized transport may contribute to sedentary lifestyles, which have detrimental implications for cardiovascular health.[4]

The Global Burden of Ischemic Heart Diseases data extracted from the GBD 2010 Study[1] charts the risk factor profile of the WHO global regions. In the high-income, advanced economies in North America, Western Europe, the Asia Pacific region, and Australasia, the profiles are of a decreasing risk factor burden, with the exception of obesity. In all other regions, the profile is increasing.

In order to address these challenges, a broad array of nutrition-specific and collateral initiatives will be required to provide appropriate food to the growing populations worldwide. Key stakeholders must interact and align with one another to overcome the nutritional challenges of societies as they change. An enabling environment should be created to encourage food manufacturers to produce a wide array of affordable, nutritious food products with reduced fat, sugar and calories in combination with appropriate levels of essential (micro)nutrients. Governments need to collaborate with the food industry and:

1 provide incentives (such as regulatory frameworks that stimulate innovative solutions);

2 make sure that the required standards are met in order to protect consumers; and

3 provide education to stimulate consumers to make more health-conscious choices.

2 Contemporary drivers of NCDs and their risk factors

Whereas diet and exercise are preventable risks factors of NCDs, the hard-to-prevent and major drivers of NCDs are increasing wealth, urbanization, air pollution, the information revolution, and global marketing. With the exception of urbanization, none of these have been given much space on the palette of public health, and they are rarely covered in the academic public health curriculum.

Urbanization is a global trend which is also evident in the emerging economies as their populations become wealthier.[5] Increasing national wealth is initially an urban phenomenon which then seeps back to the countryside via remittances, increased travel, and an increasingly well informed rural population. In the city, women join the work force, further disrupting the traditional family dynamics beyond the effects caused by the migration itself. Employment rather than farming becomes the norm. With the growing tendency toward urbanization, it can be anticipated that the dietary profile will significantly change, and an adaptation to a more Western pattern appears likely.[6] The situation for significant parts of the population will change from one of too little food to one of too much food rich in energy and poor in nutrients, and with a high component of processed foods. Disposable income is attracted to readily available fast food, sugary drinks, and tobacco. As there is less and less opportunity

for communal family meals, out-of-home outlets become increasingly utilized and important, their role being enhanced by effective and innovative marketing. Physical activity and calories burned by physical work plummet and, coupled with the altered dietary patterns, can lead to rapid rises in overweight and obesity.

While health data support the observation that urban life is healthier for children than rural life and that vaccines and primary healthcare are more readily available, children are more exposed to television, computers, and other sedentary activities, all at the expense of physical activity. These distractions may exacerbate the likelihood of overweight and obesity, and these conditions then drive their associated comorbidities, contributing in a major way to increased prevalence of insulin resistance and metabolic syndrome, DM, respiratory diseases, nonalcoholic fatty liver disease (NAFLD), and CVD.

Layered on to these local transitions and exposures are up-stream forces that further fuel NCD risk factors. Regional trade agreements often, if not always, increase the availability of processed food.[16] As urban expectations and experiences migrate back to the countryside, the risk factor profile for NCDs begins to imitate the urban patterns.

3 Costs of non-communicable diseases

We are indebted to the World Economic Forum and investigators at the Harvard School of Public Health for a thoughtful compilation of cost data for these diseases.[8] The data are based on recent cost assessments and are projected forward to 2025, and they include lost opportunity costs. The fiscal burden is grim. In aggregate, the cumulative cost of 5 NCDs (including mental illness) to 2025 is US$46.8 trillion, with the annual cost in the final year, 2025, anticipated to be in excess of US$7T (**Table 1**, overleaf).

Excluding high-income countries and the contribution of mental illness, lower- and middle-income countries are facing an NCD bill of US$14T for diabetes, heart disease, chronic lung disease, and cancer over a 15-year period, of which nearly US$8T is due to diabetes and heart disease, the most diet-sensitive of these diseases.

The fiscal burden of HIV/AIDS and acute communicable diseases is expected to fall rapidly. Control mechanisms, vaccine initiatives, and infrastructure are improving, and are becoming more and more affordable at the same time. The community-based interventions are well understood and are

more and more broadly applied. None of this can be said for NCD prevention, and as we have pointed out in Section 2 and will highlight in Section 5, the drivers of these diseases are less well controlled. Much of the burden relates to diet-responsive drivers of social behavior and diet-specific risk factors.

The more advanced the country – i.e., the greater its wealth – the higher the burden will be. Although high-income countries currently bear the biggest economic burden of NCDs, this burden is shifting to low/middle-income countries, which are expected to assume an ever larger share as their economies and populations grow. One can look at these data and conclude that the poorest countries will be spared. However, the number of countries in the least wealthy category – low-income countries by WHO categorization – took up 58% of the wealth pie chart in 1990, but this had fallen to 11% in 2010.[9] In essence, all countries except failed states are rapidly developing, accumulating wealth, and becoming subject to the same societal pressures that have traditionally fostered a receptive milieu for non-communicable diseases

Table 1 | **Economic burden of NCDs, 2011–2030 (trillions of US$ 2010)**

Country income group	Diabetes	CVD	Chronic Respiratory Diseases	Cancer	Mental illness*	Total
High	0.9	8.5	1.6	5.4	9.0	25.5
Upper middle	0.6	4.8	2.2	2.3	5.1	14.9
Lower-middle	0.2	2.0	0.9	0.5	1.9	5.5
Low	0.0	0.3	0.1	0.1	0.3	0.9
LMIC	**0.8**	**7.1**	**3.2**	**2.9**	**7.3**	**21.3**
World	**1.7**	**15.6**	**4.8**	**8.3**	**16.3**	**46.7**

*The numbers for mental illness were obtained by relating the economic burden of all other diseases to their associated numbers of DALYs. Then the burden for mental illness was projected using the relative size of the corresponding DALY numbers to all the other conditions.

Source: Bloom DE, Cafiero ET, Jané-Llopis E et al. The Global Economic Burden of Non-communicable Diseases. Geneva: World Economic Forum, 2011.

4 Innovative programmatic interventions

As we have demonstrated above, NCDs are embedded in the social, political, economic, and cultural interstices of a society and as such are very difficult to alter or manage with traditional public health measures. Moreover, as most non-communicable diseases have long, asymptomatic incubation periods, the person with precursor risk factors only infrequently sees himself or herself as a patient. However, even if in possession of that understanding, making the time and effort to visit a clinic at the expense of work or child-rearing is all too often beyond the capacity of this insightful patient. Additionally, the clinic is not designed to handle chronic, asymptomatic disease. We explore some of these factors in more detail in Section 5.

Since the routine doctor/nurse/community health worker-patient relationship is infrequently relevant in managing people with asymptomatic, precursor risk factors, and since traditional public health interventions have proved ineffective at a population level, solutions need be found in innovative ways. Before describing four contemporary approaches in different countries, we will describe a model that has worked and stands as a beacon for all who contemplate this dilemma.

Finland transformed the national mortality pattern from the highest CVD mortality in the world to near the mean of Western Europe in 35 years, and did so primarily by modifying the national risk factor profile. What did Finland do, and how did the Finns do it? The environment was unique, but many of the pieces can be transferred; the story offers hope.

Finland is a wealthy, educated, strife-free, homogenous country. Young, primarily male sudden death mortality became a disturbing reality for the population and the government. Being an open society – a crucial factor – there was a bottom-up groundswell of interest in solving the problem, giving enlightened civil servants and political leaders a permit to engage with the problem. One key to success (and one that is rarely discussed) was an economic intervention that was probably essential. Finland has had a salt reduction program (including mandatory high-salt labeling) in place since 1975, and the average salt intake among adult Finns has declined in the interim from 12 g per day to 9.3 g per day in men and 6.8 g per day in women. Also a "healthy choice" label is available for products with lower salt content and improved fat composition. Finland also developed a cold-climate rapeseed and as such could produce its own canola oil while reducing imports of foreign vegetable oil. While the animal fat producers were negatively impacted, the Finnish agricultural sector as a whole was not. Economic considerations are never far from any healthcare intervention, and this salient agricultural development was an important factor in Finland's success story.

Sesame Street in Bogota, Colombia

It is well established that health behaviors initiated in childhood, particularly those related to diet, frequently extend into adulthood. In an elegant and carefully constructed study, investigators in Bogota, Columbia designed a series of interventions to influence the dietary patterns of preschool children 3–5 years of age.[10] The investigation included health messages embedded in Sesame Street (a popular TV program), posters, video games, and songs. Teachers and parents were engaged. At 36 months, the intervention group of children showed a significant improvement in markers of a healthy life style. A much larger study involving a broad cross-section of the region is under way.

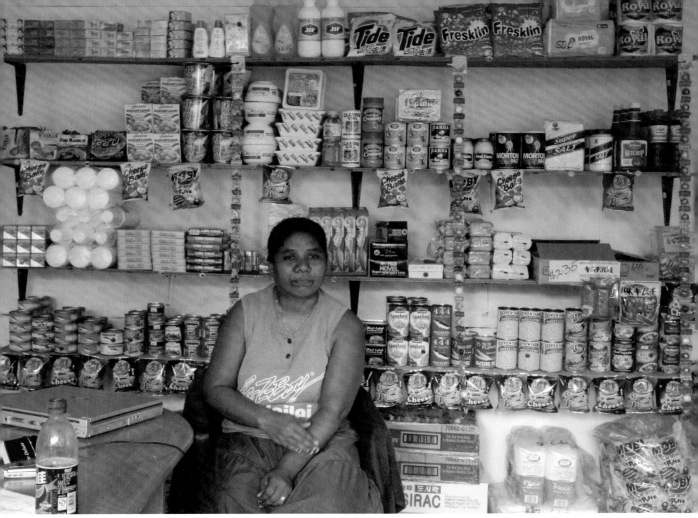

A store owner in Pohnpei, Federated States of Micronesia. Note the predominance of processeed foods on the shelves.
Source: Sight and Life.

Mass media programs have been carried out with probable success in Ethiopia, Cambodia and India, but all the studies conducted had methodological flaws. A large randomized radio-based saturation program is currently under way in Burkina Faso with high hopes for a positive outcome.[11] These studies, all of which require government buy-in, point to a future in which public health aims to improve children's access to better nutrition.

Agita São Paulo

The rapid increase in obesity in Latin America in general, and specifically in the catchment area of São Paulo, Brazil, caught the attention of the leaders of multiple societal actors. Global data indicate that 31% of people do not meet minimal levels of physical activity and that the attributable mortality rate of inadequate physical activity is 6–10%. The public health leadership realized that a series of partnerships engaging nearly all aspects of society would be essential to effectively promote physical activity in the 40 million people of greater Sao Paulo.[12] The goal was not to make everyone a runner, but to move as many people as possible up one stage in their physical activity level: the

sedentary became walkers; occasional walkers became regular walkers; regular walkers became programmed brisk walkers, etc. In addition to enlisting the support of the global academic community, the leadership engaged multiple partners from non-governmental organizations, industry, media, and multiple government ministries. A strategic decision was to encourage partnerships without requiring financial support or buy-in. This emerged voluntarily. For example, partners such as the metropolitan transport company, the Truck Drivers Radio Station, and the State Secretariat of Environment were all able to design programs for specific constituencies. From 2002–2008, sedentarism declined by about 70% in the state of São Paulo. The World Bank estimated that the program represented a saving of US$310 million a year at cost orders of magnitude less than this. There are now many similar programs around the world – Agita Mundo and Physical Activity Networks of the Americas, for example. Another innovative approach – new and as yet unvalidated as this book goes to press, and US based, but worthy of mention here – is "The Way to Wellville",[13] a national challenge founded by angel investor Esther Dyson. The Way to

Wellville involves five US communities and aims to make significant, visible and lasting improvement in respect of five measures of health and economic vitality over the course of five years. It is hoped that this will permit the mapping of new paths that will enable for entire communities to make changes that result in healthier people and places.

Traditional diet in South Korea

South Korea participated in the nutritional transition, and did so very rapidly. Obesity increased by nearly 40% between 1990 and 2010. However, the Koreans have been spared the usual ravages of this transition. Given the normal limitations on the attribution of causation, one key social phenomenon stands out. School lunches are universally available in South Korea, and while initially inexpensive, were quickly offered at zero cost to the student. From the late 1990s onward, the nutritional guidelines were to preserve the traditional Korean diet, consisting essentially of vegetables, *kimchi*, and lean meats with a variety of grains, fruits, and beans. Salt, oil, and fat were not to be "overused." In a 2010 survey, 50% of South Koreans followed this traditional diet, 10% a "Western" style diet (down from 35% in 1998), and 40% a "new diet" which is similar to a Mediterranean diet.[14] This deliberate program of extolling the national tradition is presumably a major reason why the obesity epidemic has been muted in South Korea. Both government policy entities and key non-governmental organizations participated in this effort. It's not just that the diet was healthy – which was an important message – but that it was a traditional *Korean* diet that seemingly resonated with the population. Initiated with a universal school lunch program that extolled respect and appreciation of a national tradition to be revered, a nutritional pattern was established that has served the country well.

Social network targeting

While open societies allow the dispersal of ideas, fashions, and aspirations, guiding this dispersal is not a traditional component of the public health armamentarium. Social network targeting is a new and innovative concept that targets influential members of a social group with the message and allows natural community dynamics to create the widespread dispersal necessary to influence behavior. Identification of "influential" subsets is neither obvious nor straightforward and occupies a substantial part of the inaugural research effort. The work of Christakis and his colleagues has demonstrated the potential of this approach in isolated, poor, rural communities in Honduras.[15]

The methodology will require more widespread application before it can be unconditionally endorsed, but the initial studies offer great promise.

Commonalities

These five innovations have much in common: they all include multiple partners from multiple societal sectors, one of which is the government. Each program worked hard to define core goals that all participants could accept. They all included children in their formative years, although Agita São Paulo and social network programming directed their appeal to everyone, and they all had modest budgets supported by a variety of partners.

There is one other key attribute that is common to all these studies: all possess a large and important bottom-up structure. These interventions were not created by fiat; they emerged from an engaged discussion with the participants, or their parents, who then gave the support essential for carrying out the intervention. The central ingredient in Colombia, Brazil, South Korea, and Honduras was an open society. All of these attributes existed in Finland, which in this light does not now seem so remote, and nor do its results seem so categorically unattainable in less wealthy and more troubled lands.

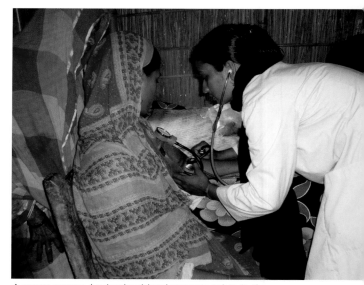

A young woman having her blood pressure taken in the People's Republic of Bangledesh. Source: JiVitA/Sight and Life.

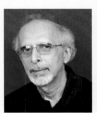

Chittaranjan S Yajnik

Director, Diabetes Unit, King Edward Memorial Hospital Research Centre (KEM-HRC), Maharashtra, India

The Rise of Non-Communicable Diseases (NCDs) in India

There is an unprecedented epidemic of non-communicable diseases (NCDs) in India. There were an estimated 69 million people with diabetes in 2013, and 77 million with pre-diabetes. Thus, India is regarded as one of the world's capitals of diabetes. Prevalence of coronary artery disease (CAD) is similarly high. NCDs contribute to 60% of all deaths and an estimated loss of 20 million productive life years annually.[16]

The epidemic is usually ascribed to rapid transition due to socioeconomic development. However, this is only a precipitating factor. Epidemiology of diabetes is somewhat different in Indians, who develop diabetes and CAD at a younger age and at a lower level of obesity (BMI) compared with Europeans. The rate of progression from normal glucose tolerance to pre-diabetes, and from pre-diabetes to diabetes, is faster in Indians compared with other populations; the rate at which long-term complications occur may also be faster.

These facts suggest a higher susceptibility to NCDs compared with Europeans. This could be genetic, but there is only scanty information on this. On the other hand, the heightened susceptibility can be partly ascribed to the "thin-fat" phenotype (higher body fat percent at lower BMI), which reflects in higher insulin resistance and a lower "disposition index" (B-cell function). This phenotype originates *in utero*, and is influenced by mother's small size, poor nutrition (protein and micronutrient deficiencies) and gestational hyperglycemia. Indian babies are among the smallest in the world, and low birth weight is an independent risk factor for future diabetes, coronary artery disease and related disorders. Dietary deficiency and imbalance of nutrients which

regulate 1-C metabolism (vitamin B_{12}, folate and others) and maternal hyperglycemia are common amongst adolescents and pregnant women in India and have been linked with an increased risk of diabetes in the offspring. This is thought to operate through epigenetic programming, and results of trials to improve adolescent nutrition so as to reduce susceptibility in the offspring are awaited.

NCDs place a huge burden on the economy and could hamper the nation's development in coming decades. Indian diabetes prevention trials have demonstrated a reduction in progression from pre-diabetes to diabetes by simple lifestyle adjustment or a small dose of metformin. Mobile telephonic messages have also been used to promote lifestyle changes. These efforts could help curtail the escalating epidemic. India could lead the way in the "primordial" (intergenerational) prevention of the NCD epidemic.

Further reading

WHO, Burden of NCDs and their risk factors in India (Excerpted from Global Status Report on NCDs, 2014) http://www.searo.who.int/india/topics/non-communicable_diseases/ncd_situation_global_report_ncds_2014.pdf?ua=1.

International Diabetes Federation. Diabetes Atlas, 7th edition, 2015.

Yajnik CS. The insulin resistance epidemic in India: fetal origins, later lifestyle, or both? Nutr Rev 2001; 59: 1–9.

Yajnik CS, Fall CH, Coyaji KJ et al. Neonatal anthropometry: the thin-fat Indian baby. The Pune Maternal Nutrition Study. Int J Obes Relat Metab Disord. 2003 Feb;27(2):173–80.

Ramachandran A, Snehalatha C, Mary S et al. The Indian Diabetes Prevention Programme shows that lifestyle modification and metformin prevent type 2 diabetes in Asian Indian subjects with impaired glucose tolerance (IDPP-1). Diabetologia 2006;49:289–97.

Yajnik CS, Transmission of obesity-adiposity and related disorders from the mother to the baby. Ann Nutr Metab. 2014;64 Suppl 1:8–17.

5 Challenges

The epidemiological transition to chronic, progressive, debilitating diseases was identified decades ago and has been well documented everywhere. Were it an easy problem to confront and manage, this would have been done already. There are many challenges – challenges beyond the cultural and demographic obstacles that we and others have identified. Two seem of particular relevance to nutrition-based up-stream drivers.

The first is the difficulty of engaging asymptomatic people, i.e., people who do not view themselves, or their children, as being patients or having an illness. The second is the absence of engagement in policy by the public health establishment. Achieving cost reductions or cost-effectiveness by reducing the prevalence of behavioral risk factors is only demonstrable in the long term, and the fiscal impact cannot be anticipated or budgeted for at the onset of the intervention. Other than tobacco in past generations, public health plays little role in generating or shaping public policy as it relates to health. Reacting to policy established by others is always a catch-up game, and is rarely successful.

Both in the developed and in the developing world, medical clinics are designed to treat and manage sick people. They function more like an emergency room in the United States. People go there when they or their children are sick, are in pain, or develop frightening symptoms. No-one shows up to have their blood pressure checked; no-one gives up a half day or full day in the fields or caring for the children to find out if their blood sugar level is well controlled; no-one closes the shop to get a blood draw for their annual cholesterol or glucose check, or for a mammogram. These are major barriers in the advanced, well-insured economies in which out-of-pocket expenses are eliminated; they are nearly insurmountable elsewhere. Population-based healthcare will have to go to the individual; the

asymptomatic person will not go to healthcare. This barely recognized reality has yet to be converted to a widespread set of healthcare delivery policies. However, there are many innovative programs being developed, such as those that utilize mobile phones with an ever-increasing number of new technological apps for modifying nutrition or physical activity behaviors, and those that engage community health workers as the bridge to care. These approaches need to be more widely incorporated in the public health community and curriculum.

Public health needs to develop a capacity and willingness to participate in the generation and shaping of public policy that influences health. The opportunity of addressing the modifiable risk factors (such as diet) of NCDs by public policy, involving multiple public-private partners, is an exciting challenge. When the relationship between policy and health is obvious, such as the promotion of universal healthcare, public health does play a role. When subtlety is required, public health is nowhere to be found. The cautionary tale of the Trans Pacific Partnership Agreement – a trade agreement between 12 countries of the Pacific Rim, concluded on October 5, 2015 after five years of negotiations – needs to be incorporated into the public health conscience. The American public health community missed this entirely and yet it posed a huge threat to global health.[17] Agricultural subsidies are another policy area where public health has been absent, only belatedly attempting to influence aspects of its impact, such as limits or taxes on sugary beverages,[18] but not engaging in the generation of the policy itself. While it is encouraging to see now an engagement with climate change, extractive industries, chemical products such as insecticides and pollutants, and television advertising to children,[19] public health needs a much more vigorous and vigilant engagement with public policy.

Our personal view

Henry Greenberg and Richard J Deckelbaum

The planet is now in the era of the "Double Burden of Nutrition," whereby over 1 billion people are hungry and undernourished while over 2 billion are overweight or obese. Coupled with the Double Burden are the adverse effects of global warming and climate change, which lead to unexpected increases in disasters such as floods and drought. These events increase the frequency of non-seasonal, as well as seasonal, hunger and starvation. In addition to affecting many adults and children, starvation during pregnancy can lead to increases the incidence of infants with low birth weight – which in turn is a risk factor for increased risk of cardiovascular disease and other NCDs in adulthood.

There is growing evidence that severe undernutrition in pregnancy and infancy, as well as overnutrition during these periods, can have epigenetic effects which will adversely affect adult outcomes. Thus, as we have described in this chapter, while cardiovascular disease and other NCDs are "taking over" in low- and middle-income countries, investments in their prevention and treatment are only a small fraction of what is currently directed towards the more classical forms of undernutrition, e.g., maternal and child malnutrition and infectious diseases.

There are many open questions relating to the root causes of cardiovascular disease and other NCDs in developed countries. Are the root causes different in the South than in the North? Clearly, there must be much more investment in research as well as in prevention and treatment programs relating to cardiovascular disease in less developed populations.

With the decreasing contribution of infectious disease and undernutrition, we are seeing increases in life expectancies in many lower- and middle-income countries. Thus we can these NCDs to place an increasing burden on human health and economic systems in the coming decades. We need to consider the costs of *not investing in the fight against NCDs* in the 21st century. As we move into the next period of the SDGs, we should ask ourselves whether enough is invested in the attempt to counter NCDs to have the necessary impact on sustainable development.

References

1   Moran A, Roth GA, Narula J et al, Eds. The global burden of cardiovascular diseases. Global Heart 2014;9:1–91.

2   Ibid.

3   Yusuf S, Hawken S, Ôunpuu S et al. Effect of potentially modifiable risk factors associated with myocardial infarction in 52 countries (the INTERHEART study): case-control study. Lancet 2004; 364: 937–52.

4   World Health Organization. Health in 2015: from MDGs, Millennium Development Goals to SDGs, Sustainable Development Goals. WHO. 2015.

5   UNFPA. "UN State of the World Population". 2014.

6   Allender S et al. Quantification of urbanization in relation to chronic diseases in developing countries: a systematic review. Urban Health 2008;85(6):938–51.

7   Moran A, Roth GA, Narula J et al, Eds. The global burden of cardiovascular diseases. Global Heart 2014;9:1–91.

8   World Economic Forum and World Health Organization. From Burden to Best Buy: Reducing the economic impact of non-communicable diseases in low and middle income countries. 2011; www.who.int/nmh/publications/best_buys_summary. Accessed 14 September 2015.

9   Jamison DT et al. Global health 2035: a world converging within a generation. Salud Publica Mex 2015;57:444–467.

10 Cespedes J, Briceno G, Farkouh ME et al. Promotion of cardiovascular health in preschool children: 36-month cohort follow-up. Am J Med 2013 126;12:1122–6.

11 Head R, Murray J, Sarrassat S et al. Can mass media interventions reduce child mortality? Lancet 2015;386:97–99.

12 Matsudo V. The role of partnerships in promoting physical activity: the experience of Agita São Paulo. Health and Place 2012;18:121–2.

13 http://www.hiccup.co.

14 Yoon J, Kwon SK, Shim JE. Present status and issues of school nutrition programs in Korea. Asia Pac J Clin Nutr 2012;21:128–33.

15 Kim DA, Hwong AR, Stafford D et al. Social network targeting to maximize population behavior change: a cluster randomized controlled trial. Lancet 2015;386:145–53.

16 WHO, Burden of NCDs and their risk factors in India (Excerpted from Global Status Report on NCDs, 2014) http://www.searo.who.int/india/topics/non-communicable_diseases/ncd_situation_global_report_ncds_2014.pdf?ua=1.

17 Greenberg H, Shaiu S. The vulnerability of being ill-informed: the Trans-Pacific Partnership Agreement and global public health. J Pub Health 2014;36:355–357.

18 Moodie, R, Stuckler, D, Monteiro, C et al. Profits and pandemics: prevention of harmful effects of tobacco, alcohol, and ultraprocesssed food and drink industries. Lancet 2013;381:670–79.

19 Mozaffarian D, Afshin A, Benowitz NL et al. Population approaches to improve diet, physical activity, and smoking habits. A scientific statement from the American Heart Association. Circulation 2012;126-1514–1563.

Further reading

Obesity Series 1–6. Lancet 2015;385:2400, 2410, 2422,2510, 2521,& 2534.

Physical Activity Series 1–5. Lancet 2012;380: 247,258.272,282,&294.

Frenk J,Chen L, Bhutta ZA et al. Health professionals for a new century: transforming education to strengthen health systems in an interdependent world. Lancet 2010;376:1923.

Marmot, M. Social determinants of health inequalities. Lancet 2005;365:1099–1104.

"Except the vine, there is no plant which bears a fruit of as great importance as the olive."

Pliny the Elder (AD 23–AD 79), *Roman author, naturalist, and natural philosopher, and military commander of the early Roman Empire*

Key messages

- The Mediterranean diet offers a range of potential health benefits, reducing susceptibility to cardiovascular disease (CVD) and supporting the prevention and/or treatment of a variety of non-communicable diseases (NCDs).

- The Mediterranean diet is a convenience phrase: not all inhabitants of the Mediterranean nowadays consume this type of diet on a regular basis.

- The benefits of the Mediterranean diet were first attested in the "Seven Countries Study" (SCS) an epidemiological longitudinal study directed by the American scientist Ancel Keys during the 1950s.

- The traditional Mediterranean diet (typical of the Mediterranean countries 50 years ago, but not now) is characterized by regular use of olive oil and high consumption of vegetables, fruits and nuts, legumes, and unprocessed cereals; low consumption of meat and meat products; and moderate consumption of dairy products.

- When compared with other "healthy" diets, two elements of the Mediterranean diet are unique: 1) fat intake is allowed, provided that it comes from virgin olive oil, tree nuts and fatty fish, and 2) moderate intake of red wine during meals.

The term "Mediterranean diet"

The concept of the "Mediterranean diet" has enjoyed considerable currency since the 1970s, when research first indicated that a diet low in trans fats and high in polyphenols might reduce susceptibility to cardiovascular disease (CVD). Since that time, the potential health benefits of the Mediterranean diet have been explored in greater detail, revealing additional links between this dietary regimen and the prevention and/or treatment of a variety of non-communicable diseases (NCDs).

The Mediterranean diet is in some senses a convenience phrase: not all inhabitants of the Mediterranean nowadays consume this type of diet on a regular basis, while a diet of this description may be found in certain other parts of the world beyond the strict confines of the Mediterranean itself. It was the typical diet of Crete and other Mediterranean countries 50 years ago, but unfortunately it is no longer so. Nevertheless, the widely attested benefits of this form of diet amply justify the continued use of this term. The Mediterranean diet has been linked to a number of health benefits, including reduced mortality risk and lower incidence of cardiovascular disease. Definitions of the Mediterranean diet vary across some settings, and scores are increasingly being employed to define Mediterranean diet adherence in intervention and epidemiological studies. Some components of the Mediterranean diet overlap with other healthy dietary patterns, whereas other aspects are unique to this particular diet.

Opposite: Some of the key ingredients of the Mediterranean diet, including the "hallmark" ingredient olive oil.

The Seven Countries Study

The traditional Mediterranean diet entered the medical literature following publication in 1970 of the results from the "Seven Countries Study" (SCS) conducted by the legendary Ancel Keys and his colleagues during the 1950s.[1] This epidemiological ecological study was conducted at what today is the University of Minnesota Laboratory of Physiological Hygiene & Exercise Science (LPHES).

Keys's interest in the relationship between diet and CVD was triggered by his observation that well-fed American business executives in the years following World War II had high rates of heart disease, while rates of CVD had declined in Europe, where diets were still heavily restricted in the wake of that conflict. Keys postulated a possible link between cholesterol levels and CVD, and he embarked on a study of the cardiovascular health of businessmen in Minnesota – the first of its kind. Noticing that the population of Southern Italy had the highest levels of centenarians worldwide, Keys explored the possibility that a diet low in animal fat might protect against CVD.

As the world's first ever multi-country epidemiological study at that time, the Seven Countries Study systematically examined the relationships between lifestyle, diet, coronary heart disease and stroke in different populations from different regions of the world. It directed attention to the causes of coronary heart disease and stroke, but also showed that an individual's risk can be changed.

Initiated in 1956, the Seven Countries Study was the first major study to investigate the risk factors for CVD and stroke across cultures and over a long period of time, paying special attention to diet and lifestyle. Ancel Keys was the first researcher to associate the traditional Mediterranean diet with a low risk of coronary heart disease (CHD). However, the design was weak for causal inference, because it used only aggregated, and not individual, data.

Climate, flora and hardship

In purely descriptive terms, the traditional Mediterranean diet is the dietary pattern prevailing among the people of the olive tree-growing areas of the Mediterranean basin before the mid-1960s – that is, before globalization made its influence on lifestyle, including diet. Essential determinants of the traditional Mediterranean diet have been climate, flora and hardship, the latter discouraging import or consumption of expensive (at that time, red) meat.[2]

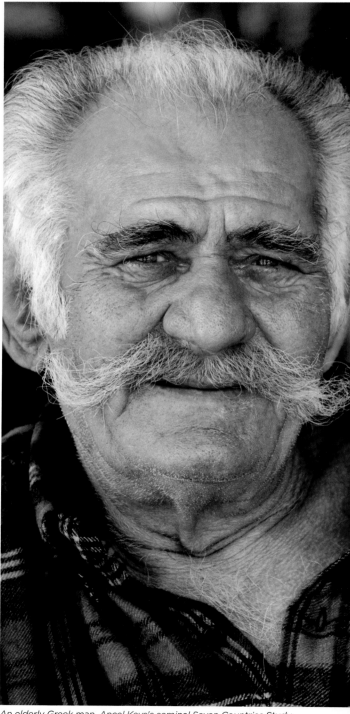

An elderly Greek man. Ancel Keys's seminal Seven Countries Study postulated a link between the Mediterranean diet and longevity.

Health benefits of the Mediterranean diet

The traditional Mediterranean diet is characterized[3] by high consumption of olive oil – its hallmark – and vegetables, fruits and nuts, legumes, and unprocessed cereals; low consumption of meat and meat products; and low consumption of dairy products (with the exception of types of cheese that keep for long periods). Alcohol consumption was common in the traditional Mediterranean diet, but generally in moderation and in the form of wine and, as a rule, during meals – in the spirit of the word "symposium," which is derived from the Ancient Greek *sumposion* and means a drinking party or convivial discussion. Total intake of lipids could be high (around 40% of total energy intake, as in Greece), or moderate (around 30% of total energy intake, as in Italy) but, in all instances, the ratio of the beneficial monounsaturated to the non-beneficial saturated lipids is high, because of the high monounsaturated content of the liberally used olive oil. Finally, levels of fish consumption have in the past been determined by greater or lesser proximity to the sea, but have been moderate overall.

In a somewhat reductionist approach, the traditional Mediterranean diet can be considered as a mainly, but not entirely, plant-based dietary pattern. Of note, olive oil is a plant product (in fact a fruit juice), and so is wine.

The definition of "Mediterranean"

Strictly speaking, the Mediterranean diet as such does not exist. The Mediterranean Sea borders 18 countries that differ markedly in geography, economic status, health, lifestyle and diet. Nevertheless, the term has gained universal currency, on account of the central role played in the study by four Mediterranean regions of the Seven Countries Study: Crete and Corfu in Greece, Dalmatia in Croatia, and Montegiorgio in Italy. In the 1960s, the Greek diet had the highest olive oil content, and was high in fruit; the Dalmatian diet was highest in fish; and the Italian diet was highest in vegetables. In line with their diet, participants from these regions were characterized by low mortality rates from CHD. Climatic conditions conducive to the Mediterranean diet are also found in Chile, California, South Africa, and the west coast of Australia.

On the basis largely of ecological evidence, Ancel Keys concluded that low content of saturated lipids in the Mediterranean diet could explain the low incidence of coronary heart disease in Mediterranean countries, through the reduction of blood cholesterol, a recognized major risk factor for this disease. It should be noted that the distinction between high (HDL) and low (LDL) density lipoprotein cholesterol was not known at that time. Later work, however, has shown that the traditional Mediterranean diet is not simply, or mainly, a cholesterol-lowering diet, but has a range of beneficial health effects on many other parameters associated with heart disease.

Two developments in the early 1990s led to an explosion of interest in the Mediterranean diet. The first of these was the recognition that high intake of carbohydrates, particularly simple carbohydrates, may not be beneficial to health because they constrain the levels of the "good" HDL cholesterol and increase the metabolically undesirable glycemic load. This has shifted interest to innocuous, indeed beneficial, lipids, like those from olive oil.[4] The second development was the operationalization of adherence to the traditional Mediterranean diet through a simple scoring system that has been used in a multitude of analytical studies to evaluate the health effects of adherence to this diet.[5] It should be made clear that, in contrast to scores and diet pyramids developed in order to point to "optimal" diets, the Mediterranean diet score is purely operational of the traditional Mediterranean diet. The fact that this diet has considerable beneficial health effects constitutes a "natural experiment" that investigators try to understand and people benefit from.

Collectively, these studies have indicated convincing inverse associations with overall mortality[6] and with the incidence of coronary heart disease[7] and thrombotic stroke,[8] compelling inverse associations with incidence of cancer overall[9,10] (including, possibly, incidence of breast[11] and colorectal[12] cancer), likely inverse association with the incidence of adult-onset diabetes mellitus[13] and possibly with the incidence of hip fractures and obesity.[14] There have also been randomized trials supporting a beneficial role of the Mediterranean diet on the incidence of cardiovascular events[15] and of survival from CHD.[16]

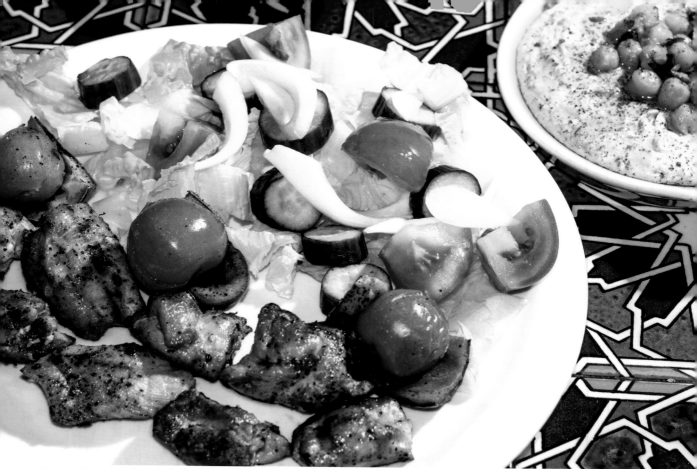

Chicken shish kebab (tavuk şiş *or* şiş tavuk) *with a salad of fresh vegetables and hummus – a typical Mediterranean dish.*

The Mediterranean Dietary Score (MDS)

More recently, the Mediterranean diet has been operationally defined in order to assess its role in analytical epidemiologic studies. The operational definition of "Mediterranean diet" most commonly used is the Mediterranean Dietary Score (MDS) proposed by Trichopoulou et al. in 1995[5,17] and updated thereafter. The MDS is built by assigning a value of 0 or 1 to each of nine components with the use of the sex-specific median as the cut-off. For five beneficial components (vegetables, legumes, fruits & nuts, cereal, and fish), persons whose consumption is below the sex-specific median of the sample are assigned a value of 0, and persons whose consumption is at or above the median are assigned a value of 1. A sixth beneficial component is the ratio of monounsaturated lipids to saturated lipids, in order to reflect the principal role of olive oil consumption in the traditional Mediterranean diet. A value of 1 is assigned to persons whose consumption is at or above the sample-specific median and a value of 0 is assigned to persons who are below the median. For components presumed to be detrimental (all meats, and all dairy products, which are rarely non-fat or low-fat in Mediterranean countries), persons whose consumption is below the median are assigned a value of 1, and persons whose consumption is at or above the median are assigned a value of 0. For alcohol, a value of 1 is assigned to men who consume between 10 and 50 g per day and to women who consume between 5 and 25 g per day. Thus, the total Mediterranean-diet score ranges from 0 (minimal adherence to the traditional Mediterranean diet) to 9 (maximal adherence).[2] The MDS is based on sample medians and, therefore, its score is highly dependent on the specific characteristics of the sample. This fact may represent a limitation for the transferability of results to other samples. An alternative is to build scores according to absolute/normative cut-off points for the consumption of specific food groups (pre-defined servings/day or servings/week). This is the approach followed by the screener which was instrumental in performing the dietary intervention with the Mediterranean diet in the successful PREDIMED trial.[15,18,19]

When compared with other "healthy" diets, two elements of the Mediterranean diet are unique: 1) a high fat intake is allowed provided that it comes from virgin olive oil, tree nuts and fatty fish, and 2) moderate intake of red wine during meals. Other components (fish instead of red meats, abundance of plant-based foods) are common with other "healthy" diets. Alcohol should be included in the definition of the Mediterranean diet. The Mediterranean alcohol drinking pattern seems a key element for reducing total mortality.[20]

The PREDIMED trial[15,19,21]

The PREDIMED trial (*Prevención con Dieta Mediterránea*) was a parallel-group, multicenter, randomized trial.

Background

Observational cohort studies and a secondary prevention trial have shown an inverse association between adherence to the Mediterranean diet and cardiovascular risk. A randomized trial of this diet pattern was conducted for the primary prevention of cardiovascular events.

Methods

In a multicenter trial in Spain, participants who were at high cardiovascular risk, but with no cardiovascular disease at enrollment, were randomly assigned to one of three diets: a Mediterranean diet supplemented with extra-virgin olive oil, a Mediterranean diet supplemented with mixed nuts, or a control diet (advice to reduce dietary fat). Participants received quarterly individual and group educational sessions and, depending on group assignment, free provision of extra-virgin olive oil, mixed nuts, or small nonfood gifts. The primary end-point was the rate of major cardiovascular events (myocardial infarction, stroke, or death from cardiovascular causes). On the basis of the results of an interim analysis, the trial was stopped after a median follow-up of 4.8 years.

Results

A total of 7447 persons were enrolled (age range, 55 to 80 years); 57% were women. The two Mediterranean-diet groups had good adherence to the intervention, according to self-reported intake and biomarker analyses. A primary end-point event occurred in 288 participants. The multivariable-adjusted hazard ratios were 0.70 (95% confidence interval [CI], 0.54 to 0.92) and 0.72 (95% CI, 0.54 to 0.96) for the group assigned to a Mediterranean diet with extra-virgin olive oil (96 events) and the group assigned to a Mediterranean diet with nuts (83 events), respectively, versus the control group (109 events). No diet-related adverse effects were reported.

Conclusions

Among persons at high cardiovascular risk, a Mediterranean diet supplemented with extra-virgin olive oil or nuts reduced the incidence of major cardiovascular events.

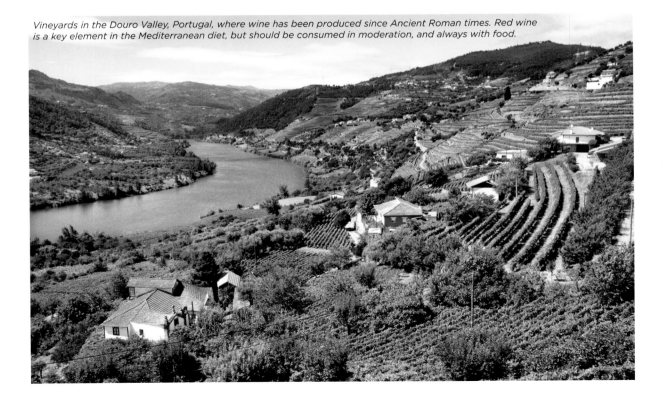

Vineyards in the Douro Valley, Portugal, where wine has been produced since Ancient Roman times. Red wine is a key element in the Mediterranean diet, but should be consumed in moderation, and always with food.

Figure 1 | PREDIMED study design: participants

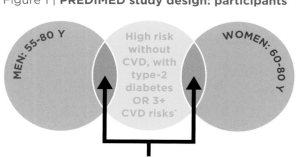

Participants are selected from these groups, then randomly assigned into 1 of 3 interventions:

MeDiet + EVOO
N = 2543

MeDiet + Nuts
N = 2454

Control Diet (low fat)
N = 2450

* 1. Smoking; 2. Hypertension; 3.↑LDL-cholesterol; 4.↓HDL-cholesterol; 5. Overweight/obesity; and 6. Family hisory of early-onset CVD.

KEY:
CVD: Cardiovascular disease
EVOO: Extra-virgin olive oil
HDL: High-density lipoprotein
LDL: Low-density lipoprotein
MeDiet: Mediterranean diet

Source: Ros et al. Adv Nutr. 2014;5:330S–6S

Figure 2 | The PREDIMED 14-point score

Food	Portion	Frequency
Olive oil	≥4 tablespoons	per day
Vegetables	≥2 servings	per day
Fruit	≥3 servings	per day
Red Meat	<1 portion	per day
Butter, margarine	<1 portion	per day
Soda drinks	<1 drink	per day
Wine	≥7 glasses	per week
Legumes	≥3	per week
Fish and seafood	≥3 portions	per week
Cakes, sweets	<3 portions	per week
Nuts	≥3 portions	per week
Poultry > red meats		
Sofrito		

Figure 3 | 14-item score of adherence to the Mediterranean diet

1	Do you use olive oil as the principal source of fat for cooking?	Yes
2	How much olive oil do you consume per day (including that used in frying, salads, meals eaten away from home etc.)?	≥4 tbsp.
3	How many servings of vegetables do you consume per day? (One serving = 200 g, count garnish and side servings as 0.5 portion)	≥2
4	How many pieces of fruit (including freshly squeezed juice) do you consume per day?	≥3
5	How many servings of red meat, hamburger or sausages do you consume per day? (One serving = 100–150 g)	<1
6	How many servings of butter, margarine or cream do you consume per day? (One serving = 12 g)	<1
7	How many carbonated and/or sugar-sweetened beverages do you consume per day?	<1
8	Do you drink wine? How many glasses do you consume per week?	≥7 glasses
9	How many servings of pulses do you consume per week? (One serving is 150 g)	≥3
10	How many servings of fish/seafood do you consume per week? (One serving = 100–150 g fish, 4–5 pieces or 200 g seafood)	≥3
11	How many times do you consume commercial (not homemade) pastry, such as cookies or cakes, per week?	<2
12	How many times do you consume nuts per week? (One serving = 30 g)	≥3
13	Do you prefer to eat chicken, turkey or rabbit instead of beef, pork, hamburgers or sausages?	Yes
14	How many times per week do you consume boiled vegetables, pasta, rice or other dishes with a sauce of tomato, garlic, onion or leeks sautéed in olive oil?	≥2

Source: Martinez-Gonzalez et al. Int J Epidemiol 2012; 41-377–385,doi:10.1093/ije/dyq250

Source: Zazpe et al for the PREDIMED group, J Am Diet Assoc 2008;108:1134–44.

Figure 4 | **PREDIMED – Primary end-point (MI, stroke or CV death)**

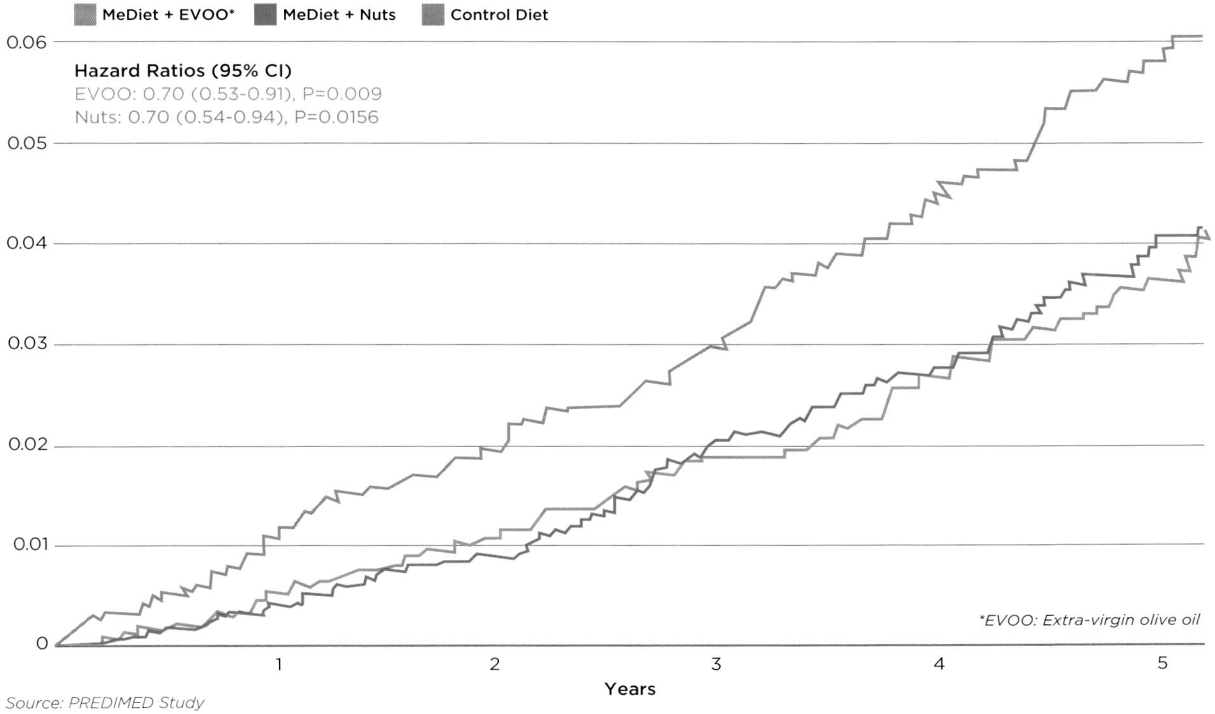
MeDiet + EVOO*
MeDiet + Nuts
Control Diet
Hazard Ratios (95% CI)
EVOO: 0.70 (0.53-0.91), P=0.009
Nuts: 0.70 (0.54-0.94), P=0.0156
0.06
0.05
0.04
0.03
0.02
0.01
0
1
2
3
4
5
Years
*EVOO: Extra-virgin olive oil

Source: PREDIMED Study

High-fat Mediterranean diet does not cause weight gain, study finds

Researchers found that people whose diets were rich in olive oil and nuts lost more weight than those on low-fat regime

Sarah Boseley Health Editor, *The Guardian*, Monday 6 June 2016

The Mediterranean diet, with a high fat content from olive oil and nuts, does not cause people to gain weight, a major study has found.

Fear of fat is misplaced and guidelines that restrict it in our diets are wrong, say the Spanish researchers who have followed more than 7,000 people, some eating 30 g of nuts (≥50% fat) or 50 ml of extra virgin olive oil (100% fat) a day while others were put on a standard low-fat diet. Their research, they say, should put healthy fats – from vegetables, nuts and fish – back on the menu, changing attitudes and the way we eat.

The publication of data on fats and weight loss from the respected Predimed randomized controlled trial, comes in the wake of a furor over a paper published by the UK's National Obesity Forum. The campaigning document attacked Public Health England's guidance on diet, claiming that eating saturated fats including butter and meat would enable people to lose weight. A damning response from Public Health England said this was "irresponsible and misleads the public". Four members of the NOF resigned, saying they did not support publication of the paper.

The fats and the furious: how the row over diet heated up

Latest battle in food wars shows how passionate debate can be and how hard it is to reach any sort of simple truth.

The Mediterranean diet in the Predimed study, however, though high in fats does not include red meat or butter. Participants ate fish, nuts, vegetables, fruits, and whole grains. "It does not include many foods and beverages that have been associated with long-term weight gain, such as fast foods, sweets and desserts, butter, red meat and processed meat, and sugar-sweetened beverages," write the authors in the Lancet Diabetes and Endocrinology journal.

Those who took part were randomly assigned to one of three groups. Some ate an unrestricted-calorie Mediterranean diet with added extra virgin olive oil (they were given 1 liter a week for themselves and their family), while others ate an unrestricted-calorie Mediterranean diet with added nuts – they got 15g of walnuts, 7.5g of almonds, and 7.5g of hazelnuts, with an additional 1kg sachet of mixed nuts every three months to account for family needs, says the paper. The third group were put on a low-fat diet and given small non-food gifts every three months, such as a kitchen clock or spoons.

More than 90% of those who took part, aged between 55 and 80, were obese or overweight. Weight loss was not substantial, but was greatest in the Mediterranean diet with olive oil group – 0.88 kg compared with 0.60 kg on the low-fat diet. All the groups increased their waist measurement, which tends to happen as people age, but the smallest increase was among those eating a Mediterranean diet with added nuts (0.37 cm compared with 1.2 cm in the low-fat group).

The belief that fat is always going to make people fat, because it is calorie-dense, led four decades ago to mass sales in supermarkets of low-fat and fat-free foods. It had the unfortunate effect of contributing to the obesity epidemic, as food manufacturers substituted sugar and other carbohydrates for fat in everything from yoghurts to ready meals.

"More than 40 years of nutritional policy has advocated for a low-fat diet but we're seeing little impact on rising levels of obesity," said lead author Dr Ramon Estruch from the Spanish Biomedical Research Centre in Physiopathology of Obesity and Nutrition, Spain.

"Our study shows that a Mediterranean diet rich in vegetable fats such as olive oil and nuts had little effect on bodyweight or waist circumference compared with people on a low-fat diet. The Mediterranean diet has well-known health benefits and includes healthy fats such as vegetable oils, fish and nuts. Our findings certainly do not imply that unrestricted diets with high levels of unhealthy fats such as butter, processed meat, sweetened beverages, desserts or fast-foods are beneficial."

Obesity is a global concern and puts people at risk of heart disease, cancers, strokes and diabetes. Standard advice on losing weight is to eat a low-fat diet, say the researchers, while health bodies including the World Health Organization recommend fat should make up no more than 30% of our diet.

Mediterranean diet may help stop breast cancer coming back, study says

Out of 199 women asked to eat lots of fruit, vegetables, fish and olive oil in an Italian trial, none suffered recurrence in three years.

"Dietary guidelines should be revised to lay to rest the outdated, arbitrary limits on total fat consumption," writes Prof. Dariush Mozaffarian, from the Friedman School of Nutrition Science & Policy at Tufts University, Boston, US, in a comment piece in the journal.

"Calorie-obsessed caveats and warnings about healthier, higher-fat choices such as nuts, phenolic-rich vegetable oils, yoghurt, and even perhaps cheese, should also be dropped. We must abandon the myth that lower-fat, lower-calorie products lead to less weight gain."

We should be focusing on the quality of our food rather than the calorie content on restaurant menus, and it is paradoxical to ban whole milk but allow sugar-sweetened fat-free milk, he writes.

"The fat content of foods and diets is simply not a useful metric to judge long-term harms or benefits. Energy density and total caloric contents can be similarly misleading. Rather, modern scientific evidence supports an emphasis on eating more calories from fruits, nuts, vegetables, beans, fish, yoghurt, phenolic-rich vegetable oils, and minimally processed whole grains; and fewer calories from highly processed foods rich in starch, sugar, salt, or trans-fat. We ignore this evidence – including these results from the Predimed trial – at our own peril."

Prof Simon Capewell, vice-president for policy of the Faculty of Public Health, said the study and commentary, "provide clear dietary messages; we need to promote a Mediterranean diet with olive oil and nuts, and cut our intake of meat, animal fats, refined carbohydrates, junk food and sugary drinks."

Source: http://www.theguardian.com/society/2016/jun/06/ high-fat-mediterranean-diet-does-not-cause-weight-gain-study-finds (slightly adapted).

What we can learn from the Mediterranean diet: 10 healthy foods to eat

Writing in The Huffington Post of May 7, 2013 and referencing a study involving thousands of participants in Spain, Lisa R Young, adjunct professor of nutrition in the Department of Nutrition, Food Studies, and Public Health at New York University (NYU), provided culinary tips on 10 foods found in the Mediterranean diet.

Olive oil

Olive oil is rich in monounsaturated fat, a heart-healthy fat. Diets high in olive oil have been associated with heart health. Olive oil is also rich in antioxidants, including vitamin E, polyphenols, and beta-carotene, which protects blood vessels and other components of the heart. Drizzle olive oil on salads and steamed veggies.

Tuna

Tuna is high in omega-3 fatty acids, which have been associated with a decrease in the risk of heart disease risk. The American Heart Association recommends including at least two servings of fish per week, in particular fatty fish. Tuna is affordable, convenient, and versatile. Throw canned tuna on a salad, make a sandwich, or toss it into whole wheat pasta, to get a dose of omega-3s.

Broccoli

Broccoli is one of my favorite vegetables as it is chock-full of the antioxidant vitamins A and C. It is a cruciferous vegetable, and part of the Brassica family, rich in phytochemicals, known to have antioxidant properties. Sautee broccoli in olive oil and enjoy it as a side dish.

Raspberries

Raspberries contain the antioxidant quercetin – which contains anti-inflammatory benefits – and the phenolic compound ellagic acid, and can help fight heart disease. And even more good news: One cup contains only 105 calories and eight grams of fiber. Throw some berries into your morning yogurt for added color, taste, and a healthy dose of antioxidants and fiber.

Walnuts

Walnuts not only taste great, but also provide a heart-healthy addition to your diet. Rich in the plant-based omega-3 fatty acid alpha-linolenic acid, and antioxidants such as selenium, walnuts also provide protein, fiber, magnesium and phosphorus to the diet. Include a handful of walnuts as a snack or toss a few tablespoons into your breakfast oatmeal.

Chickpeas

Chickpeas are a great option for plant protein and fiber. They also contain magnesium, manganese, iron, and folate. Hummus, which is made from chickpeas, is delicious with crackers or veggies as an afternoon snack.

Brown Rice

Brown rice contains fiber, B-vitamins, and a variety of minerals. It contains nearly three times the fiber of white rice. A half-cup serving of cooked brown rice contains nearly a half-day's worth of the mineral manganese, which works with various enzymes facilitating body processes. Brown rice makes a healthy grain to include with a meal of grilled fish and vegetables.

Spinach

Spinach contains the minerals iron and potassium, as well as vitamins A, C, K, and the B-vitamin folate. Spinach also contains flavonoids, which have antioxidant properties that may prevent against certain diseases. For good news, it is available year-round, offering a readily available source of many vitamins and minerals. A fresh spinach salad drizzled with olive oil and a handful of nuts tastes great.

Blueberries

Blueberries are rich in antioxidants and vitamin C and may benefit heart health. Consuming blueberries may keep your blood pressure in check. Blueberries contain anthocyanins, which may reduce the risk of heart disease in women. Snack on these tasty berries or throw a handful into your cereal.

Lentils

Lentils contain soluble fiber, protein, and complex carbohydrates and also offer the added benefit of being a significant source of iron. Consider beginning your lunch or dinner with a hot lentil soup.

Source: http://www.theguardian.com/society/2016/jun/06/ high-fat-mediterranean-diet-does-not-cause-weight-gain- study-finds (slightly adapted).

129 ## Mediterranean mackerel with a tomato panzanella salad

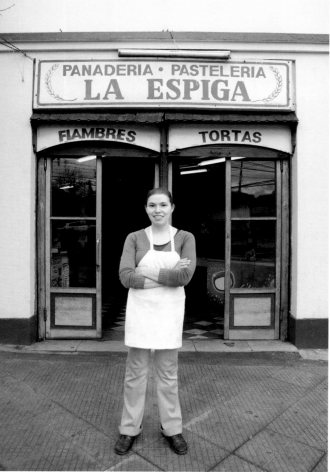

Restaurant owner in Santiago de Chile. The Mediterranean diet is found in parts of the world that have a Mediterranean climate, and not just in the Mediterranean itself.

This example of a Mediterranean dish comes from the Irish food writer, food photographer and television presenter Donal Skehan.

Ingredients

- 4 Mackerel Fillets
- Juice of 1 lemon
- 4 cloves of garlic, finely chopped
- 1/2 loaf of ciabatta bread, torn into rough pieces
- 1/2 red onion, finely sliced
- 1 punnet of cherry tomatoes
- 150 g of sunblush tomatoes
- 1 tablespoon of red wine vinegar
- 3 tablespoons of extra virgin olive oil
- 1 clove of garlic, finely chopped
- A good handful of basil, roughly chopped

Directions

Preheat the oven to 200°C/ 400°F/ Gas mark 5.

Toss the bread chunks in a roasting tray with a generous drizzle of olive oil. Season with sea salt and ground black pepper and then place in the oven until toasted and golden for about 8 minutes. Give them a good toss half way through. Remove from the oven and feed with an extra drizzle of olive oil.

In a large bowl whisk together the red wine vinegar, olive oil, and garlic and then add in the onion, cherry tomatoes, sunblushed tomatoes, toasted bread and toss until completely coated. Leave to soak up the dressing while you get on with the fish.

Place the mackerel on a plate and drizzle with a little olive oil, a squeeze of lemon juice and sprinkle with sea salt, black pepper and a little of the dried oregano.

Heat a large frying pan over a medium high heat and then place the mackerel flesh side down for 2–3 minutes, then turn over squeeze over lemon juice and cook for further 2–3 minutes.

Serve straight away alongside the panzanella salad.

Source: *http://www.donalskehan.com/recipes/crispy-med-mackerel-with-a-tomato-panzanella-salad, accessed June 7, 2016.*

Our personal view

J Alfredo Martinez and Miguel Martinez-Gonzalez

No other dietary pattern has such a strong evidential base as the Mediterranean diet to support its benefits on cardiovascular disease, diabetes and other major chronic diseases.

Current Mediterranean-based trials (PREDIMED, RESMENA, etc.) did not use energy restriction (total energy intake was ad libitum), but in the context of the current epidemics of obesity and diabetes, a combined energy-MedDiet would probably be the most sensible option to combat obesity, type 2 diabetes and cardiovascular disease (the huge epidemics of the 21st century).

The issue for weight loss is not the fat, but rather the *subtypes* of fat (butter and meat contain saturated fats, whereas olive oil contains monounsaturated, and nuts mainly polyunsaturated, fats). The PREDIMED trial showed that the intervention with the Mediterranean diet and olive oil or nuts did not of itself lead to substantial weight loss (the diet was not restricted in calories).

The PREDIMED 14-item assessment tool does not take long to complete, but it can validly appraise adherence to MedDiet, predict future incidence of CVD, and be used for immediate feedback in intervention studies.

The consumption of foods belonging to the Mediterranean dietary patterns has been associated with multiple healthy outcomes and improved life quality, including anti-inflammatory response, immunocompetence, oxidative stress balance, etc., with benefits on homeostatic functions as well as on disease prevention and body wellness related to excessive adiposity and glucose regulation.

References

1   Keys A, Arvanis C, Blackburn H: Seven Countries: A Multivariate Analysis of Death and Coronary Heart Disease. Cambridge, MA: Harvard University Press; 1980:381.

2   Trichopoulou A, Lagiou P: Healthy traditional Mediterranean diet: an expression of culture, history, and lifestyle. Nutr Rev 1997, 55:383–389.

3   Trichopoulou A, Costacou T, Bamia C, Trichopoulos D: Adherence to a Mediterranean diet and survival in a Greek population. N Engl J Med 2003, 348:2599–2608.

4   Sacks FM, Willett WW: More on chewing the fat. The good fat and the good cholesterol. N Engl J Med 1991, 325:1740–1742.

5   Trichopoulou A, Kouris-Blazos A, Wahlqvist ML et al: Diet and overall survival in elderly people. BMJ 1995, 311:1457–1460.

6   Trichopoulou A, Orfanos P, Norat T et al: Modified Mediterranean diet and survival: EPIC-elderly prospective cohort study. BMJ 2005, 330:991.

7   Martinez-Gonzalez MA, Bes-Rastrollo M. Dietary patterns, Mediterranean diet, and cardiovascular disease. Curr Opin Lipidol 2014, 25:20-6.

8   Misirli G, Benetou V, Lagiou P et al: Relation of the traditional Mediterranean diet to cerebrovascular disease in a Mediterranean population. Am J Epidemiol 2012, 176:1185–1192.

9   Benetou V, Trichopoulou A, Orfanos P et al: Conformity to traditional Mediterranean diet and cancer incidence: the Greek EPIC cohort. Br J Cancer 2008, 99:191–195.

10 Couto E, Boffetta P, Lagiou P et al: Mediterranean dietary pattern and cancer risk in the EPIC cohort. Br J Cancer 2011, 104:1493–1499.

11 Toledo E, Salas-Salvadó J, Donat-Vargas C, et al. Mediterranean Diet and Invasive Breast Cancer Risk Among Women at High Cardiovascular Risk in the PREDIMED Trial: A Randomized Clinical Trial. JAMA Intern Med 2015, 175:1752–60.

12 Bamia C, Lagiou P, Buckland G et al: Mediterranean diet and colorectal cancer risk: results from a European cohort. Eur J Epidemiol 2013, 28:317–328.

13 Rossi M, Turati F, Lagiou P et al: Mediterranean diet and glycaemic load in relation to incidence of type 2 diabetes: results from the Greek cohort of the population-based European Prospective Investigation into Cancer and Nutrition (EPIC). Diabetologia 2013, 56:2405–2413.

14 Benetou V, Orfanos P, Pettersson-Kymmer U et al: Mediterranean diet and incidence of hip fractures in a European cohort. Osteoporos Int 2013, 24:1587–1598.

15 Estruch R, Ros E, Salas-Salvado J et al, PREDIMED Study Investigators: Primary prevention of cardiovascular disease with a Mediterranean diet. N Engl J Med 2013, 368:1279–1290.

16 de Lorgeril M, Renaud S, Mamelle N ET AL: Mediterranean alpha-linolenic acid-rich diet in secondary prevention of coronary heart disease. Lancet 1994, 343:1454–1459.

17 Bach A, Serra-Majem L, Carrasco JL et al: The use of indexes evaluating the adherence to the Mediterranean diet in epidemiological studies: a review. Public Health Nutr 2006, 9:132–146.

18 Schroder H, Fito M, Estruch R et al: A short screener is valid for assessing Mediterranean diet adherence among older Spanish men and women. J Nutr 2011, 141:1140–1145.

19 Martinez-Gonzalez MA, Corella D, Salas-Salvado J et al: Cohort profile: design and methods of the PREDIMED study. Int J Epidemiol 2012, 41:377–385.

20 Trichopoulou A, Bamia C, Trichopoulos D: Anatomy of health effects of Mediterranean diet: Greek EPIC prospective cohort study. BMJ 2009, 338:b2337.

21 Martinez-González MA, Salas-Salvadó J, Estruch R, et al. Benefits of the Mediterranean Diet: Insights From the PREDIMED Study. Prog Cardiovasc Dis 2015, 58:50-60.

131

Further reading

Anand SS, Hawkes C, de Souza RJ et al. Food Consumption and its Impact on Cardiovascular Disease: Importance of Solutions Focused on the Globalized Food System: A Report From the Workshop Convened by the World Heart Federation. J Am Coll Cardiol. 2015 Oct 6;66(14):1590-614.

Martinez-Gonzalez MA, Bes-Rastrollo M, Serra-Majem L et al Mediterranean food pattern and the primary prevention of chronic disease: recent developments. Nutr Rev. 2009 May;67 Suppl 1:S111–6.

Trichopoulou A, Martínez-González MA, Tong TY et al. Definitions and potential health benefits of the Mediterranean diet: views from experts around the world. BMC Med. 2014;12:112.Willett WC, Stampfer MJ. Current evidence on healthy eating. Annu Rev Public Health. 2013;34:77–95.

García-Calzón S, Martínez-González MA, Razquin C et al. Mediterranean diet and telomere length in high cardiovascular risk subjects from the PREDIMED-NAVARRA study. Clin Nutr. 2016 Apr 1. pii: S0261-5614(16)30001-2.

San-Cristobal R, Navas-Carretero S, Celis-Morales C et al. Analysis of Dietary Pattern Impact on Weight Status for Personalised Nutrition through On-Line Advice: The Food4Me Spanish Cohort. Nutrients. 2015 Nov 17;7(11):9523-37.

Marques-Rocha JL, Milagro FI, Mansego ML et al. Expression of inflammation-related miRNAs in white blood cells from subjects with metabolic syndrome after 8 wk of following a Mediterranean diet-based weight loss program. Nutrition. 2016 Jan;32(1):48-55.

Babio N, Becerra-Tomás N, Martínez-González MAet al; PREDIMED Investigators. Consumption of Yogurt, Low-Fat Milk, and Other Low-Fat Dairy Products Is Associated with Lower Risk of Metabolic Syndrome Incidence in an Elderly Mediterranean Population. J Nutr. 2015 Oct;145(10):2308-16.

Garcia-Arellano A, Ramallal R, Ruiz-Canela M et al; Predimed Investigators. Dietary Inflammatory Index and Incidence of Cardiovascular Disease in the PREDIMED Study. Nutrients. 2015 May 29;7(6):4124-38.

Eguaras S, Toledo E, Buil-Cosiales P et al; PREDIMED Investigators. Does the Mediterranean diet counteract the adverse effects of abdominal adiposity? Nutr Metab Cardiovasc Dis. 2015 Jun;25(6):569-74.

Bondia-Pons I, Martinez JA, de la Iglesia R et al. Effects of short- and long-term Mediterranean-based dietary treatment on plasma LC-QTOF/MS metabolic profiling of subjects with metabolic syndrome features: The Metabolic Syndrome Reduction in Navarra (RESMENA) randomized controlled trial. Mol Nutr Food Res. 2015 Apr;59(4):711-28.

Sayón-Orea C, Santiago S, Cuervo M et al. Adherence to Mediterranean dietary pattern and menopausal symptoms in relation to overweight/obesity in Spanish perimenopausal and postmenopausal women. Menopause. 2015 Jul;22(7):750-7.

Lopez-Legarrea P, Fuller NR, Zulet MA et al. The influence of Mediterranean, carbohydrate and high protein diets on gut microbiota composition in the treatment of obesity and associated inflammatory state. Asia Pac J Clin Nutr. 2014;23(3):360-8.

Livingstone KM, Celis-Morales C, Navas-Carretero S et al. Food4Me Study. Effect of an Internet-based, personalized nutrition randomized trial on dietary changes associated with the Mediterranean diet: the Food4Me Study. Am J Clin Nutr. 2016 Jun 29. pii: ajcn129049. [Epub ahead of print] PubMed PMID: 27357094.

Santiago S, Sayón-Orea C, Babio N et al. Yogurt consumption and abdominal obesity reversion in the PREDIMED study. Nutr Metab Cardiovasc Dis. 2016 Jun;26(6):468–75.

Approaches to Fixing Broken Food Systems

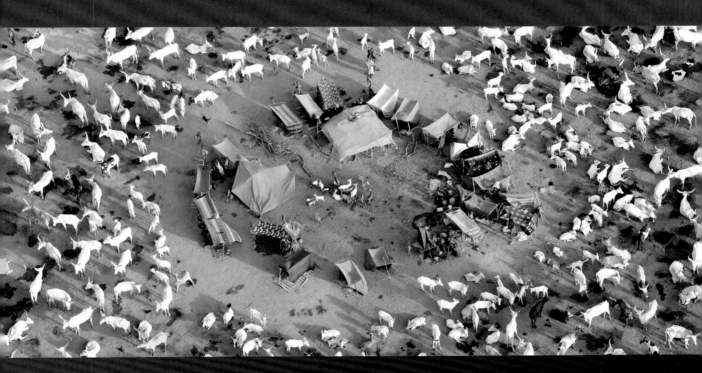

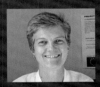

Robyn Alders

Faculty of Veterinary Science, University of Sydney, Australia. *Healthy Food Systems: Nutrition, Diversity, Safety* Project Node, Charles Perkins Centre and Marie Bashir Institute (CPC/MBI), University of Sydney, Australia. Kyeema Foundation, Brisbane, Australia and Maputo, Mozambique

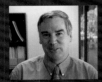

Mike Nunn

Healthy Food Systems: Nutrition, Diversity, Safety Project Node, Charles Perkins Centre and Marie Bashir Institute (CPC/MBI), University of Sydney, Australian. Australian Centre for International Agricultural Research, Canberra

Brigitte Bagnol

Faculty of Veterinary Science, University of Sydney, Australia. *Healthy Food Systems: Nutrition, Diversity, Safety* Project Node, Charles Perkins Centre and Marie Bashir Institute (CPC/MBI), University of Sydney, Australia. Kyeema Foundation, Brisbane, Australia and Maputo, Mozambique. The University of the Witwatersrand, Department of Anthropology, Johannesburg, South Africa

Julian Cribb

Healthy Food Systems: Nutrition, Diversity, Safety Project Node, Charles Perkins Centre and Marie Bashir Institute (CPC/MBI), University of Sydney, Australia. Julian Cribb and Associates, Canberra, Australia

Richard Kock

Healthy Food Systems: Nutrition, Diversity, Safety Project Node, Charles Perkins Centre and Marie Bashir Institute (CPC/MBI), University of Sydney, Australian. Royal Veterinary College, University of London, Hatfield, Hertfordshire, United Kingdom

Jonathan Rushton

Healthy Food Systems: Nutrition, Diversity, Safety Project Node, Charles Perkins Centre and Marie Bashir Institute (CPC/MBI), University of Sydney, Australian. Royal Veterinary College, University of London, Hatfield, Hertfordshire, United Kingdom

"Sustainable development is not an option! It is the only path that allows all of humanity to share a decent life on this, one planet. Rio+20 gives our generation the opportunity to choose this path."

Sha Zukang, *Secretary-General of the Rio+20 Conference.*

Key messages

Everyone on the planet belongs to one and the same ecosystem. Improved health and wellbeing for the world's population and better stewardship of the planet can be achieved by recognizing that adequate food and nutrition is a human right. Improved nutrition can be achieved by a variety of means. These include:

- Developing diets that are appropriate for individuals, taking into account a variety of factors such as age, gender and health status

- Increasing food resilience and counteracting losses in biodiversity by promoting greater diversity in the range of foods produced and consumed

- Playing a more active part in curating efficient nutrient cycling (or ecological recycling)

- Taking steps to maintain soil fertility, soil availability and the quality of fresh water.

- Encouraging the development of nutrition-sensitive value chains that deliver food with a high "cost-to-nutritional-benefit" ratio and support sustainable agricultural and distribution systems and

- Defining and facilitating sustainable and ethical food systems that contribute to human and planetary health – among the greatest challenges facing our world today.

1. Sustainable agricultural production

Between 2016 and 2050, when the world's population is expected to reach 9 billion, it will be necessary to produce as much food as has been produced during the entire existence of *Homo sapiens* on this planet. However, the "broken" food systems of today have delivered the double burden of under- and overnutrition, led to the degradation of ecosystems, and reduced many farming families to impoverishment. Within these broken systems, women carry most of the burden of health problems and poverty. Focusing on good nutrition and the encouragement of efficient nutrient cycles can help strengthen interrelationships between farmers, traders, regulators, consumers and policy-makers, thereby helping to generate policies that support food systems that deliver sustainable, diverse and nutritious diets that meet the individual needs of everyone and limit negative agricultural effects on biodiversity and ecosystem health. This chapter reviews the West's historical and physiological relationship with food, examines how food is produced and distributed, and presents a range of options for making food choices that are beneficial both for people and for the planet.

Previous page: Pastoralism shows a remarkable degree of integration between livestock and people, with the welfare of animals on a par with that of the people. The nutritional benefits to the South Sudan tribes are obvious, with some of the most physically well developed human beings on the planet.

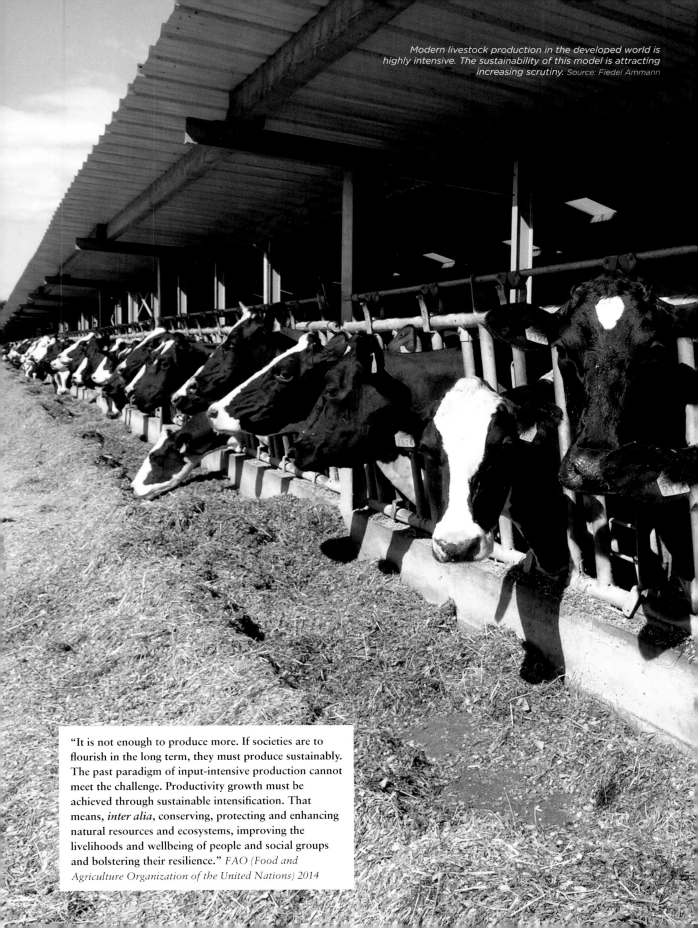

Modern livestock production in the developed world is highly intensive. The sustainability of this model is attracting increasing scrutiny. *Source: Fiedel Ammann*

"It is not enough to produce more. If societies are to flourish in the long term, they must produce sustainably. The past paradigm of input-intensive production cannot meet the challenge. Productivity growth must be achieved through sustainable intensification. That means, *inter alia*, conserving, protecting and enhancing natural resources and ecosystems, improving the livelihoods and wellbeing of people and social groups and bolstering their resilience." *FAO (Food and Agriculture Organization of the United Nations) 2014*

135 Figure 1 | **Global dietary patterns among men and women in 187 countries in 2010**
Values represent degrees of adherence to each dietary pattern, ranging from 0 (least healthy) to 100 (most healthy).

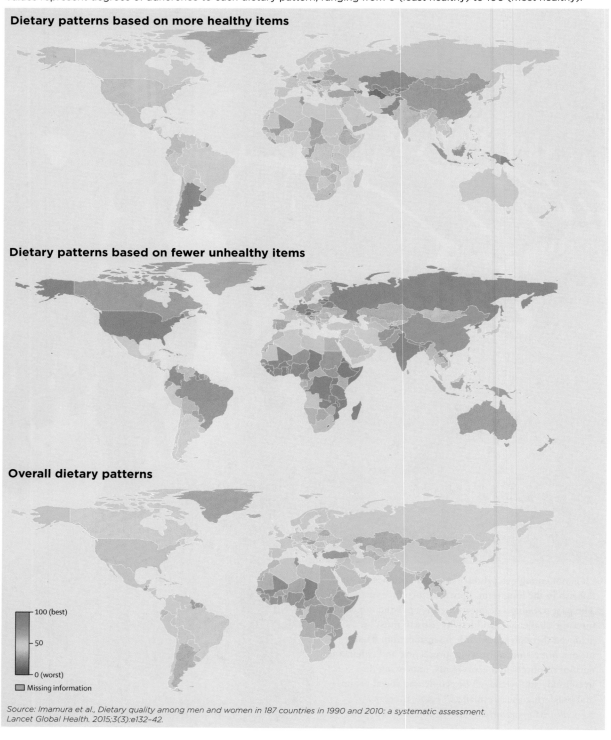

Dietary patterns based on more healthy items

Dietary patterns based on fewer unhealthy items

Overall dietary patterns

100 (best)

50

0 (worst)

☐ Missing information

Source: Imamura et al., Dietary quality among men and women in 187 countries in 1990 and 2010: a systematic assessment. Lancet Global Health. 2015;3(3):e132–42.

2. Sustainable food systems for the planet's dominant consumers

From earliest times, wildlife played a critical role in the emergence of earth's most successful mammalian species, *Homo sapiens*. Exploitation of wild food by means of hunting and gathering was the main evolutionary driver for humans, and was critical to our species' nutritional health and growth.

During the past 10,000 years, the growing human population has been sustained through the domestication of various animal species and the development of agricultural systems, as well as by continued hunting, fishing and foraging. These activities have been industrialized to a greater or lesser extent in the effort to achieve increased food output per unit of scarce resource. The economic logic of this approach has major unintended consequences for the planet, particularly where key resources are inappropriately valued. Many aspects of the world's current food systems are less than optimal. In some instances, they are actually undermining the long-term food security and health of the Earth and the people who inhabit it.

A number of new trends give cause for concern, including an unprecedented loss of biodiversity; a concomitant reduction in ecological resilience; the emergence of newly identified infectious and non-infectious diseases; and a rise in global ambient temperatures that is triggering climate change worldwide. Directly and indirectly, human behavior has driven many of these trends, underpinned by widespread adoption of Western-style consumption patterns across vast swathes of the globe. People have become increasingly estranged from nature through a process of

urbanization that has disconnected urban communities from rural food-producing communities, and wealthier nations have become disassociated from poorer nations, despite the fact that the world is more interconnected than ever by modern technology and transport. Food producers have lost their link to both food consumers and the environment, and vital, nutrient-rich foods have been debased to the status of commodities to be traded in a highly volatile global marketplace.

Gender inequities are also increasingly being recognized as a major social determinant of health and nutritional outcomes, as well as of reduced agricultural production. For example, in Sub-Saharan Africa women play a dominant role in the production, processing and post-harvest storage of food, yet only 15% of landholders are women. Women are also less likely than men to benefit from credit and extension services.

Figure 2 | **The yield gap between men and women farmers and its impact on productivity**

The yield gap between male and female farmers averages about **20–30%**, mostly due to differences in resource use.

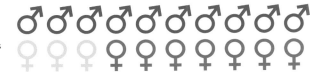

Given equal access to resources as men, women would achieve the same yield levels, boosting total agricultural output in developing countries by **2.5–4%.**

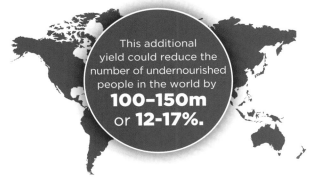

This additional yield could reduce the number of undernourished people in the world by **100–150m** or **12–17%.**

Source: FAO (2014).

Human beings are the world's dominant consumers.
Source: Mike Bloem

Food systems include the governance and economics of food production, the sustainability of food production, the degree to which food is wasted, and the way in which food production affects the natural environment. In many countries, governments in the 20th century largely ceded responsibility for food production, marketing and distribution to industry-funded organizations that set standards for food production, processing, distribution and sale. The Sustainable Development Goals are reinstating a role for nation-states in food system governance with an emphasis on nutrition and bio-sensitive food systems (i.e., food systems that deliver nutritious food in harmony with natural ecosystems), human security systems (i.e., systems that protect the vital core of all human lives in ways that enhance human freedoms and human fulfillment), and

social protection systems (i.e., systems that protect and help those who are poor and vulnerable, such as children, women, older people, those living with disabilities, the displaced, the unemployed, and the sick). Yet there are still conflicts within these goals with respect to the environment and biodiversity conservation.

The production and distribution of food has become increasingly complex as our food systems have evolved from the distribution of seasonally available natural produce to the manufacture of a wide range of highly processed foods. With globalized food systems, few countries are self-sufficient in food supply, creating complex interdependencies, with some benefits to diversity on the plate, but also with increasing social, economic and political tensions.

Figure 3 | **Examples of Australian, Tanzanian and US households and where their food originates**

USA

117.5m households with an average of: **2.6** people.
Of pet owners: **37%** own a **dog**
29% own a **cat**.
The **blue** area estimates the origin of American food.

Australia

7.8m households with an average of: **2.6** people.
Of pet owners: **39%** own a **dog**
29% own a **cat**.
The **yellow** area estimates the origin of Australian food.

Tanzania

9.16m households with an average of: **4.9** people.
Of pet owners: **14%** own a **dog**
<1% own a **cat**.
The **pink** area estimates the origin of Tanzanian food.

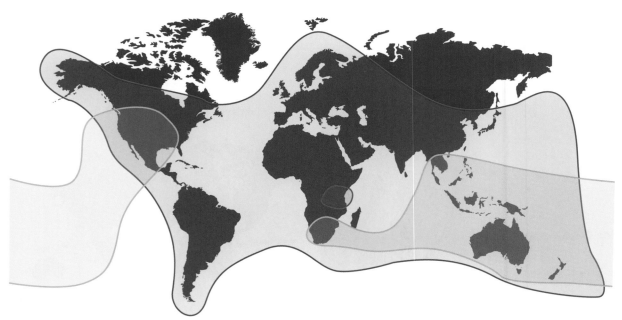

Source: Household data compiled from Animal Health Alliance (2013), American Veterinary Medicine Association (2012), Australian Bureau of Statistics (2006), Knobel et al. (2008), UNFPA (2013), US Government (2009). Graphical representation of origin of food estimated by authors.

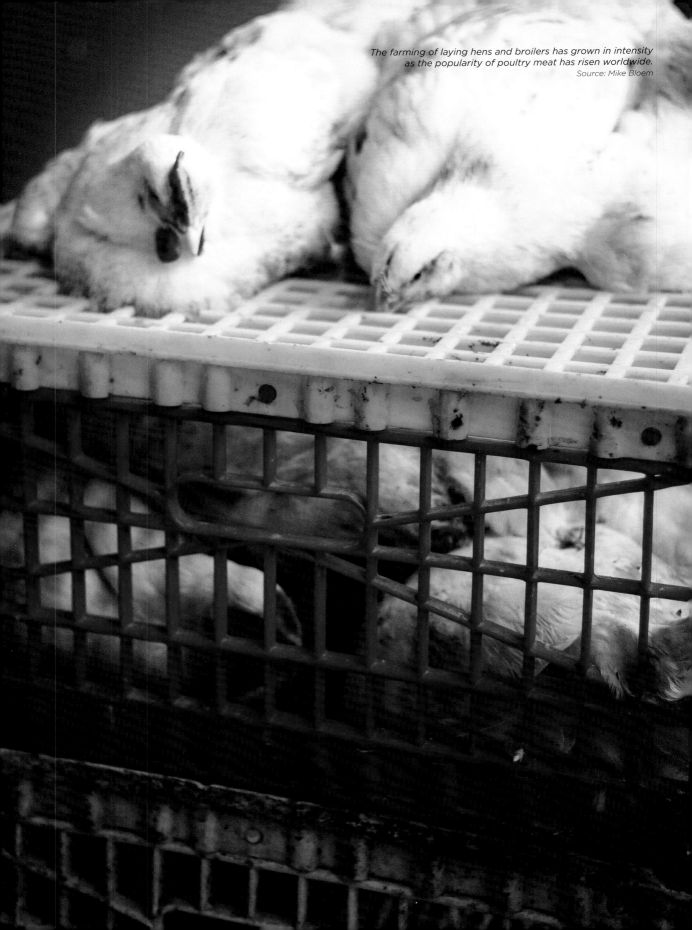

The farming of laying hens and broilers has grown in intensity as the popularity of poultry meat has risen worldwide.
Source: Mike Bloem

3. Building resilient and sustainable food systems

Sustainable food systems require a collective effort to tailor and integrate food production, processing, distribution, consumption and waste management to enhance environmental, economic and social health in harmony with agro-ecological systems.

There is no single, universally appropriate food system. Across the globe, food production and distribution continue to occur in myriad ways. There is no such as thing as global best practice, as all food systems can have unexpected and unintended consequences. These consequences need to be better documented and critically evaluated to help pave the way to more sustainable and environmentally supportive approaches. Hunting and gathering still exist in some parts of the world, and non-cultivated foods and the landscapes that produce them require greater attention. Such attention is critical if these landscapes are to maintain their capacity to renew themselves and the food sources they provide. At the same time, extensive or intensive production systems that harness science and technology may be the most appropriate means of making food available in most parts of the world. Full accounting of the comparative ecological costs of different systems is needed to identify best practice to inform effective nutrition policy. This should take into consideration a range of factors, including soil and water security, subsidies (e.g., fuel, fertilizer, pesticides, herbicides), and nutrition-sensitive value chains.

Currently few examples exist of truly sustainable food systems that can support the world's growing human population. Food underpins population growth, and the sustainability of the world's food systems in their present state depends on a slowing of the current rate at which the global population is growing. If such a deceleration is to occur, it will require the education and empowerment of women in particular, and the adoption of a range of family planning measures.

Nevertheless, there are examples of sustainable food systems in the making. These include agro-ecologically managed smallholder farms such as Latin America's *Campesino* and Zapotec agroforestry movements that increase yields, conserve soil, water, and biodiversity, and capture carbon to cool the planet. Kenya's Northern Rangeland Trust is another example where ecosystem services benefit communities through a balanced livestock wildlife-integrated livelihood system providing sustainable food, natural resources and tourism income. Urban farms from Havana to Bangkok are steadily increasing food production and improving the livelihoods of local communities. Community-supported agriculture groups around the world are providing fresh, healthy food for members – and, at the same time, a living income for local family farmers. Hundreds of municipal Food Policy Councils and Food Hubs are implementing citizen-driven initiatives to keep the "food dollar" in the community, where it can be recycled up to five times, thereby creating jobs and stimulating local economic development.

Healthy land that can support healthy people requires sustained fertility and functionality of the soil as the basis for biomass production. Soil is the "foundation" for the ecosystem, and healthy soil ensures renewable water reserves and captures carbon. In the case of Europe, for instance, eight main threats to the quality of soil have been identified, including erosion; local and diffuse contamination; loss of organic matter; loss of biodiversity; compaction and other physical soil deterioration; salinization; floods and landslides; and sealing. These threats are endangering soil quality, and cause millions of euros of damage every year. They remain a continued source of concern, and require urgent attention.

Maintaining natural and agricultural biodiversity will help absorb the inevitable shocks that occur in the more industrialized food-producing systems, which are the main systems now serving the world's population. This involves, among other interventions, identifying genetic traits that endow resistance to changing environmental conditions and encouraging natural and sustainable methods of harvesting.

The world's future food systems will need to:

- Provide full socio-ecological accounting;

- Assess nutrient recycling;

- Minimize or eliminate all forms of tillage;

- Prevent over-grazing and over-cropping;

- Make systems equitable, sustainable (environmentally, socially and economically), and resilient to weather variability;

- Provide diets suitable to the life stages and cuisines of sub-populations;

- Be based on ecosystem, human and animal health needs dictating production levels using sustainable systems adapted to local agro-ecological zones; and

- Contribute to evidence- and rights-based policy-making on access to food for humans and animals (domestic as well as wild).

4. Three key food production challenges

To deliver sustainable food systems, three challenges need to be overcome. These are to:

- move from "commodity-based" to "gender- and nutrition-sensitive" value chains;

- improve food processing, packaging and distribution; and

- ensure food safety.

4.1. Maximizing the nutritional benefits of food production: gender- and nutrition-sensitive, sustainable and safe value chains

Despite increases in agricultural production during the past two decades, undernutrition in children has not diminished significantly in many developing countries, and obesity is now causing significant mortality and morbidity across the globe. High levels of undernutrition, lack of education among adult women (who frequently play a key role in agricultural production), and gender inequality have also shown a strong positive association with the prevalence of child undernutrition. Accessing sufficient calories is important, but calories alone are not sufficient to deliver optimal nutrition; the proper balance of micronutrients is also essential for both short- and long-term health. This has become clear as obesity and related health concerns are becoming significant issues in individuals and communities adopting Western diets worldwide.

4.2. Food processing: the freshness challenge

In almost all cases, fresh food is more nutritious than highly processed food.[1] In many parts of the world, household food preservation techniques such as salting and pickling traditionally enabled generation upon generation to store perishable food for consumption during lean periods. However, the processed products now manufactured and distributed by large corporations are reducing the diversity of many people's diets. Processed food products are also transported and presented for sale in packaging such as plastics that consume significant natural resources and present major issues in terms of disposal or recycling and chemical leaching. Delivering sustainable, safe, nutritious, and fresh food to people across the globe is central to the concept of good nutrition in one world. In many parts of the world, meals prepared using locally sourced natural ingredients tend to have a higher nutritional value than their highly processed counterparts,[2] and sourcing produce locally supports small farmers and other traders in the food chain. In the future, food processing will promote food safety while also incorporating agents, such as phytase, that reduce anti-nutritional factors. Phytase inhibits the action of phytates (which occur naturally to varying levels in most plants) that bind minerals in the gut before they are absorbed and reduce the digestibility of starches, proteins, and fats. Phytase can be promoted by fermentation and soaking of grains and these processes could be incorporated into food processing to enhance phytases naturally occurring in the raw material as well as the addition of isolated phytases. Interestingly, phytase is already a common ingredient in feed produced for intensive chicken and pig production.

Figure 4 | **Comparing "gender- and nutrition-sensitive" with "commodity-based, processed" food value chains**

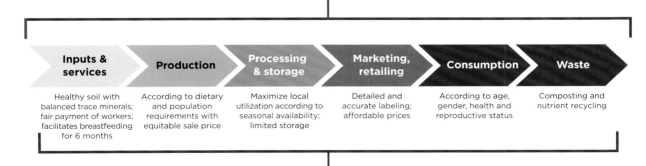

Commodity-based, processed food value chain

Inputs & services	Production	Processing & storage	Marketing, retailing	Consumption	Waste
Healthy soil with balanced trace minerals; fair payment of workers; facilitates breastfeeding for 6 months	According to dietary and population requirements with equitable sale price	Maximize local utilization according to seasonal availability; limited storage	Detailed and accurate labeling; affordable prices	According to age, gender, health and reproductive status	Composting and nutrient recycling

Nutrition- and gender-sensitive value chain

Source: Alders (2016).

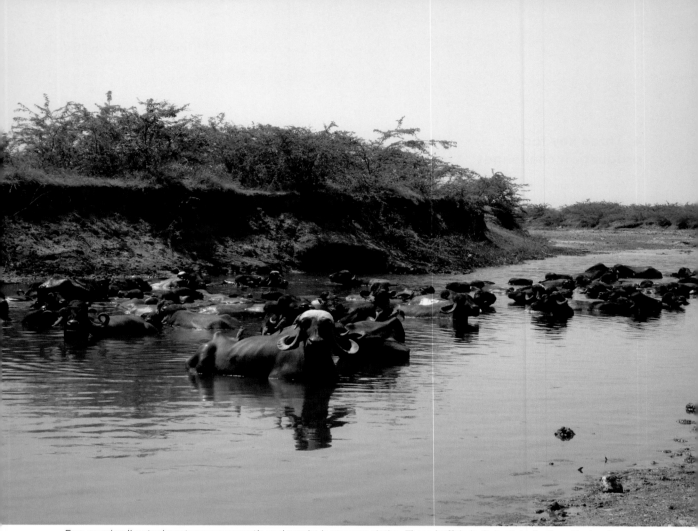

Free-ranging livestock systems vary greatly and persist in many societies. These buffalo in Gujarat, India show the level of welfare and good health of these traditional free-ranging systems, which also contribute to healthy human diets.
Source: R Kock

4.3. Food packaging and distribution

One concept that would be of global benefit is the development of a simple rating system that can be used in the labeling of any food, to enable consumers to gauge the sustainability of the system that produced it and the healthiness of the food itself. At present there is no easy way for consumers, governments and donors to know any of this – although in many countries they can now choose their refrigerator, washing machine and car according to various detailed criteria. The anomaly is striking. It would be extremely beneficial to develop an algorithm that encompasses the main elements of sustainability – such as virtual water content, energy content, soil erosiveness index, and carbon emissions – and combines this with consumer health and ethical ratings.

To deliver fresh and safe food to our tables, value chains need to be shorter, and a greater proportion of the world's burgeoning population needs to start taking responsibility for producing at least some of its own food and for consuming diets that are optimal in terms of nutrient content and environmental impact. This involves, among other things, ensuring that nutrients are recycled. Although not practicable for inhabitants of cities, deserts and icy regions, for instance, it would generally be beneficial for as great a percentage of the world's food as possible to be both produced and consumed locally.

4.4. Food safety

Food safety is both vital and complex, and food safety standards usually touch all parts of the value chain. Much of the focus of food safety has hitherto been on pathogens and toxins. The intensification of livestock industries has contributed to the emergence and spread of zoonotic pathogens such as highly pathogenic avian influenza and campylobacteriosis, which are found in in highly intensive commercial poultry production, for example. Increasing attention is also being given to the potential risks associated with modern processing and packaging procedures, the use of additives in processed foods and beverages, and the use of genetically modified foods.

Figure 5 | **Components of intensive commercial poultry production and the unintended consequences observed since the 1990s**

These consequences include the global spread of highly pathogenic avian influenza (HPAI), very virulent Newcastle disease (ND) and very virulent Marek's disease.

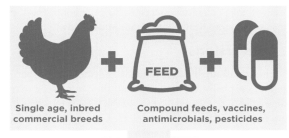

Single age, inbred commercial breeds + Compound feeds, vaccines, antimicrobials, pesticides

NEWCASTLE DISEASE, SALMONELLA, CAMPYLOBACTER, HPAI & MAREK'S
Resulting in
Amplification of pathogen in aberrant host (HPAI), biocontaminants (i.e., Salmonella, Campylobacter) and new resistant & virulent strains

HEALTH RISK

Source: Adapted from Kock, Fornace, Alders and Wallace (2012).

One popular way of preserving certain foods has for centuries been by using high concentrations of sugar. It is now clear that the inclusion of high levels of sugar in processed foods is a significant contributor to the obesogenic environment that is evident in many parts of the world today. Similarly, the traditional use of high levels of salt for the preservation of certain types of food is now recognized as being associated with elevated blood pressure and an increased likelihood of stroke and cardiovascular disease.

There is a need for new ways of preparing and preserving foods that make them attractive to consumers while at the same time reducing the levels of sugar and artificial additives that they contain. Refrigeration as a strategy for preserving food should also be revisited, as it does not always help reduce food wastage at the household level and can delay the disposal of food that has passed its use-by-date. Refrigeration has also helped distance urban consumers from the seasons and the agricultural calendar, reduced diversity by encouraging the cultivation of cool-tolerant fruits and vegetables, increased energy usage, and driven up greenhouse gas emissions (in cases where hydrofluorocarbons are used as refrigerants).

Innovative methods of preserving food include:

- **Biopreservation/fermentation**
  The use of non-toxic and beneficial microorganisms to ferment foods and beverages is an ancient form of biopreservation that was, and still is, used to produce foods such as beer, wine, vinegar, bread, yoghurt, and cheese. This technique can be applied in small and large food preservation ventures.

- **Solar drying**
  Based on thermal energy storage materials, exposure to sunlight is quite effective for continuously drying agricultural and food products at a steady state in the temperature range of 40 °C to 60 °C.

- **Ultra-high pressure hydrostatic processing**
  This approach eschews the use of chemical additives, and there is no contamination, or alteration to the taste of, the food. The bacteria in the food remain intact but are deactivated due to the pressure-induced dismantlement of their nucleic acid. With the exception of some fruits and vegetables, most foods can be pressurized without losing their structure.

- **Packaging innovations**
  Modified atmosphere packaging (e.g., the insertion of a mixture of gases usually including oxygen, carbon dioxide and nitrogen) retards microbial spoilage and provides fresh and safe products.

Conducting effective risk assessments has its challenges, not least because the negative effect of a particular factor may not become apparent for many years. For example, it has been known for a long time that cooking food eliminates many pathogens. However, cooking will not necessarily eliminate all the pathogens that may be present in food. In the case of "mad cow" disease (bovine spongiform encephalopathy, or BSE), for example, agents such as prions are not inactivated by normal cooking, and their presence in the food chain can take years to become evident (e.g., the occurrence of a case of BSE in the United Kingdom in 2015, more than 25 years after rigorous controls were put in place following identification of the first cases in 1986).[3]

143

4.5. Food retailing

In a relatively short time, food retailing has become a massive global industry through which high-quality food finds its way to those who can pay for it, wherever they are in the world. With modern technology, even highly perishable goods such as fruit and vegetables can be transported vast distances. However, the existence of this technology, and of the accompanying infrastructure, has not delivered high-quality food to all communities. For example, in remote communities in Australia, food retailers generally offer highly processed foods, containing high amounts of salt and sugar, to younger generations who are no longer able to recognize and make use of wild foods (even in places these foods have not been decimated by feral animals or invasive weeds). Similarly in many cities, communities of low socioeconomic status also depend heavily on cheap highly processed foods. In both situations, "food deserts" are having long-term negative effects on society in relation to physical wellbeing, immunity, obesity, cognition, and mental status. The impact of poor nutrition on such communities contributes to the poverty cycle, with children failing to reach their genetic potential and the cumulative negative effects across generations leading to a vicious spiral of increasing health problems and diminishing productivity.

Our changing relationship with companion animals

At the same time, in more affluent societies, where dogs and cats are in some cases considered members of the family even though they make no contribution to hunting or pest control, the content of pet food has changed due to the anthropomorphic manner in which pets are viewed by their owners. The dietary requirements of companion animals are increasingly met by commercial pet foods of growing sophistication or by specially prepared home food. The irony whereby specially formulated diets are marketed to pet owners while human beings subsist on an inadequate, industrially produced diet is profound.

The new status of companion animals was highlighted in the aftermath of Hurricane Katrina in 2006, when many people refused to be evacuated unless they could take their pets with them. In response, the United States Congress passed the *Pets Evacuation and Transportation Standards (PETS) Act* with near-unanimous support. This act compels rescue agencies to save pets as well as people during natural disasters and marks a legal turning-point in our relationship with companion animals, as it made them members of society. A number of food companies now run parallel operations that cater for humans and their companion animals. This association is important both in terms of how

and to whom food is distributed and in terms of nutrition security and food safety. Currently, market forces tend to dictate food distribution systems. With increasing human population and decreasing land for food production, those tasked with ensuring good nutrition in urban and rural areas will take increased interest in how nutritious food is allocated geographically and within households.

5. Conclusions

To achieve sustainable food systems and adequately nourish 9 billion people by 2050, a paradigm shift is required that will involve action at every stage of the food value chain from the level of the soil to the plate. Such a shift would see sustainable, nutritious and safe food produced and delivered worldwide with minimal waste, with consumers being intimately reconnected to the environment and to the origins of the food that they consume.

Our personal view
Robyn Alders, Mike Nunn, Brigitte Bagnol, Julian Cribb, Richard Kock & Jonathan Rushton

The authors of this chapter have a vision for the future whereby we all actively engage in designing our diets according to our individual needs in harmony with agro-ecological and political systems. Food has to regain center stage in our attention.

In this vision, people will seek out nutritious fresh food that meets our dietary requirements in an efficient and tasty manner. They will actively engage with food systems and nutrient cycles by having a kitchen garden or a herb pot on a window-sill, and chickens in the backyard. They will purchase food that has been grown sustainably by farmers who are treated ethically and paid a fair price for their labour, enabling them to tend their land and sustain natural ecosystems.

Research suggests that this approach is good not only for our planetary ecosystems but also for our internal systems, because it allows "good" microbes to flourish in our microbiome, leading to improved physical and mental wellbeing, increased capacity to make a positive contribution to society, and reduced dependence on medicines and healthcare systems.

Further reading

Alders RG. (2016) Peak food and our quest for an ethical and ecologically sustainable human diet. Proceedings of the Australian Poultry Science Symposium, Sydney, Australia, Volume 27, pp.9-13.

Bennegouch N, and Hassane M. (2010) Mooriben: l'expérience d'un système de services intégrés au bénéfice des paysans nigériens. Dynamiques paysannes, 23, p. 8.

CBO and WHO. (2015) Connecting Global Priorities: Biodiversity and Human Health. The Communication of the European Commission (COM(2006)231 final), entitled Towards a Thematic Strategy for Soil Protection.

Fanzo J, Hunter D, Borelli T and Mattei F, eds. (2013) Diversifying Food and Diets: using agricultural biodiversity to improve nutrition and health. Earthscan, London and New York. Available online at: http://www.bioversityinternational.org/uploads/tx_news/Diversifying_food_and_diets_1688_02.pdf.

FAO (2014) The female face of farming. Available online at: http://www.fao.org/gender/infographic/en/

Frank Fenner Foundation. Biosensitivity: comprehensive and indispensable. Frank Fenner Foundation, Canberra. Available online at: http://www.natsoc.org.au/our-projects/biosensitivefutures/part-3-our-place-in-nature/3.-biosensitivity-a-vision.

Holt-Giménez E. (2015) First Sustainable Food Systems for Security and Nutrition: the need for social movements. World Food Day USA. Available: http://www.worldfooddayusa.org/sustainable_food_systems_for_security_and_nutrition_the_need_for_social_movements.

Imamura F, Micha R, Khatibzadeh S Fahimi S, Shi P, Powles J and Mozaffarian D . (2015) Dietary quality among men and women in 187 countries in 1990 and 2010: a systematic assessment. Lancet Glob Health 3: e132–42.

Kock R, Alders R, Wallace R. (2011) Wildlife, wild food, food security and human society. Proceedings of the OIE Global Conference on Wildlife: Animal Health and Biodiversity – Preparing for the Future; 23–25 February 2011, Maison de la Chemie, Paris, France. p 23. (Full paper).

Kock, R, Fornace, K, Alders, R. and Wallace, R. (2012) Is industrial husbandry an ecosystem disservice driving pathogen emergence? And can sovereign conservation agriculture fix the problem? Proceedings of the EcoHealth Conference, Kunming City, 15-18 October 2012, p. 106.

Leiss W and Powell DA. (2014) Mad Cows and Mother's Milk: the perils of poor risk communication , 2nd edition. McGill-Queen's Press, Toronto.

McMichael A. (2014) Earth as humans' habitat: global climate change and the health of populations. International Journal of Health Policy Management 2: 9–12., Available online at www.ijhpm.com/pdf_2809_f2b642ffecf3ddcdecc906dca08b46dc.html.

McMichael AJ and Lindgren E. (2011) Climate change: present and future risks to health, and necessary responses. Journal of Internal Medicine 270; 401–413. Available online at http://onlinelibrary.wiley.com/doi/10.1111/j.1365-2796.2011.02415.x/pdf.

Otte J, Costales A, Dijkman J Pica-Ciamarra U, Robinson T, Ahuja V, Ly C and Roland-Holst D (2012) Livestock sector development for poverty reduction: an economic and policy perspective – livestock's many virtues. FAO, Rome. Available (open access at http://www.fao.org/docrep/015/i2744e/i2744e00.pdf via http://www.fao.org/docrep/015/i2744e/i2744e00.htm.

Roesel K and Grace D, eds. (2015) Food Safety and Informal Markets: animal products in Sub-Saharan Africa. Earthcsan, London and New York. Available online at https://cgspace.cgiar.org/bitstream/handle/10568/42438/Food%20Safety%20and%20Informal%20Markets.pdf?sequence=4 via https://cgspace.cgiar.org/handle/10568/42438.

Sherman M. (2002) Tending Animals in the Global Village: a guide to international veterinary medicine. Lippincott Williams and Wilkins, Philadelphia.

Swanson KS, Carter RA, Yount TP, Aretz J and Buff PR. (2013), Nutritional sustainability of pet foods. Advances in Nutrition 4: 141–150.

Wang Y, Lehane C, Ghebremeskel K and Crawford MA. (2009) Modern organic and broiler chickens sold for human consumption provide more energy from fat than protein. Public Health Nutrition: 13(3): 400–408.

References

1   Moubarac J-C, Bortoletto Martins AP, Moreira Claro R et al. (2012) Consumption of ultra-processed foods and likely impact on human health. Evidence from Canada. Public Health Nutrition: 16(12), 2240–2248

2   Monteiro CA. (2009) Nutrition and health. The issue is not food, nor nutrients, so much as processing. Public Health Nutrition: 12(5), 729–731.

3   http://www.oie.int/animal-health-in-the-world/bse-specific-data/number-of-cases-in-the-united-kingdom/.

Nutrition and Climate: Requirements for mitigating the influence of climate change

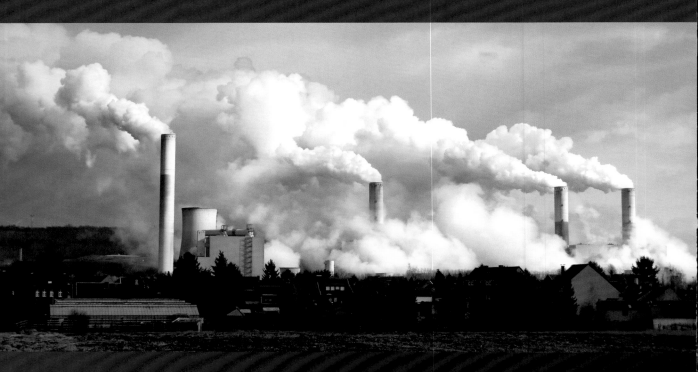

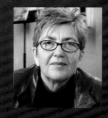

Madeleine Thomson
Senior Research Scientist, International Research Institute for Climate and Society, Palisades, NY, USA; Senior Scholar, Mailman School of Public Health, Department of Environmental Health Sciences, Columbia University, NY, NY USA; Director of the IRI/PAHO-WHO Collaborating Center (US 306) for Early Warning Systems for Malaria and Other Climate Sensitive Diseases, Columbia University, NY, NY USA

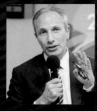

Lawrence Haddad
Senior Research Fellow, Poverty, Health and Nutrition Division, IFPRI (International Food Policy Research Institute), Washington DC, USA

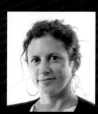

Jess Fanzo
Bloomberg Distinguished Associate Professor of Ethics and Global Food and Agriculture Policy in the Berman Institute of Bioethics and the School of Advanced International Studies at Johns Hopkins University, Baltimore, MD, USA

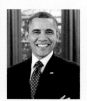

"No challenge poses a greater threat to future generations than climate change."

Barack Obama, *44th President of the United States of America.*

Key messages

- Climate change has been identified as one of the biggest global health and food security threats of the 21st century.

- Both directly and indirectly, climate influences the four environments, which underpin nutrition: our food, social, health, and living environments.

- The co-existence of under- and overnutrition in many countries, especially low- and middle-income countries, makes affected populations increasingly susceptible to multiple forms of climate-related health risks.

- Better management of seasonal and year-to year-changes in climate today may help future policy-makers to better address the climate-related nutrition and health risks of tomorrow.

- Nutrition also influences climate by means of people's dietary choices and energy consumption.

- An evidence-based advocacy and public health movement is needed to encourage decision-makers from governments, business and civil society to support new policies and personal actions to reduce greenhouse gas emissions from food systems while adapting to the effects of climate change on nutrition.

The relationship between nutrition and climate change

The Sustainable Development Goals (SDGs), which were adopted by the UN General Assembly in 2015 after three years of global consultation, build on the progress of the Millennium Development Goals (MDGs). The SDGs contain a commitment to "end hunger and ensure access by all people to safe and nutritious food all year round" (Goal 2) and to "take urgent action to combat climate change and its impacts" (Goal 13). In this chapter, we explore the linkages between nutrition and climate and the potential for identifying and implementing viable strategies, policies and programming opportunities that serve both to improve nutrition and to help societies mitigate and, where necessary, adapt to climate change.

The connection between climate change and nutrition is multifaceted. The common expectation is that climate change will have an effect on nutrition outcomes through its impact on the underlying drivers of nutritional status. The seasonality of the climate, climate and weather shocks (floods, droughts, heat-waves), year-to-year variability and longer-term shifts (climate, sea level rise and increased atmospheric CO_2 etc.) all influence, both directly and indirectly, the four environments which underpin nutrition – namely our food, social, health and living environments (**Figure 1**).[1] For example, climate influences the seasonality of food production and consumption, epidemics of diarrheal disease, and the time utilization of mothers whose ready access to clean drinking-water in coastal regions declines as sea-levels rise. The multiple burdens of nutrition-related diseases (including under- and overnutrition and associated nutritional deficiencies) may make affected populations increasingly susceptible to multiple forms of climate-related nutritional and health risks. The economic impacts can be potentially devastating to the incomes of smallholder farmers.

However, the literature regarding the specific interaction of climate and nutrition is relatively small. What exists is often a conceptual exploration of pathways from climate change to nutrition status, and from nutrition status to adaptive capacity – for example, drawing out the links between climate change and food security on the one hand and between climate change and undernutrition on the other. We also note that dietary choices and actions have major impacts on resource use and on global greenhouse gas emissions. A literature detailing this alternative pathway – how food production and dietary choices affect greenhouse gas emissions – is now emerging (see, for example, Tilman and Clark 2014).

Figure 1 | **Conceptual links between climate change and nutrition**

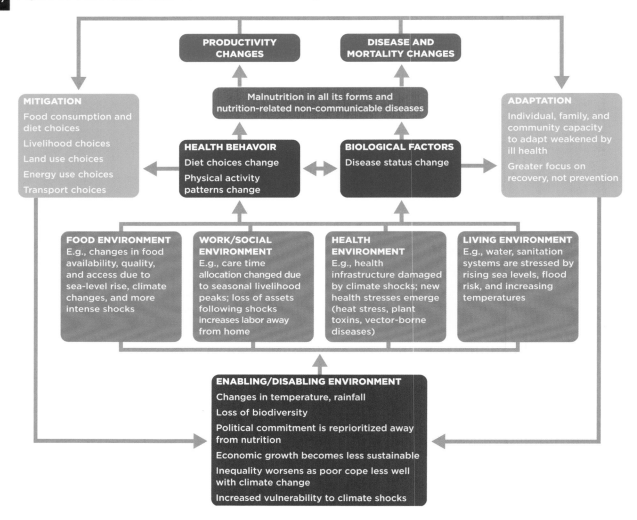

Source: IFPRI (International Food Policy Research Institute). 2015. Global Nutrition Report 2015:Actions and Accountability to Advance Nutrition and Sustainable Development. Figure 6.1.Washington, DC.http://dx.doi.org/10.2499/9780896298835.

Climate: Human-induced change and natural variability

Human-induced changes in climate occur as a result of changes in the water cycle, atmospheric circulation, and ocean currents, driven by changes in the global energy cycle associated with anthropogenic activities.[2] These activities, such as burning coal, oil and gas to power our homes, factories and transport systems, have released huge quantities of carbon dioxide into the atmosphere, causing an enhanced warming or "greenhouse" effect. Changes in land use (e.g., cutting down forests to create farmland or grazing areas) also directly impact greenhouse gases. One consequence of the general warming associated with climate change is the melting of the icecaps and the associated rise in the sea level.

Anthropogenic climate change is superimposed on natural climate variability, which has always been important in human development. Throughout history, societies have modified their environment to manage seasonal variations in rainfall and cope with climate shocks such as floods and droughts. Terracing in Nepal, irrigation along the Nile, the use of drought-resistant crops such as cassava, and the pursuit of drought-resistant livelihoods such as pastoralism are all means by which humans have managed climate-related risks and created new opportunities for development.

Hence to understand the likely impact of climate change on nutrition, we must first understand how seasonality and natural climate variability impact nutritional drivers, and then consider how projected changes in the climate might exacerbate (or reduce) current risks or create new ones.

The impact of changes in climate on nutrition: A seasonal lens

Climate-related food and nutrition crises often make the headlines. However, they represent only 10% of global hunger. Approximately 75% of undernourished people live in low-income rural areas within developing countries, principally in farming areas. Here, chronic hunger usually occurs prior to the harvest season, when food stocks are low, food prices high, and jobs scarce. Thus we can see that climate drives the seasonal patterns of human food security – including the availability of micronutrient-rich foods, the presence of infectious disease, and patterns of human behavior[3] – to generate a complex series of interacting effects. This is particularly acute in regions where the rains are highly seasonal and agriculture is rain-fed. Here, the period between planting and harvesting is widely known as the "hungry season."

For example, studies have shown that seasonal food insecurity can lead to low diet diversity (and a concomitant insufficiency in dietary iron).[4] When combined with seasonal malaria (which causes iron losses), the consequence can be seasonal anemia from iron deficiency and associated pre-eclampsia[5] in pregnant women. Epidemic malaria concomitant with anemia has also been shown to contribute to a poorly developed fetal immune system and an increase in the incidence babies of low birth weight[6] – both of which increase the likelihood of child and adolescent mortality. The health consequences of anemia may be exacerbated by the seasonally impassable roads or the pre-harvest gap in disposable household income.[3]

The renowned development researcher Robert Chambers once wrote that "seasonal hunger is the father of famine," and that "any development professional serious about poverty has…to be serious about seasonality."[3] In the context of climate, seasonal hunger may be the primary indicator of population vulnerability to climate change.

However, some years are worse than others. Climate and weather shocks may further intensify these recurrent seasonal nutritional crises. The successive failure of the East African short rains (October–December) and subsequent long rains (March–May) in 2010–11 plunged much of the Horn of Africa into severe drought, impacting millions of people and triggering a humanitarian crisis reminiscent of the catastrophic droughts of 1983–85 (Ethiopia) and 1972–73 (the Sahel).[7] The high mortality rates, often due to acute severe malnutrition, also known as "wasting", associated with these drought-related famines highlight the role of vulnerability in turning a problem into a disaster. These catastrophic short-term events are often part of a longer natural decadal cycle of dryer or wetter conditions which are then superimposed upon longer-term trends which may be associated with anthropogenic change. While some human-made climate change now seems inevitable, the way it is likely to manifest itself at the local level remains highly uncertain. This is in part due to the fact that these natural climate cycles confound the measurement of change resulting from anthropogenic forcing alone.

The current plethora of analysis of downscaled climate change models for projections of future food security or health events rarely indicate the level of uncertainty associated with natural variability in rainfall. The results for most regions of the world are consequently highly speculative at shorter timeframes (<20 years). Understanding variability and change at multiple timescales is critical to ensuring that decisions are informed by relevant climate information.

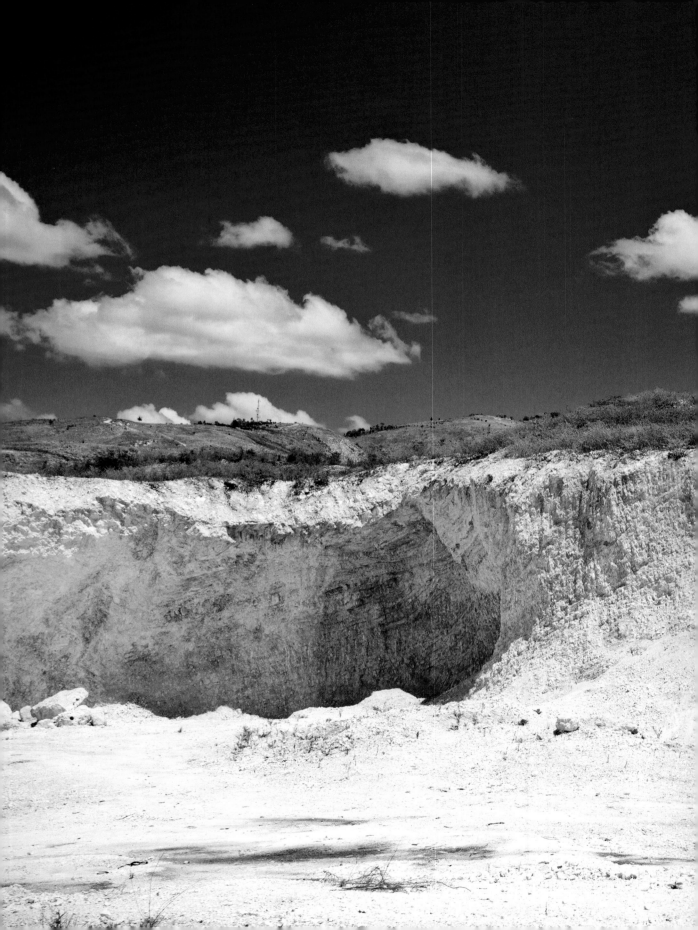

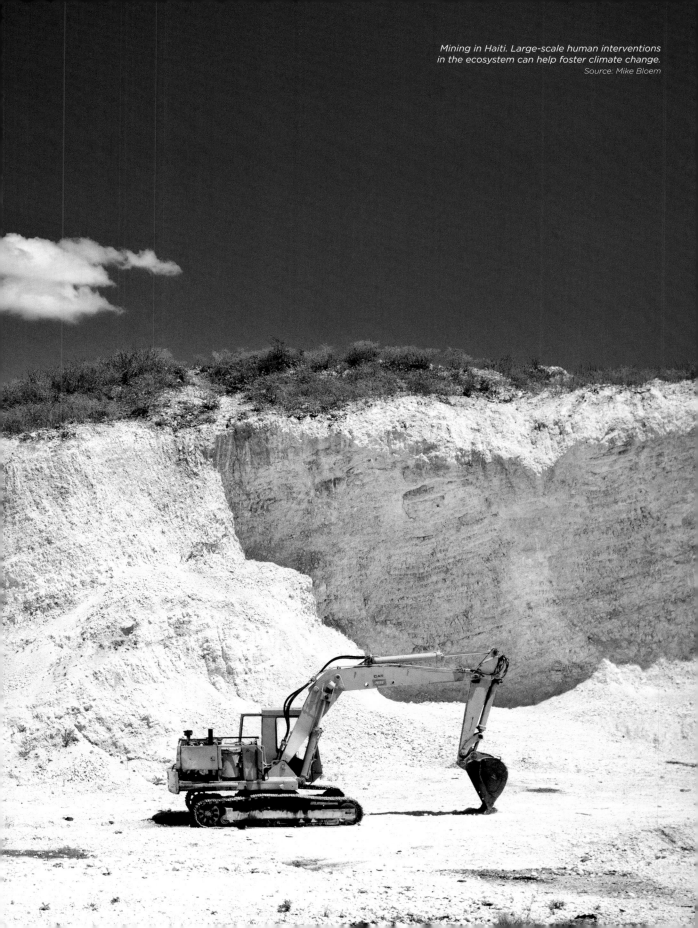

Mining in Haiti. Large-scale human interventions in the ecosystem can help foster climate change.
Source: Mike Bloem

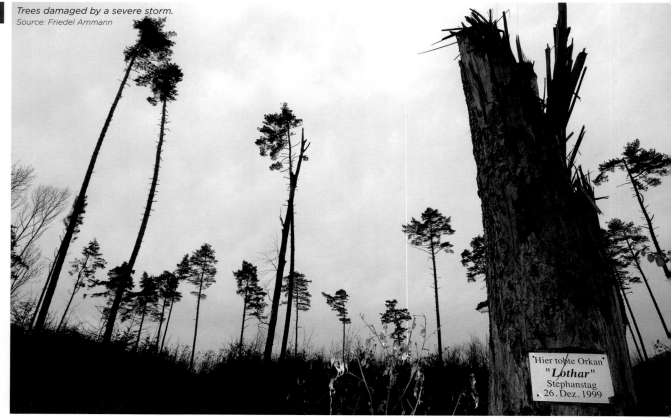

Trees damaged by a severe storm.
Source: Friedel Ammann

"Hier tobte Orkan
"Lothar"
Stephanstag
26. Dez. 1999

Climate: Human-induced change and natural variability

At the seasonal to inter-annual timescale, the El Niño-Southern Oscillation phenomenon (both El Niño and La Niña) is the most significant natural driver of variability in the climate system. Recurring every 2–7 years, ENSO events bring predictable drought or floods to many regions of the world (**Figures 2** and **3**) and increase temperatures across the tropics.

Because ENSO events improve the ability of climate scientists to forecast the seasonal climate, considerable attention has been paid by the agricultural community to the role that ENSO plays in determining the agricultural yield and nutritional quality of staple crops across the globe. The 2015–16 El Niño had significant impact around the world, resulting in failed rainy seasons in Ethiopia, Indonesia and Northern Brazil. Unlike the 1984 drought and associated famine, the 2015 June–September severe drought in Ethiopia was well predicted by the National Meteorological Agency, and the government was thus forewarned and better prepared to respond.

Increasing evidence suggests that ENSO impacts on the yield of global food staples both positively and negatively, although the overall global impact is negative.[8] ENSO impacts on some of the key rice-producing/exporting and rice-importing countries, with extreme and predictable effects on rainfall in the Philippines and Indonesia during the main monsoon season. Variations in average July–September El Niño sea surface temperatures explain approximately 29% of the inter-annual variations in the total January–June (dry season) rice production.[9]

El Niño events are also associated with a short-term dramatic increase in global temperatures around the tropics. The 1997–98 El Niño was the hottest year on record, and global temperatures in 2015 (also an El Niño year) also broke the global temperature records. These short-term temperature anomalies are superimposed on longer warming trends and may impact agricultural output, food safety, the incidence of infectious disease, and health outcomes associated with heat-waves.

Figure 2 | **El Niño and rainfall**

El Niño conditions in the tropical Pacific are known to shift rainfall patterns in many different parts of the world. Although they vary somewhat from one El Niño to the next, the strongest shifts remain fairly consistent in the regions and seasons shown on the map below.

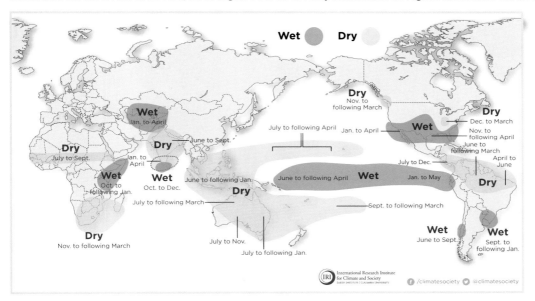

Figure 3 | **La Niña and rainfall**

La Niña conditions in the tropical Pacific are known to shift rainfall patterns in many different parts of the world. Although they vary somewhat from one La Niña to the next, the strongest shifts remain fairly consistent in the regions and seasons shown on the map below.

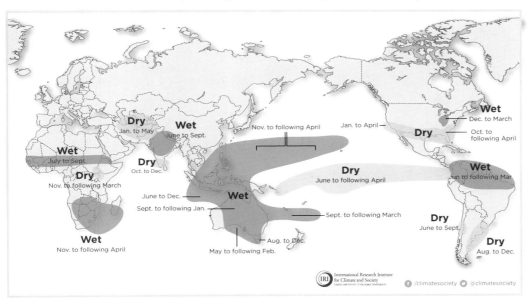

Source: International Research Institute for Climate and Society http://iridl.ldeo.columbia.edu/maproom/IFRC/FIC/elninorain.html
For more information on El Niño and La Niña, go to: http://iri.columbia.edu/enso
Sources:
1 Ropelewski, C. F. and M. S. Halpert. Precipitation patterns associated with the high index phase of the Southern Oscillation. J Climate. 1989;2:268-284.
2 Mason and Goddard. Probabilistic precipitation anomalies associated with ENSO. Bull Am Meteorol Soc 2001;82:619-638

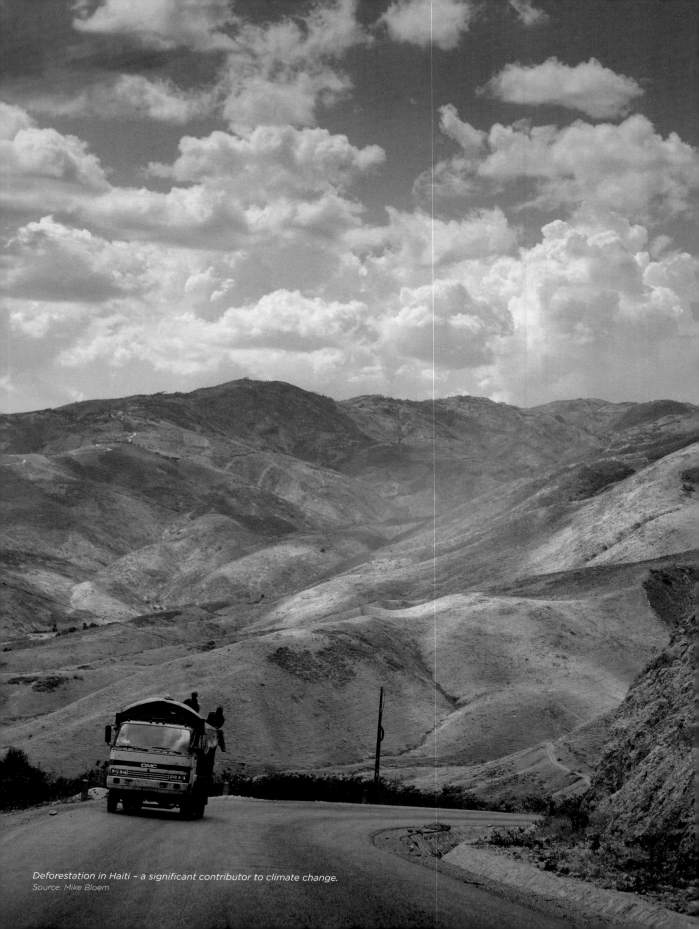

Deforestation in Haiti – a significant contributor to climate change.
Source: Mike Bloem

Bangladesh and rice: At the intersection of climate and nutrition

While a staple of low nutritional value, rice is central to the food security of more than half the world's population. As a "strategic" commodity in many Asian countries, it is subject to a wide range of government controls and interventions. In addition, rice production is also sensitive to drought and extreme flooding.

Bangladesh is a rice-growing country, and more than 70% of the calories consumed by rural Bangladeshis come from rice.[10] While seasonal river flooding is essential to the rice farming system, major floods cause substantial losses. When the rice crop fails because of excessive flooding in the Aman season or regional drought in Boro season, Bangladesh responds by

importing from neighboring countries and increasing production in the following season. However, such transitions are not smooth, they interact with regional and global shocks, and they can lead to rapid increases in rice prices that may affect consumers. In turn, rice prices have a direct impact on child nutrition. High rice prices following production shocks have been shown to be strongly associated with a decline in spending on non-rice foods (essential for good nutrition given the low micronutrient value of rice) and an associated increase in underweight children.[10]

Source: Madeleine Thomson, Global Nutrition Report 2015, International Food Policy Research Institute (IFPRI) (abridged).

Climate and nutrition

A number of studies have shown that risks and shocks that happen at the population level (including climate shocks) can perpetuate poverty and aggravate vulnerability to livelihood failure by inducing income losses and forcing the sale of assets – sometimes with consequences that perpetuate themselves over several generations. It is not surprising that poverty itself is an important determinant of poor nutritional status. A multi-country study on poverty and nutritional status covering Ethiopia, Peru, India and Vietnam revealed that the poorest 20% of those surveyed had a significantly increased likelihood of being stunted in comparison to children residing in the households within the highest wealth quintile.[11]

While climate change predictions for rainfall are much less certain than those for temperature, the general expectation for many regions of the world is an increase in the occurrence and intensity of droughts, with impacts on agriculture and water supply exacerbated by increases in evapotranspiration associated with higher temperatures.

Droughts affect human nutrition not only by seriously reducing crop harvests but also by reducing grazing and fodder for livestock, thus lessening the availability of milk and meat. The use of drought-resistant crops is a long-standing strategy for coping with climate risks. Drought inhibits plant growth and development by disturbing the uptake and absorption of essential minerals. This is reflected in the final crop yield, and may also affect the

nutritional content of roots/tubers, foliage and seeds. The impacts of drought on crop yield and nutritional content are complex as well as species- and cultivar-specific, and they invariably depend on the severity and duration of stress and the stage of the plant's life-cycle at which the stress occurs.[12]

Drought-tolerant plants such as the cowpea (widely grown in semi-arid areas of the tropics and extra-tropics) have long been used to manage climate risks to food supply. However, drought tolerance may also come at a nutritional cost. For instance, cassava is widely used in Africa as a staple and, in marginal regions or during drought periods, as a survival crop that will grow under the harshest of conditions. While providing a good source of energy, cassava has low protein and poor essential nutrient density. It also has anti-nutritional and toxic cyanogens which are made worse by drought but whose effect is reduced through appropriate preparation and cooking. Excessive use of cassava under distressed circumstances may result in severe neurological disorders and other toxicity-related issues.

So far, we have focused on seasonality and climate variability, which are part of the normal climate baseline to the changes that are being observed in longer-term trends. As the climate system warms, variability and extreme events may increase, and seasonal patterns may change. The following section focuses on the longer-term trends in temperature and other key climate variables.

Increases in temperature and CO_2 effects

The impact of higher minimum and maximum temperatures on crop yields has been demonstrated in both the laboratory and the field. For instance, higher-than-optimal minimum and maximum temperatures have been shown to decrease yields, making rice highly vulnerable to the increased temperatures predicted to occur as a result of climate change.[13] Warming temperatures may also have an impact on the occurrence of contamination and food safety at various stages of the food chain, from primary production through to consumption.

As well as driving up global temperatures, carbon emissions have also been contributing significantly to the elevation of CO_2 levels in the atmosphere. A wide range of agricultural experiments have been undertaken in CO_2-enhanced environments. Results suggest that crops will grow faster, with slight changes in development, such as flowering and fruiting, depending on the species. This is known as the "CO_2 fertilization effect." However, the beneficial direct impact of this "fertilization effect" will probably be offset by the influence of climate change. Vitally important for nutrition, the increased CO_2 associated with climate change is projected to significantly reduce the nutritional content (especially the zinc and iron content) of the grains and legumes that form the basic diet of the world's most vulnerable populations.[14] Countries that have growing seasons constrained by cold weather may benefit from climate change, whereas others at the upper temperature limit for successful crop production may have their food security or production of export crops compromised. There will always be winners and losers in global change, but the most significant losers are developing countries in the tropics which have contributed least to greenhouse gas emissions.

Links between nutrition choices, outcomes and climate mitigation

Nutrition also matters directly in the achievement of the SDG goal to reduce greenhouse gas emissions below dangerous levels. It is estimated that food systems contribute 19%–29% of global anthropogenic greenhouse gas emissions, and that they released 9,800–16,900 megatonnes of carbon dioxide equivalent into the atmosphere in 2008.[15] Agricultural production, including indirect emissions associated with land-cover change, accounts for 80%–86% of total food system emissions, with significant regional variations.[15] One third of agricultural emissions come from the production of meat and milk. Relative to animal-based foods, plant-based foods have lower greenhouse gas emissions. Tilman and Clark (2014) calculated that ruminant meats (beef and lamb) are responsible for emissions per gram of protein that are about 250 times those of legumes. Thus ruminants contribute a significant proportion of the greenhouse gas emissions from food systems (including enteric methane from ruminant digestion).

Although in marginal lands ruminants play a unique role in food production because of their ability to turn non-human food into edible protein and nutrients, ruminant meat-centered diets can have a much higher emission impact when compared with more sustainable vegetarian or vegan diets.[16] In addition, while meat can provide a vital source of protein and nutrients, the current global trend towards the excessive consumption of meat, fats and sugar poses major health risks for both people and planet. Encouraging a global transition to more environmentally sustainable diets may be a win-win opportunity for a reduction in emissions plus improved public health.

Impact of poor diets on health and energy consumption

According to a report commissioned by the Sustainable Development Unit of the United Kingdom National Health Service (NHS) the NHS is responsible for approximately 5% of the UK's combined greenhouse gas emissions.[17] Greening the NHS is an important part of the UK's efforts to reduce CO_2 emissions. According to Scarborough and colleagues,[18] 46% of total NHS costs (over £43 billion) in 2006–07 were due to diseases related to poor diet, physical inactivity, smoking, alcohol and overweight/obesity (although not all of these costs were due to the associated risk factors). High levels of obesity are not only a health and economic burden; they may also be associated with higher than normal CO_2 emissions.[19] Thus lifestyle characteristics that promote ill health may also foster climatic risk.

Enhancing National Climate Services (ENACTS): A critical development for improving the use of climate information in nutrition planning

Natural climate variability and long-term changes in rainfall and temperature are expected to have major impact in Africa, where most of the population depends on rain-fed agriculture for their food and livelihood. Reliable climate information will be crucial in efforts to build resilience against the negative impact of climate change and to maximize the benefits of favorable conditions.

Currently, the primary source of climate data is observation by ground-based weather stations across the continent. The main strength of these station observations is that they give the true measurements of the climate variable of interest. However, in many parts of Africa stations are sparse, declining in number, and unevenly distributed.

The ENACTS (Enhancing National Climate Services) initiative, led by the International Research Institute for Climate and Society (IRI) of Columbia University, is a unique, multifaceted initiative designed to bring climate knowledge into national decision-making by improving availability, access to, and use of climate information. Availability of climate data is improved by combining quality-controlled data from national observation networks with satellite estimates for rainfall, elevation maps, and reanalysis products for temperature. Access to information products is enhanced by making derived information products available online. The use of climate information is facilitated by engaging and collaborating with potential users.

For an example, please see the information for Ethiopia at: *http://www.ethiometmaprooms.gov.et:8082/maproom/*

Source: *Dinku TR, Cousin J, del Corral P et al "THE ENACTS APPROACH: Transforming climate services in Africa one country at a time." World Bank Policy, 2016.*

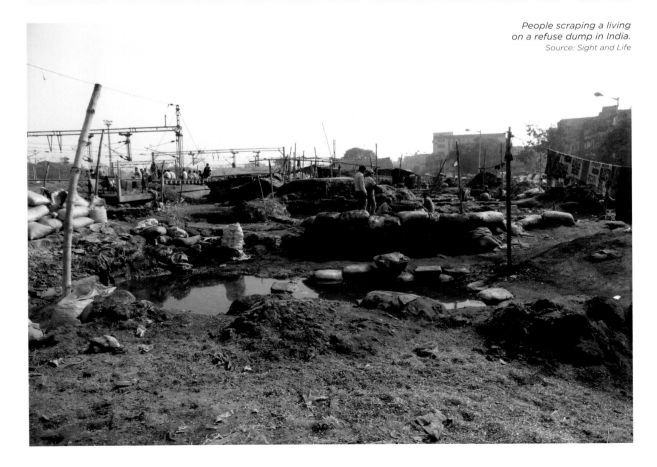

People scraping a living on a refuse dump in India.
Source: Sight and Life

The 2015 United Nations Climate Change Conference and the invisibility of nutrition in climate documents

The 2015 United Nations Climate Change Conference, also known as COP 21, was held in Paris, France, from November 30 to December 12, 2015. It was the twenty-first annual session of the Conference of the Parties (COP) to the 1992 United Nations Framework Convention on Climate Change (UNFCCC) and the eleventh session of the Meeting of the Parties to the 1997 Kyoto Protocol.

The conference aimed, for the first time in over 20 years of UN negotiations, to achieve a legally binding and universal agreement on climate, with the aim of keeping global warming below 2 °C. The result was the Paris Agreement – a global agreement on the reduction of climate change which represented a consensus of the representatives of the 195 participating countries.

In the days following the conference, the Paris COP21 Agreement was described by several influential commentators as an agreement that was "better than expected," but "less than hoped for." On the plus side, all 195 countries showed they can come together to actually reach an agreement – it was, after all, the first deal to cover every major polluter. In addition, the 187 countries responsible for 95% of the world's pollution put forward plans that would cut the growth of emissions. The emissions would not be cut nearly enough, but at least the ideal maximum temperature increase was lowered from 2 °C to 1.5 °C.

On the negative side, the national targets were not sufficiently ambitious and not legally binding, and the financing commitments from developed countries lacked transparency. Food was mentioned three times in the Agreement, in the sense that food security must not be compromised by climate change or by climate action. Agriculture and nutrition were not mentioned explicitly, but both were probably considered to be adequately subsumed under food security.

The invisibility of nutrition in climate documents is illustrated by the fact that few of the Intended Nationally Determined Contributions mentioned nutrition (GloPan). The reverse is also true: too few national nutrition plans mention climate (Global Nutrition Report, Chapter 6).[1] The nutrition and climate communities need to come together more purposefully. Why? On the adaptation side, climate already affects nutrition status through seasonality and shocks, and these fluctuations in nutrition outcomes will only become more unpredictable with a changing climate. Nutrition programs need to become more climate-proof. On the mitigation side, improved nutrition could be one of the best opportunities for reducing greenhouse gas emissions. The production of foods that promote good health tends to have a lower emissions footprint, although there are exceptions.

To realize some of these connections, the nutrition community should get more involved in the health group of the Intergovernmental Panel on Climate Change (IPCC); NGOs that work on both climate and nutrition should connect up their efforts; nutrition plans and programs need to take shifting seasonality into account; and those responsible for the collection of data con nutrition need to be more mindful of the season in which their work is undertaken.

Recommended action on climate change

By the time of the UN Conference on Climate Change (COP21) in November 2015, the climate change and nutrition communities should form alliances to meet common goals. The Intergovernmental Panel on Climate Change (IPCC) should form a group comprising nutrition and climate-health experts to assess the climate-nutrition literature and define new research and policy agendas. Governments should build climate change explicitly into their national nutrition and health strategies. And civil society should use existing networks to build climate change–nutrition alliances to advocate for nutrition at the COP21 and other leading climate change events and processes.

1   **Governments** should build climate change more explicitly into existing and new national nutrition strategies. Reviews of nutrition policies show that many countries do not yet incorporate climate change into their nutrition policies.

2   **The Intergovernmental Panel on Climate Change** should develop a nutrition subgroup to ensure that climate policy-makers take advantage of climate-nutrition interactions and community adaptation. The four major UN nutrition agencies – FAO, UNICEF, World Food Programme (WFP), and WHO – should work with the IPCC to add nutrition experts to IPCC Working Groups 2 (vulnerability to climate change) and 3 (options for mitigation) in time for them to make a meaningful contribution to the next IPCC assessment report, anticipated to be published in four to five years' time.

3   **Civil society** should lead the formation of climate-nutrition alliances to identify new opportunities for action on both fronts. Civil society groups should then present these new opportunities at side meetings at the 2016 COP in Marrakesh. Civil society groups concerned with nutrition should build climate change into their own activities.

Source: Global Nutrition Report 2015

Dietary choices that are good for both health and the planet

The 2015 Global Nutrition Report noted that countries are only now beginning to incorporate climate into their national nutrition strategies. As the world's climate change and nutrition communities have overlapping agendas, this situation should improve. More collaboration between the two communities could generate a better understanding of climate-related risks to nutrition while also engaging the nutrition community in concerns about the impact of food systems and dietary choices on greenhouse gas emission pathways. The ideal is to identify dietary choices that are both good for health and good for the planet. However, the requisite data, methodologies and tools for making such assessments are poorly developed. To ameliorate the situation, the following are necessary:

• Better data on nutritional status is required – particularly longitudinal studies that can identify seasonal nutritional deficiencies and the impact of local and global shocks.

• Higher-quality climate data should be generated at appropriate temporal and spatial scales for global and local analysis and made available for use in climate impact analysis.

• Tools are needed that can sensitively measure the influence of food systems and dietary choices on greenhouse gas emissions (and other climate/environment indicators) in a holistic and comparative way.

• An awareness and understanding of climate (including the relevant data, methodologies and tools) should be incorporated into training programs for nutritional epidemiologists.

• The climate and nutrition communities should engage in dialogue that can stimulate collaboration between them and improve the coherence of their respective policy agendas.

• Personnel and institutional capacity development is necessary, accompanied by appropriate training measures, to help create greater awareness of the issues and get action-oriented ideas onto the table.

159

My personal view

Madeleine Thomson

Climate variability and change acts as an additional stressor for those suffering from poor nutrition and related health issues by increasing food insecurity, reducing food quality, and exacerbating ongoing health risks. Globally, the problem is not yet the *availability of food resources*, but the *allocation of food*, given that at the local level too many people are unable to access, safe, nutritious food on a regular basis. Dietary choices are increasingly seen as a means to combat climate change as well as to tackle under- and overnutrition, but what constitutes a good and sustainable diet (both from a nutritional and a climate perspective) for a particular community in a given locality is not well defined at present. More empirical, place-based research is needed, along with better tools. Processes that can connect the science to policy and practice are also essential.

Further reading

IFPRI. *Global Nutrition Report 2015: Actions and Accountability to Advance Nutrition and Sustainable Development.* Washington DC: IFPRI; 2015.

Haddad L, Cameron L, Barnett I. *The Double Burden of Malnutrition in SE Asia and the Pacific: Priorities, Policies and Politics.* 2014: czu110.

Devereux S, Sabates-Wheeler R, Longhurst R. *Seasonality, rural livelihoods and development:* Routledge; 2011.

Zebiak SEB. Orlove AG, Muñoz, C et al *Investigating El Niño-Southern Oscillation and society relationships.* WIRES Climate Change, 2014. doi: 10.1002/wcc.294. doi: 10.1002/wcc.294

Vermeulen SJ, Campbell BM, Ingram SJI *Climate Change and Food Systems. Annual Review of Environment and Resources* 2012;37: 195–222.

United Nations Sustainable Development Goals website: https://sustainabledevelopment.un.org/topics/sustainabledevelopmentgoals.

Website of the International Research Institute for Climate and Society, Earth Institute, Columbia University: http://iri.columbia.edu.

References

1   IFPRI. *Global Nutrition Report 2014: Actions and Accountability to Accelerate the World's Progress on Nutrition. Washington D.C. : IFPRI, 2015.*

2   IPCC. *IPCC, 2012: Change Adaptation. A Special Report of Working Groups I and II of the Intergovernmental Panel on Climate Change. Cambridge UK and New York, USA: Cambridge University Press, Cambridge, UK; 2012.*

3   Devereux S, Sabates-Wheeler R, Longhurst R. *Seasonality, rural livelihoods and development:* Routledge; 2011.

4   Savy M, Martin-Prével Y, Traissac P et al. *Dietary diversity scores and nutritional status of women change during the seasonal food shortage in rural Burkina Faso. Journal of Nutrition* 2006; 136(10): 2625-32.

5   Hlimi T. *Association of anemia, pre-eclampsia and eclampsia with seasonality: A realist systematic review. Health Place* 2015; 31C: 180–92.

6   Moore SE, Cole TJ, Poskitt EME et al. *Season of birth predicts mortality in rural Gambia. Nature* 1997; 388(434).

7   Batterbury S, Warren A. *The African Sahel 25 years after the great drought: assessing progress and moving towards new agendas and approaches. Global Environmental Change* 2001; 11(1): 1–8.

8   Iizumi T, Luo J-J, Challinor AJ et al. *Impacts of El Niño Southern Oscillation on the global yields of major crops. Nature Communications* 2014; (5): 3712.

9   Roberts MG, Dawe D, Falcon W et al. *El Niño–Southern Oscillation Impacts on Rice Production in Luzon, the Philippines. . Journal Applied Meteorology and Climatology* 2009; 48: 1718–24.

10 Torlesse H, Kiess L, Bloem MW. *Association of Household Rice Expenditure with Child Nutritional Status Indicates a Role for Macroeconomic Food Policy in Combating Malnutrition. Community and International Nutrition* 2003: 1320.

11 Petrou. S, Kupek. E. *Poverty and childhood undernutrition in developing countries: a multi-national cohort study. Social Science and Medicine* 2010; 71(7): 1366–73.

12 Prasad PVV, Staggenborg SA, Ristic Z. *Impacts of drought and/or heat stress on physiological, developmental, growth, and yield processes of crop plants. In: Ahuja LH, Saseendran SA, eds. Advances in Agricultural Systems Modeling.* Madison, WI, USA,; 2008: 301–55.

13 Welch JR, Vincent JR, Auffhammer M et al. *Rice yields in tropical/subtropical Asia exhibit large but opposing sensitivities to minimum and maximum temperatures. Proceedings of the National Academy of Sciences* 2010; 33: 14562–7.

14 Myers SS, Zanobetti A, Kloog I et al. *Increasing CO2 threatens human nutrition. Nature* 2014; 510: 139–42.

15 Vermeulen SJ, Campbell BM, Ingram JSI. *Climate Change and Food Systems. Annual Review of Environment and Resources* 2012; 37: 195–222.

16 Tilman D, Clark M. *Global diets link environmental sustainability and human health. Nature* 2014; 515(518–522).

17 NHS. *sustainable development commission NHS England Carbon Emissions Carbon Footprinting Report.* 2008.

18 Scarborough P, Bhatnagar P, Wickramasinghe KK et al. *The economic burden of ill health due to diet, physical inactivity, smoking, alcohol and obesity in the UK: an update to 2006–07 NHS costs. Journal of Public Health* 2011; 33(4): 527–35.

19 Edwards P, Roberts I. *Population adiposity and climate change. International Journal of Epidemiology* 2009.

Sustainable Diets for Nutrition and Environmental Health: The impact of food choices, dietary patterns and consumerism on the planet

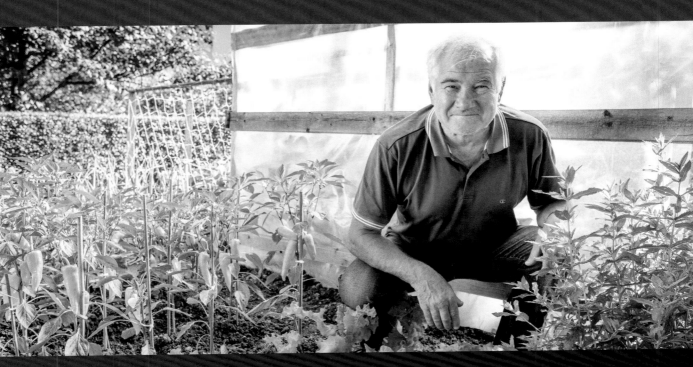

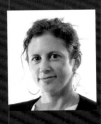

Jess Fanzo
Bloomberg Distinguished Associate Professor of Ethics and Global Food and
Agriculture Policy in the Berman Institute of Bioethics and the School
of Advanced International Studies at Johns Hopkins University, Baltimore, MD, USA

"A safe and nutritionally adequate diet is a basic individual right and an essential condition for sustainable development, especially in developing countries."

Gro Harlem Brundtland, *former Prime Minister of Norway and currently a current Special Envoy with the United Nations.*

Key messages

- Current food production methods are contributing to severe environmental problems.

- Populations are being driven towards a less diverse diet.

- Diets are shifting toward more convenient, nutrient-dense products, but also toward more highly processed foods.

- Globally, we are recognizing that the health of human beings cannot be isolated from the health of ecosystems and the environment.

- Recently, the concept of sustainable food systems and diets has become increasingly important.

- There should be incentives that encourage farmers to grow food in a more sustainable way, while consumers should be educated to make informed choices about what foods are healthy both for themselves and for the planet.

The current global food system is producing enough food for the world's population. However, ensuring access to (and consumption of) a sufficient quantity of food that is culturally acceptable, affordable, nutritious and healthy for everyone on the planet presents more of a challenge. Making sure that a proportion of this food does not simply go to waste it also far from easy. Projections for the next 10 to 50 years further underline the need to improve the quality and environmental sustainability of the diet. This is especially the case given the challenges imposed by climate change and increasing population growth, in combination with a rising appetite for environmentally costly animal-source foods.

The purpose of this chapter is to introduce the impacts of different diets on planetary and human health, and to outline how the changing climate and environment will affect nutrition and health outcomes; they are, indeed, starting to do so already. The idea of sustainable diets will be introduced, and it will be shown how dietary consumption patterns must change over the coming decades if we wish to secure a sustainable future within the planetary boundaries.

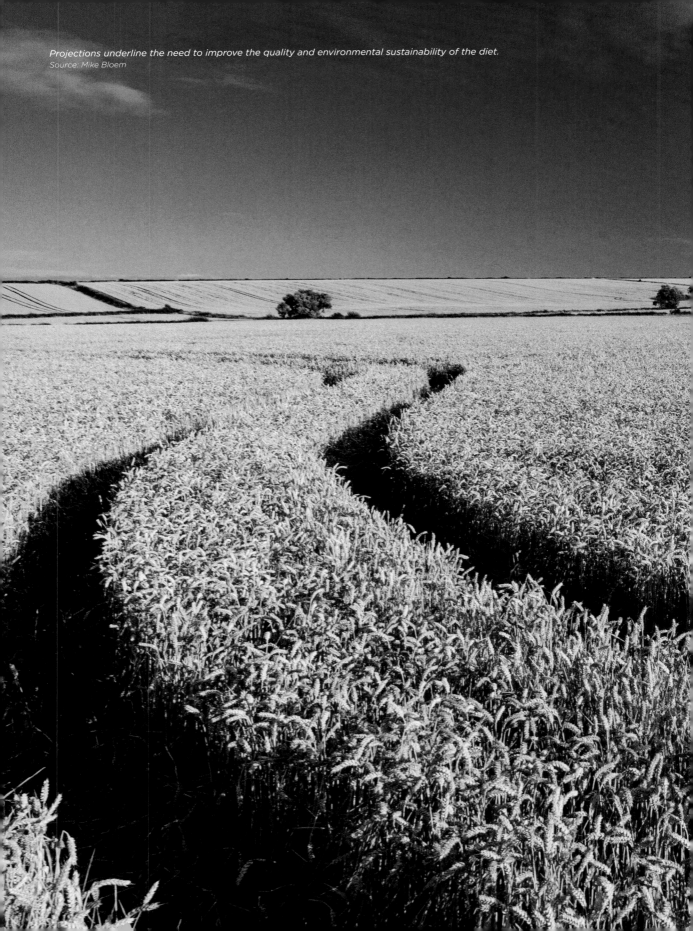

Projections underline the need to improve the quality and environmental sustainability of the diet.
Source: Mike Bloem

Trends in unsustainable production and consumption within the food system

With global demands for food changing due to a growing population and increased consumption of animal-source foods, current production methods are contributing to severe environmental problems. Agricultural intensification, poverty, population pressures, urbanization and lifestyle changes have altered the production and consumption of food in ways that profoundly affect diets, leading to an overall reduction in the recognition of seasonality and a concentration on staple food sources. In addition, the alarming pace of biodiversity loss and ecosystem degradation – together with climate change and resource extraction, and the negative impact of these developments on farming systems, livelihoods and health – makes a compelling case for re-examining the global food system from an environmentally sustainable and public health perspective.

On the production side, the challenge of improving the productivity and yields of major food crops (mainly cereal grains) has dominated the agriculture sector. The strong focus on crop yields has led agriculture to make heavy use of inputs, including fertilizers and pesticides, as the standard means of meeting demand. Less attention has been given to environmental impacts. A significant proportion of the food grown goes toward feeding the animals which we humans are increasingly demanding on our plates. The loss of food for human consumption produced from arable land (partly as a result of biofuel production) as well as the significant contributions of animal production systems to greenhouse gas (GHG) emissions are not components of a sustainable food system.

On the consumption side, much of the world's population has poor access to nutrient-rich foods from animal sources, while at the same time we are witnessing overconsumption of highly processed foods. There is increasing demand for cheap calories, and up to 30% of food purchased or cooked is wasted. Interestingly, we still do not know enough about what people eat and what informs their choices in our complex food environment. What is known is that eating is strongly influenced by behaviors determined by culture, media and information. Consumption patterns and their consequences are also a function of income, as well as of lifestyle. Demand for highly processed foods will continue to increase because of convenience, cost and taste. With the advancement in food processing methods and techniques, there is an opportunity to improve the nutritional content, quality and safety of these processed foods so that – in contrast to junk foods that are high in sugar, fat and salt – they meet the health needs of populations.

Changes to the current global food system include the locations where food is purchased and eaten, attitudes towards specific foods, the way foods taste, and the effects of marketing. Collectively, these changes are driving populations towards a more processed and convenient, and less diverse, diet. The importance of diversity and quality in foods (in terms both of what is grown and of what is eaten) is generally recognized, however. Studies have also shown that dietary diversity is associated with food security and socioeconomic status, and the links between socioeconomic factors and nutrition outcomes are well known.

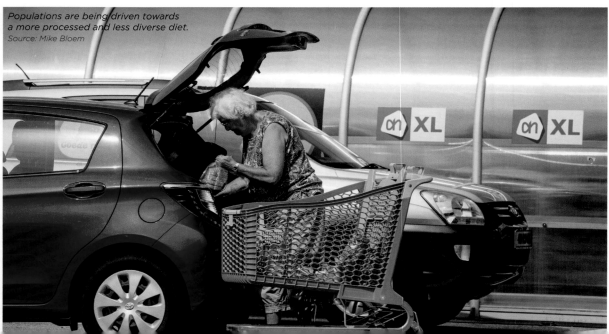

Populations are being driven towards a more processed and less diverse diet.
Source: Mike Bloem

Figure 1 | **How mothers and children are situated within the larger food system**

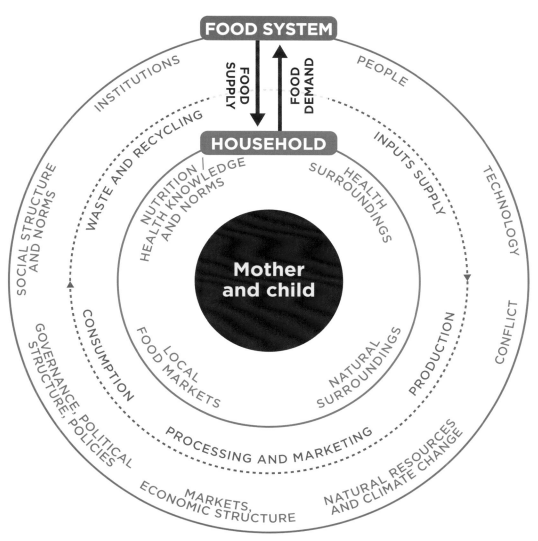

Within the food and agricultural system are people and institutions involved in the production, processing, marketing, consumption, and disposal of food. There are also the sociopolitical, economic, and technological environments associated with the food system, separate from but enveloping the households, as households and the individuals therein are part of the food system. Food system activities affect the availability and affordability of food for all food consumers, including producer households, as well as the demand for diverse, nutritious foods in the food market environment. The food system also impacts the natural resources environment; the health, water, and sanitation environment; and the knowledge and norms surrounding nutrition and health. The figure represents a conceptualization of how mothers and children within households are situated within the larger food system.

Source: Du L, Pinga V, Klein A et al. Leveraging Agriculture for Nutrition Impact in the Feed the Future Initiative. Chapter 1 In: Advances in Food and Research 2015;74:1-46.

Trends in environmental and ecosystem degradation and climate variability: Reaching our planetary boundaries

"Planetary boundaries" is the central concept in an Earth system framework designed to define a "safe operating space for humanity" as a precondition for sustainable development. This framework is based on scientific research that indicates that since the Industrial Revolution, human actions have gradually become the main driver of global environmental change. Scientists assert that once human activity has passed certain tipping points, defined as "planetary boundaries," there is a risk of "irreversible and abrupt environmental change." There are nine Earth system processes, which have boundaries that, to the extent that they are not crossed, mark the safe zone for the planet. However, because of human activities, some of these dangerous boundaries have already been crossed, while others are in imminent danger of being transgressed.[1]

Humans are rapidly influencing ecosystems, which is causing increasing risk of irreversible changes. The main drivers of these changes are demand for food, water and natural resources. This in turn accelerates the loss of biodiversity, which impacts not only ecosystems themselves but also the diversity available to humans in their diets. Land such as forests, grasslands and wetlands is being converted to farmland by humans in order to feed the hungry planet. This too, is increasing the loss of biodiversity as well as negatively affecting precious water and nutrient flows.

Food systems contribute 19%–29% of global anthropogenic greenhouse gas (GHG) emissions. Agricultural production, including indirect emissions associated with land-cover change, contributes 80%–86% of total food system emissions, with significant regional variation.[2] Modeling indicates that the impact of climate change on food systems will be widespread, geographically and temporally variable, and influenced by socioeconomic conditions. There is strong evidence that climate change will affect agricultural yields and livelihoods, food prices, reliability of delivery, food quality, and safety.[2]

Impacts of different diets on planet health

Changes in the types of food we eat are driving a new demand for certain types of food that are grown and processed in particular ways. This demand will of course be tempered by factors such as climate change and variability, dwindling ecosystem and biodiversity resources, and conflicts over ownership of, and access to, land.

While populations are increasing, so is overall wealth in some countries, particularly India, China and Brazil, as well as certain countries of Africa. Diets are increasingly shifting towards higher-quality, nutrient-dense products such as meat, dairy products, and oils – but also towards more highly processed foods. The pressure to produce more food in an environmentally sustainable way, while upholding safety and health standards, runs counter to these consumer demands. At the same time, there are profound inequities both globally and within individual countries regarding the access to, and affordability of, nutritious foods. There is no ethically simple way to reconcile these competing demands, which impact economies, trade and globalization, and ultimately nutrition.

The food system and our diets are often examined in terms of how they influence environmental outcomes such as environmental and ecosystem degradation and climate variability. For example, evidence suggests that the food system as a whole contributes 15%–28% to overall greenhouse gas emissions in high-income countries, which includes all aspects of a functional food supply chain, from agricultural production through processing, distribution, retailing, home food preparation and waste.[3]

It is also clear that the way in which animal-source foods are produced can impact environmental and climactic triggers such as the intensification of methane production, which leads to increases in greenhouse gas emissions, with ruminant animals having a bigger impact than those animals (e.g., fish and chicken) whose place is lower on the food chain. That said, ruminants have the advantage of being able to utilize pasture which would otherwise have no nutritional value. Of course they are not exclusively dependent on pastureland, and if they are fed concentrated feeds instead of being grazed, they produce relatively small amounts of the GHG methane, so the issue of their environmental impact is a complex one. Nevertheless, if current dietary trends continue at their present rate, they could by 2050 fuel an estimated 80% increase in global agricultural GHG emissions from food production and global land clearing. Moreover, these dietary shifts are greatly increasing the incidence of non-communicable diseases.[4]

Chapter 3.3 | Sustainable Diets for Nutrition and Environmental Health:
The impact of food choices, dietary patterns and consumerism on the planet

166

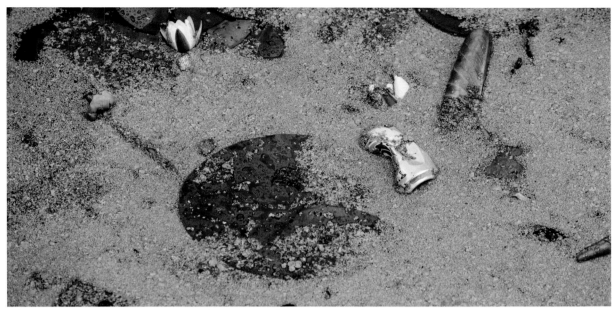

What we consume influences environmental outcomes such as environmental and ecosystem degradation.
Source: Mike Bloem

Figure 2 | **The food conversion ratio of various animal-source foods**

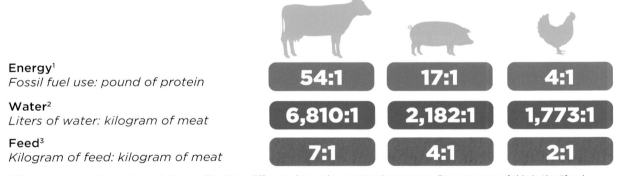

Energy[1]
Fossil fuel use: pound of protein

| 54:1 | 17:1 | 4:1 |

Water[2]
Liters of water: kilogram of meat

| 6,810:1 | 2,182:1 | 1,773:1 |

Feed[3]
Kilogram of feed: kilogram of meat

| 7:1 | 4:1 | 2:1 |

Different sources of animal protein in our diet place different demands on natural resources. One measure of this is the "feed conversion ratio": an estimate of the feed, energy or water required to gain one pound or kilogram of body mass.

Sources:

1 Pimentel D. Livestock production: energy inputs and the environment. In: Scott SL, Zhao X, eds. Canadian Society of Animal Science Montreal: Canadian Society of Animal Science 1997:17-26

2 Water Footprint Network

3 Wang Y, Beydoun MA, Caballero B et al. Trends and correlates in meat consumption patterns in the US adult population. Public Health Nutr. 2010;13(9):1333-45

Yet animal-source foods can provide a variety of micronutrients that are difficult to obtain in adequate quantities from plant-source foods alone, especially vitamin A, vitamin B12, riboflavin, calcium, iron and zinc. Negative health outcomes associated with inadequate intake of these nutrients include anemia, poor growth, impaired cognitive performance, blindness and neuromuscular deficits. Not only are these foods high in many micronutrients; the nutrients themselves are often more bioavailable. Studies have shown that consumption of milk and other animal-source foods by undernourished children improves anthropometric indices and cognitive function and reduces the prevalence of biochemical and functional nutritional deficiencies, reducing morbidity and mortality. Although animal-source foods are important sources of essential nutrients, some sources high in saturated fats are also significantly increase the risk of cardiovascular disease and colorectal cancer (see **Text box 1**).

Text box 1 | **The animal production-consumption debate**

Most countries are shifting from plant-based diets to highly refined foods, meats and dairy products, with the exception of a few poor countries that cannot afford to make this leap. This is particularly seen in the urban middle classes. Americans account for just 4.5% of the world's population, but eat approximately 15% of the meat produced globally.[10] On average, the USA consumes 124 kg/capita/year compared to the global average of 38 kg/capita/year.

The countries that consume the least meat are found in Africa and South Asia, where the highest burden of undernutrition lies, with consumption in some countries as low as 8.5 kg/person/year in Ethiopia and 3 kg/person/year in Bangladesh. Meat consumption per capita refers to the total meat retained for use in a country per person per year. Total meat includes meat from animals slaughtered in countries, irrespective of their origin, and comprises pork, beef, poultry, lamb, horsemeat, and meat from all other domestic or wild animals such as camels, rabbits, reindeer, and game animals.

Production is attempting to keep up with current demand. However, this increased demand has serious ramifications for both the climate and human health. Production of foods from animal sources is resource-intensive, and is the major contributor to greenhouse gas emissions from the agricultural sector. Overconsumption and escalating demand for livestock has created ethical conflicts over ensuring animal welfare and limiting drains on the environment. In addition, many of these animals consume grains, resulting in a significant amount of land being assigned to growing feed. One-third of global cereal crop production is fed to animals, while we know that the world still faces serious famines and seasonal hunger periods.

This in itself presents an ethical dilemma: feed people to stave off hunger, or feed animals to keep up with the luxury diets of the middle and upper classes. There are also low-resource alternative sources, including the fortification of staple foods and dietary supplementation, that should be considered in filling nutrient gaps for all countries. These sources of foods make significant contributions to nutrition, while leaving a smaller footprint for the planet. Farmed fish, mollusks, insects and protein-rich plant foods can serve as important and alternative sources of nutrient-rich foods (including protein, fatty acids, zinc, iron, vitamin B_{12} and vitamin D), as compared to muscle and organ meats from livestock.

Impacts of the changing environment on nutrition and health outcomes

Nutrition, the food system, and the environment are inextricably linked. However, measurements and indicators that assess how the environment impacts human health and nutrition are less clear. In general, natural resource measurements capture soil and water quality, biodiversity, tree and vegetation coverage, and pollutants in water streams, ocean water, ground water, soil, and air, as well as climate variability and change. How these measures relate to health outcomes is less clear. It is also not clear how changes in these indicators influence dietary patterns, "healthy" food systems and nutrition outcomes.

According to the 2014 IPCC report, the health of human populations will be impacted by shifts in weather patterns and other aspects of climate change due to alterations in temperature, precipitation and extreme weather events as well as ecological disruptions (i.e., changing patterns of disease vectors).[5] The IPCC also showed that the effects of climate change on crop and food production are currently evident in several regions of the world, particularly the abundance and distribution of harvested aquatic species and aquaculture production systems in various parts of the globe. These are expected to continue, with negative impacts on nutrition and food security for especially vulnerable people, particularly in some tropical low- and middle-income countries. "The nutritional quality of food and fodder, including protein and micronutrients, is negatively affected by elevated CO_2, but these effects may be counteracted by effects of other aspects of climate change."[5]

There are, of course, downstream negative impacts on food security, health and nutrition outcomes, with soil and water degradation, loss of biodiversity and reduction of ecosystems (including pollinators and forests). Temperature and rainfall shifts also have human health impacts due to weather extremes such as heat waves, droughts and floods. Land degradation, water issues, soil nutrient loss, and eroding crop genetic diversity threaten people's present and future livelihoods as well as their nutritional status.

Chapter 3.3 | Sustainable Diets for Nutrition and Environmental Health:
The impact of food choices, dietary patterns and consumerism on the planet

168

Figure 3 | **The effect of different diets on reducing risk of non-communicable diseases (NCDs)**

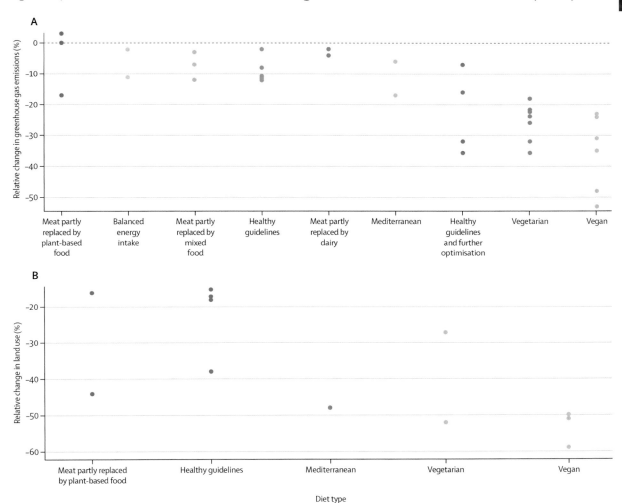

Legend in Lancet article is: Relative change of greenhousegas emissions and land use of alternative diets compared with baseline diets

(A) Point estimates of relative changes in greenhouse gas emissions from studies comparing environmental impacts of present dietary patterns with healthy and sustainable alternatives, in carbon dioxide equivalents per person per year.

An alternative diet category of switching from ruminant to monogastric meat intake was omitted because it contained only one study (–18% relative difference in greenhouse gas emissions). (B) Point estimates of relative changes in agricultural land use from studies comparing environmental impacts of present dietary patterns with healthy and sustainable alternatives, in square metres per person per year.

Source: Whitmee S, Haines A, Beyrer C et al. Safeguarding human health in the Anthropocene epoch: report of the Rockefeller Foundation-Lancet Commission on planetary health. Lancet 2015;386:1973-2028.

169

The concept of sustainability and sustainable diets

Sustainability implies a state whereby the needs of the present and local population can be met without diminishing the ability of future generations or populations in other locations to meet their needs or without causing harm to the environment and natural assets.

Globally, we are recognizing that the health of human beings cannot be isolated from that of ecosystems.[6] More debate has centered on how food insecurity and climate variability impact diets, and how our consumption patterns contribute to environmental degradation.[4] The concept of "sustainable diets" is one that promotes environmental and economic stability through low-impact and affordable foods, while at the same time improving public health through adequate nutrition.

Recently, the concept of sustainable food systems and diets has grown in importance. It is thought that while the benefit of the global food system is a safe, nutritious, and consistent food supply, that same system also places significant strain on land, water, air, and other natural resources. The idea of "sustainable diets," which combines dietary recommendations with healthier environments and consumers, was proposed in the 1980s and was recently revived. FAO[7] further defined sustainable diets as "those diets with low environmental impacts which contribute to food and nutrition security and to healthy life for present and future generations." Sustainable diets are protective and are respectful of biodiversity and ecosystems; they are culturally acceptable, accessible, economically fair and affordable, nutritionally adequate, safe and healthy while at the same time optimizing natural and human resources. However, the complex web of determinants in sustainable diets makes it challenging for policy-makers to understand the benefits and considerations for promoting, processing, and consuming such diets. Better measurements and indicators must be developed to assess the impact of the various determinants on the sustainability of a diet and the tradeoffs associated with any recommendations aimed at increasing the sustainability of our food system and, ultimately, human health.[6]

Defining sustainable diets is important, yet more work is needed on what constitutes a sustainable diet from environmental, biological, cultural and health standpoints, at the global, regional, local and individual levels. A healthy diet requires the right nutrients and bioactive health components in the right amounts (see **Text box 2**). The implications of what we eat involve more than just the known constituents of food. The sustainability implication of the diet remains elusive and undefined. There is a need to assess what quantifies or qualifies a sustainable diet that can be benchmarked over time. This includes better indicators that measure the tradeoffs between the requirements of processing and packaging on the one hand and those of food safety, food protection and nutrient density on the other. Finally, these indicators need testing, further debate, and, most importantly, a negotiation among users and disciplines so that the best that our scientists and researchers have to offer can be reflected in the work carried out.

Text box 2 | **What is a healthy diet?**

A key feature of a healthy diet is dietary diversity – consuming a variety of foods across and within food groups to ensure adequate intake of essential nutrients. Fruits, vegetables, complex carbohydrates, nuts, fish, healthy vegetable oils and modest amounts of meat and dairy products are emphasized. Sugar, trans fats, processed meats and foods should be limited.[9]

One place to start is an understanding of the key drivers or determinants of a sustainable, culturally relevant, cost-effective food system that incorporates the best of local and exotic foods and ingredients in terms of dietary diversity, dietary quality, good nutrition and health. However, how can those drivers be measured and elucidated so as to ensure environmental sustainability and the health of ecosystems, while ensuring that dietary diversity and quality for humans is not compromised? It is not enough to examine the relationships of these determinants: we need to better understand how to promote diversity so as to mitigate the negative impacts of dietary transition while at the same time highlighting the positive effects of improving the efficiency and sustainability of food systems.[8]

There has also been an emerging movement toward foods and food choices based on values, ethics and concerns for the health and wellbeing of the consumer and the environment. This has been echoed by support for measuring "food miles," "carbon costs," "slow foods," "organic foods," "fair trade" and, more recently, efforts to tax and restrict portion size along with the sale and marketing of "obesogenic foods" and foods containing high amounts of sugar, salt and saturated fats.

Figure 4 | **Sustainable diets around the world**

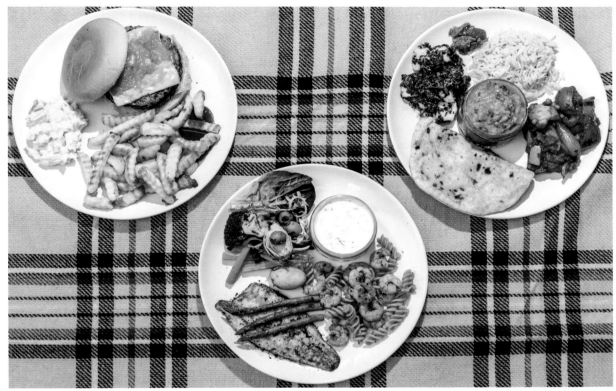

Popular meals around the world vary greatly in their composition and nutritional value. Three dishes, from North America, the Mediterranean and the Indian subcontinent (from left to right).
Source: Mike Bloem

Solutions to be taken for sustainable diets

Middle- and high-income countries are devoting more attention and publicity to the consumption of better-quality diets – both in terms of nutrition and of environmental sustainability. However, the financial cost of such diets is currently unaffordable for many.Inexpensive foods are often the least healthy: highly processed, high in sugar and fat, and high in energy content for every dollar spent.[11] In much of the world, the cost of even basic diets which meet mainly caloric needs exceeds daily wages due to escalating food prices.

Below are some examples of what policy, programs, individuals and researchers can do to begin instituting sustainable diets.

Policy levers for sustainable diets

- Governments can start by aligning food and agriculture policies with diet and nutrition policies. For example, the dietary guidelines should be better aligned with the constraints of the food system on the environment. Countries such as Brazil and Sweden have taken into account environmental indicators with their dietary guidelines. It is important, though, to ensure that these guidelines are useful, and that they are actually used by consumers.

- Governments also need to grapple with sustainability labeling, and should ensure that the food industry is not "abusing" this trend in order to sell unhealthy products.

- Governments can also encourage cooperative efforts in local and regional food system "hubs." This involves adding the necessary capacity and infrastructure to improve local food processing, distribution, and marketing so as to better reach consumers.

Program levers for sustainable diets

Chapter 3.3 | Sustainable Diets for Nutrition and Environmental Health:
The impact of food choices, dietary patterns and consumerism on the planet

171

There should be incentives that encourage farmers to grow food in a more sustainable way. Sustainable food production can be costly for some farmers or can dramatically change livelihood models away from cash cropping systems. Whether this change of focus should be effected by means of new subsidies remains a question. Farmers often grow whatever the market will take. If specific foods are in high demand, these are the foods that will be grown. This would mean changing the demand for certain foods with high environmental costs, such as beef.

There should be support for small-scale farmers in low- and middle-income countries to help them produce a greater proportion of their respective countries' own food supply, and to ensure that this food supply is diverse. Other ideas include:

- Encouraging governments to consider incorporating sustainably produced healthy foods into their food safety net programs

- Creating and incentivizing farmers' markets and community-supported agriculture (CSA) on-site farm stores and

- Moving greenbelt diversity closer to urban populations in order to reduce the distance between food production and the consumer and create "food hubs" – centralized locations for farmers to distribute farm products.

Individual levers for sustainable diets

Consumers have the right to make informed choices regarding what they consume. Navigating the complexity of what is a healthy diet and how this diet impacts on the environment is not an easy task, however. Education and access to knowledge are key. Some ideas include:

- Engaging the public health community in the evidence-based issues of sustainable food systems so that they can educate and work with the policy-makers, advocates, media, the food industry and other professionals in public health, nutrition and environment regarding potential solutions and involvement of the community

- Increasing education of the general public about the food system's contribution to climate change and the benefits of eating more locally produced food and reducing industrially produced meat consumption. Creating tools that provide information about how to choose environmentally preferable and healthy types of animal-source foods and

- Using social media to crowdsource messages that are important for the sustainable diets agenda.

Research levers

Although the need to advance commitments towards sustainable diets as a central aspect of sustainable development is clear, gaps nevertheless persist in our understanding of what constitutes a sustainable diet for different populations and contexts, and how to measure this. It also remains unclear how to assess these diets within our global food system and achieve environmental sustainability in our consumption patterns and dietary goals.[6]

- To identify approaches used to describe a sustainable diet, through specific, measurable, achievable, realistic and time-based descriptors.

- To explore options on how to measure a sustainable diet, in a systematic and reproducible way.

- To characterize what are the key determinants for a sustainable diet and how these determinants can be measured in a spatio-temporal way, perhaps using a suite of indicators and a consolidated index.

- To generate the evidence on how these determinants create opportunities as well as challenges concerning what is a sustainable diet for the future.

- To inform policy and programs with a view to improving dietary quality, nutrition and health.

Chapter 3.3 | Sustainable Diets for Nutrition and Environmental Health:
The impact of food choices, dietary patterns and consumerism on the planet

172

My personal view

Jess Fanzo

Through the act of eating, we are more than just consumers. Eating often involves moral decision-making rooted within the context of cultures, traditions and social structures that impact human nutrition and health outcomes in a globalized way. We have a responsibility as "eaters" to think about our actions and their consequences as we participate in an ever more globalized food system.

How can we still have people who go hungry? How can one-fifth of our children be chronically undernourished in body and brains most likely for the rest of their lives? How can we also have such high numbers of people living with extra weight putting them at risk of lifelong diseases that are costly for them and us and that impair quality of life?

At the same time, our planet is on the brink – with serious natural resource degradation, biodiversity loss and altered ecosystems. Diets play an important role in these multiple human and planetary burdens. It is our responsibility to ensure that the diets we consume are ones that are not only equitable, but also are healthy for our bodies and the planet. This is our task.

Further reading

Auestad N, and Fulgoni VL. What current literature tells us about sustainable diets: emerging research linking dietary patterns, environmental sustainability, and economics. Advances in Nutrition 2015;6(1):19–36.

FAO. Livestock's Long Shadow. Rome: Food and Agriculture Organization, 2006.

Garnett, T. What is a sustainable healthy diet? A discussion paper. London, UK: Food Climate Research Network, 2014.

IOM (Institute of Medicine). Sustainable diets: Food for healthy people and a healthy planet: Workshop summary.

Washington, DC: The National Academies Press 2014. Whitmee S, Haines A, Beyrer C et al. The Rockefeller Foundation–Lancet Commission on planetary health. Safeguarding human health in the Anthropocene epoch: Report of The Rockefeller Foundation–Lancet Commission on planetary health. Lancet 2015:60901-1.

References

1   1 Rockstrom J, Steffen W, Noone K et al. A safe operating space for humanity. Nature 2009;461(7263):472–475.

2   Vermeulen SJ, Campbell BM, Ingram JS. Climate change and food systems. Annual Review of Environment and Resources 2012; 37(1):195.

3   Garnett T, Appleby MC , Balmford A et al. Sustainable Intensification in Agriculture: Premises and Policies. Science 2013;341(6141):33–34.

4   Tilman D, Clark M. Global diets link environmental sustainability and human health. Nature 2014;515(7528):518–522.

5   Pachauri RK, Allen, MR, Barros VR et al. Climate Change 2014: Synthesis Report. Contribution of Working Groups I, II and III to the Fifth Assessment Report of the Intergovernmental Panel on Climate Change. 2014:151.

6   Johnston JL, Fanzo JC, Cogill B. Understanding sustainable diets: a descriptive analysis of the determinants and processes that influence diets and their impact on health, food security, and environmental sustainability. Advances in Nutrition: An International Review Journal 2014;5(4):418–429.

7   FAO. Biodiversity and Sustainable Diets: Directions and Solutions for Policy, Research and Action. Rome, Italy:FAO, 2010.

8   Fanzo JC, Cogill B and Mattei F. Metrics of Sustainable Diets and Food Systems. A Technical Brief. Bioversity International, Rome, Italy, 2012.

9   Nugent R. Bringing agriculture to the table: how agriculture and food can play a role in preventing chronic disease. Washington DC: Chicago Council on Global Affairs, 2011.

10 Stokstad E. "Could Less Meat Mean More Food?" Science 2010;327(5967):810–1.

11 Keats S, Wiggins S. Future Diets: Implications for Agriculture and Food Prices. Report, London: Overseas Development Institute, 2014. http://www.odi.org/sites/odi.org.uk/files/odi-assets/publications-opinion-files/8776.pdf. Accessed 23 June 2015.

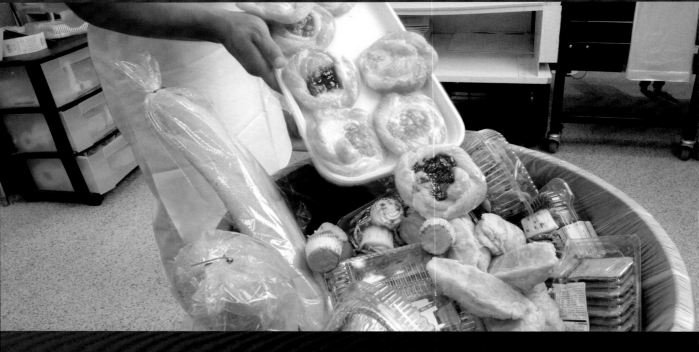

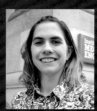

Jenifer Baxter

Head of Energy and Environment, Institution of Mechanical Engineers,
Westminster, London, UK

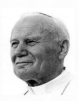

"Modern society will find no solution to the ecological problem unless it takes a serious look at its lifestyle."

Pope Saint John Paul II, *born Karol Józef Wojtyła (1920 –April 2005); Pope from 1978 to 2005.*

Key messages

- Approximately 4 billion tonnes of food is produced globally each year.

- Some 30–50% of all food produced is either lost or wasted.

- Levels of wasted food lead to overproduction in both the developed and the developing world.

- Engineering solutions can reduce food waste and protect the food-growing environment.

- Engineering solutions can use food waste for heat, power and fertilizer.

- Consumer behaviors can reduce food wastes in developed countries.

- Less food waste in combination with good engineering practices can lead to better access to food for those in developing countries.

Definitions

Food loss

The decrease in edible food mass at the production, post-harvest, processing and distribution stages in the food supply chain. These losses are mainly caused by inefficiencies in the food supply chains, like poor infrastructure and logistics, lack of technology, insufficient skills, knowledge and management capacity of supply chain actors, no access to markets. In addition, natural disasters play a role.

Food waste

Food which is fit for consumption being discarded, usually at retail and consumer level. This is a major problem in industrialized nations, where throwing away is often cheaper than using or re-using, and consumers can afford to waste food. Accordingly, food waste is usually avoidable.

Food wastage

Any food lost by wear or waste. Thus, the wastage is here used to cover both food loss and waste.

Source: Food Wastage Footprint and Environmental Accounting of Food Loss and Waste. Concept Note. Natural Resources Management and Environment Department Food and Agriculture Organization of the United Nations. March 2012.

Factors influencing the global phenomenon of food wastage

Across the globe, we currently produce around four billion metric tonnes of food per annum. The UN has projected that by 2100 the population could peak at 9–12 billion, creating an extra 3–5 billion mouths to feed.[1] Today we waste between 30–50% of all food produced: this happens at farms, in storage and transportation, and in factories and retail outlets, as well as in the home. This huge wastage is leaving people food-insecure and dependent on food banks in both the developing and the developed world.

This chapter will explore the differences between the developing and developed world and how different engineering solutions can reduce this waste. Through the application of these activities and a change in culture and attitude, the challenge of feeding the rapidly growing population may be less overwhelming than it seems.

In section 1, the developing and transitioning world will be discussed; in section 2, the potential opportunities for change in the developed world and their impact on developing and transitioning countries. Finally some general observations about engineering and the role of engineers in farming and nutrition will be offered.

The United Nations describes three types of countries: developing economies, economies in transition, and developed economies. These classifications are designed to reflect the characteristics expected with each type of economy, and some countries in the transition category will appear in more than one category.[2] This chapter will consider developing and transitioning nations together, and developed nations separately.

The Institution of Mechanical Engineers in its 2013 Global Food report[3] identified three areas where impacts will continue to cause problems for food production and climate change in the future. These are as follows:

- The area of land available for agriculture will reduce due to factors including environmental degradation, stresses related to climate change, and restrictions aimed at the preservation of ecosystems, as well as competition with other land use demands, such as biomass-derived energy initiatives, urbanization, transport, industrial activity and leisure needs.

- Increased competition for available water from urban developments and industry will reduce the quantities available for crop and livestock production. This will happen in a world of uncertain rainfall patterns, drought and flooding, due to the effects of global warming. The impact of global warming on water resources, the potential regional losses of fresh water accompanied by rising sea levels, and the subsequent consequences for

agriculture present a future global challenge whose potential extent is currently unclear.

- Energy costs, particularly for fossil fuels, are likely to rise substantially, with increasing demand and diminishing availability of easily exploitable secure supplies. This applies to fuels used directly to power agricultural machines, processing equipment, transportation and storage facilities, as well as to the significant amount of natural gas that is used in the production of fertilizers and pesticides.

Tackling these three challenges will be key to successfully reducing not only food waste, but also the associated unnecessary waste of energy, water, human resources and emissions and damage to soils and ecosystems. This will lead to more efficient food production, better access to food globally, and a reduction in the impact of food wastes.

1. Developing nations

Food loss is created in the developing world primarily through poor or low-tech approaches to the farming, harvesting, storage and transportation of crops. This can be due to inefficient farming techniques whereby food is damaged or remains unharvested and is left to rot.

This type of harvesting may be followed by inappropriate storage, in which there is insufficient cooling to keep crops fresh or early biodegradation by mold is increased through dense storage techniques that generate excess heat and humidity. Further losses can occur in the transportation of food: this may be due to lack of refrigeration or damage sustained by badly secured produce. This can be seen in rice losses in South East Asian countries: in China, a country experiencing rapid development, the rice loss figure is about 45%, whereas in less-developed Vietnam, rice losses are as high as 80%.

As nations move into the transitioning phase of development, the technologies used for efficient farming reduce the waste at production, but an increase is seen further along the food chain at the levels of transportation, storage, retail and the consumer.

In addition to this food waste being created by easier access to, and consumption of, food in transitioning nations, further packaging waste is produced. This is often unmanaged, as commercial economies experience growth faster than the transitioning nations can build the necessary infrastructure to manage wastes.

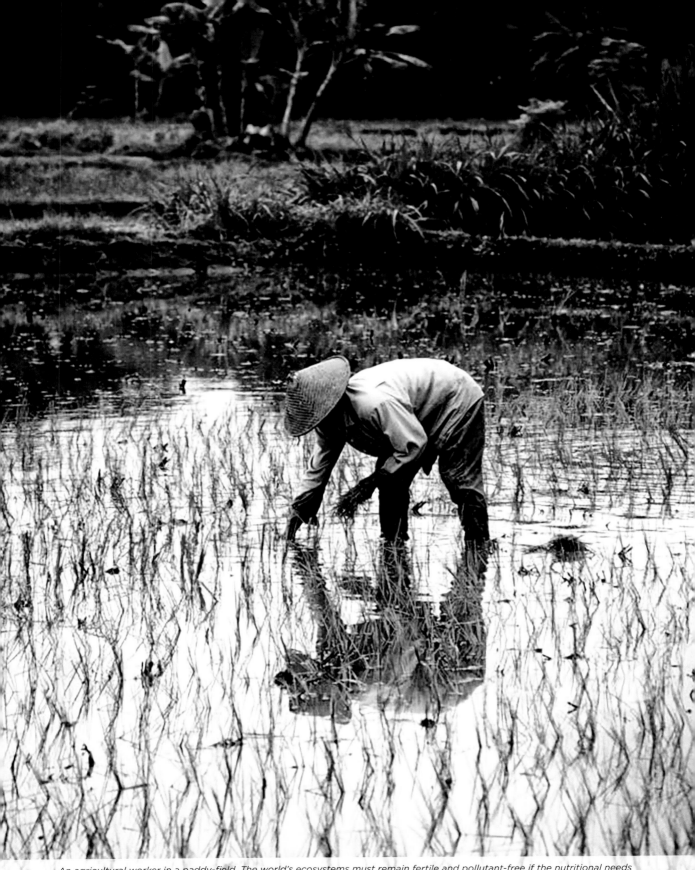

An agricultural worker in a paddy-field. The world's ecosystems must remain fertile and pollutant-free if the nutritional needs of the rapidly growing global population are to be met. Source: Institution of Mechanical Engineers

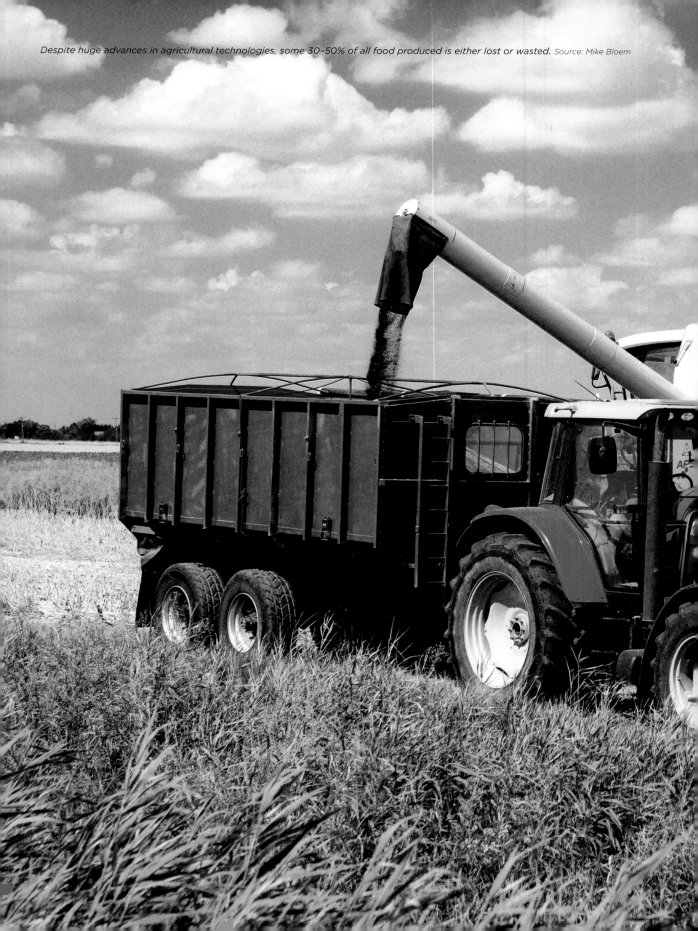

Despite huge advances in agricultural technologies, some 30–50% of all food produced is either lost or wasted. Source: Mike Bloem

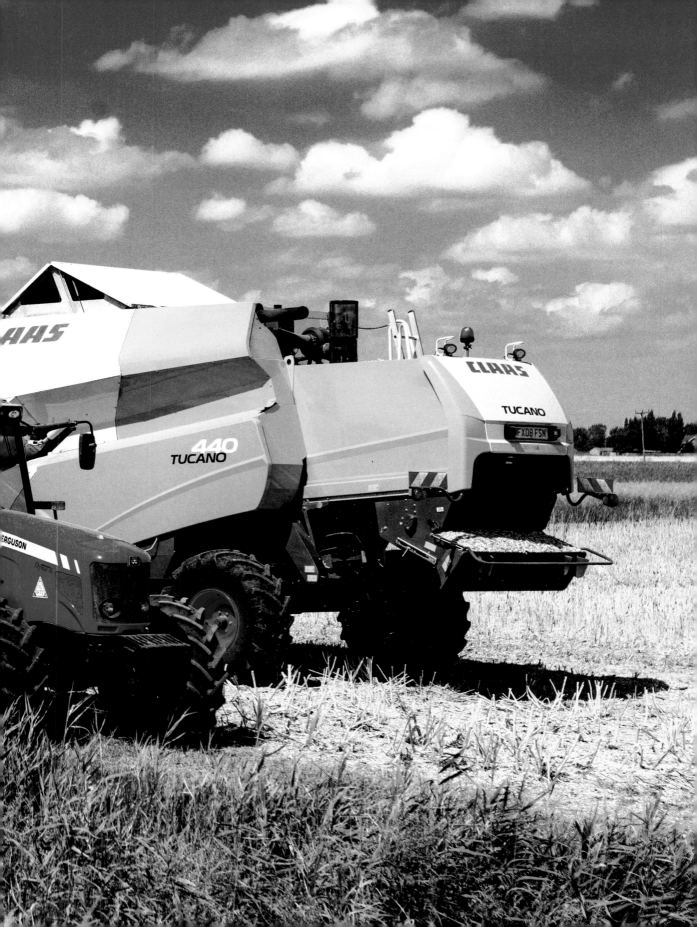

Engineering a solution in developing and transitioning nations

Across the globe, engineering has consistently provided solutions aimed at increasing food production, from the effective spreading of fertilizers and pesticides to advances in crop management techniques. Today we look to engineering to provide a low-carbon, clean solution that will help developing and transitioning nations to feed their populations without devastating the land. This is becoming increasingly important as populations grow and land space for farming decreases.

Agriculture produces greenhouse gas emissions: these emissions help to create a warmer climate that reduces access to water and fertile land areas. There is an evident need to engineer out the emissions from agricultural practices and wastes if the vicious cycle described above is to be stopped.

As the 21st century unfolds, the role of systems thinking in engineering is beginning to influence all aspects of life. From food production to consumer waste, engineering systems can be used both to reduce waste and to provide heat and power to communities. This power can then be used to create better storage and transportation for crops.

When considering systems in developing and transitioning nations, there are some technologies that are equally suitable to managing wastes and creating heat and power. The idea of combined heat and power – whereby a small gas or biomass generator provides both electricity and heating – is not a new technology, but is rarely thought of as useful in countries where there is too much heat. These technologies use anaerobic digestion: a process that digests food and sewage waste and produces a biogas can be used to generate both electricity and gas for adapted farm vehicles. Waste heat from this process can be used to produce cold from absorption chillers or electricity from the generator. Cooling can then be transported through pipes to manage storage spaces for food crops.[5]

An absorption chiller is a technology that uses heat and a concentrated salt solution to produce chilled water. Absorption refrigeration uses very little electricity compared to an electric, motor-driven refrigerator. Variable heat sources can be used to drive the absorption refrigerator.[6]

In many developing and transitioning countries where the climate is warm and sunny, the use of solar power for retail and domestic cooling is another technology that could significantly reduce food waste. There are two ways this can be achieved. Solar energy can be harvested through the heating of water on roof tops, and this water can then be used to drive an absorption chiller for air conditioning. The second approach is to use solar panels that produce electricity and can be deployed directly to drive refrigeration.

These types of technology can be particularly useful in regions where continuous mains electricity is intermittent. Taking the off-grid approach to managing cold not only reduces the food waste and maintains the nutrition value of the food; it also reduces carbon dioxide and other greenhouse gas emissions.

For this to be successful across the globe, support from developed countries will be required in terms of technology and skills transfer, along with aid to support infrastructure development. These technologies may not be successful without adequate support to help governments, at local and national level, to implement waste collection and management schemes.

2. Developed nations

In much of the developed world, food is affordable and readily available to us. But the value of food and the natural systems involved in food production are often not considered. People rarely think of the land, water and energy used to bring food to our tables, nor indeed of the related losses in terms of diminished soil quality, nitrogen depletion, the appropriation of natural land space for agriculture, water pollution, and the generation of emissions by energy production processes, fertilizers and wastes.

In high-income countries, such as those in Europe and North America, populations are stabilizing and people are generally living longer lives. In these countries, the problem of food wastage is different, often occurring further up the distribution chain as the understanding of production processes improves and access exists to appropriate storage, and to the energy required to support storage. Processing and distribution of food in developed countries is well established. However, it is at this level that food waste occurs, mainly due to behavioral characteristics associated with our "on-demand" lifestyles and increased wealth.

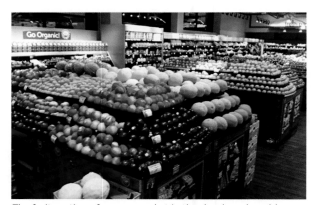

The fruit section of a supermarket in the developed world. Consumers need to become increasingly aware of their own contribution to the problem of food wastage.
Source: Ricardo Uauy

Considering first the technological improvements that can be made in developed countries, these are innovations in mature sectors. As previously discussed, the level of damage being caused to land, soil and water through intensive industrial farming in the developed world is serious. The difficulty of addressing this problem is compounded by the need for food producers to continue to produce more food to meet the high standards of retailers and to cover the wastages when crops are either ruined by weather events or else discarded by retailers for not meeting exacting standards.

So what can we do? We need to continue to raise awareness of the issue with consumers, suppliers and retailers. But we also need to look at the role of engineering in tackling this issue. **Figure 1** shows the food system in the UK and the areas where engineers can make positive change.

Figure 1 | **The cycle of production, storage & transportation, retail & consumption, and waste management**

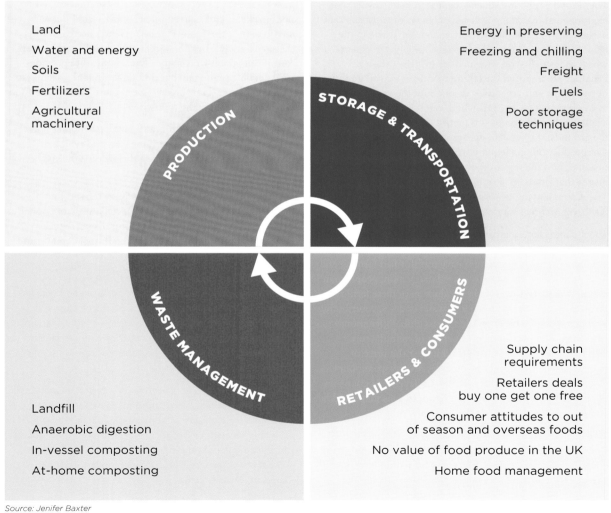

Source: Jenifer Baxter

Two changes could reduce emissions and waste from the food system shown in Figure 1. Firstly, the role of anaerobic digestion in the treatment of food waste. This is a process whereby active bacteria is added to food waste to digest it down, leaving a biogas of carbon dioxide, methane, and a liquor that is nutrient-rich and can be reused as fertilizer. This process can be combined with the treatment of sewage, creating a waste treatment and energy & heat production method. The current legislative framework around food production restricts the use of such fertilizers, however, and would need to be adjusted to accommodate new practices.

The second emission-reducing change is field wastage. As mentioned above, the purchasing policies of supermarkets in the UK, for example, actively encourage waste in the field. Produce is purchased through "supply agreements" in which the benefits are weighted against the producer. Penalties are imposed for failure to deliver agreed quantities of fresh fruit and vegetables throughout the year. This leads to overproduction in cases where suitable storage is not available. In addition to this, entire crops can be rejected on the grounds of physical appearance. The effect of overproduction, inadequate storage facilities for the extra produce, and the rejection of crops based on appearance means that up to 30% of the UK vegetable crop is wasted. The accompanying wasted resources of land, water, energy, fertilizers and fuels are not recognized in these losses.

The use of resources expands out from the field to the factories where fertilizers are produced. Manufactured nitrogen fertilizers for use in agriculture have transformed farming and food production, allowing us to feed many more people than ever anticipated. However, the production of these fertilizers involves fossil fuels that leach into water courses, contributing nitrogen oxide and carbon dioxide to global greenhouse gas emissions. The continued production of manufactured fertilizers may become cost-prohibitive if the price of natural gas increases and carbon taxes become commonplace, jeopardizing food security globally. In developed countries, there is an opportunity to explore new solutions that could be competitive for current fertilizer manufacture.

Two changes could be made to reduce the damage caused by fertilizer production. Firstly, the process of manufacture could be made even more efficient. This would include energy-efficient ammonia production and reducing the nitrogen dioxide emissions produced during the production of nitric acid for ammonium nitrate.

The second change would be to manufacture fertilizers using renewable sources, such as methane or hydrogen produced using energy from non-fossil fuel sources, such as wind or solar energy. Although this could be perceived as a relatively easy approach to reducing the emissions and pollution from fertilizer production and use, there is little or no sign that the fertilizer industry will move toward renewables. The main reason behind this is financial: changes would have to be made in the technology used for production and application, and the level of investment required to bring these changes is immense.[7]

In developed countries, significant amounts of food are transported long distances using refrigerated vehicles, and the food is then stored in refrigerated warehouses and supermarkets. This cold supply chain is a vital but energy-intense part of the food chain that creates access to food and keeps prices low. The recent Doing Cold Smarter report from Birmingham University's Energy Institute provides some details of innovative technologies that are beginning to tackle food and resource waste in these parts of the food chain. These include the following:

- Camfridge has created a novel magnetic cooling cycle that dispenses with refrigerant gases, and which the manufacturer claims will raise the energy efficiency of domestic fridges by 40%.

- Simply Air has developed a system to refrigerate supermarket display cabinets that makes use of cool air from outside, which the manufacturer says reduces energy consumption by 25% in the British climate, and by far more in colder ones.

- Sure Chill has developed a fridge that keeps its contents cool at a steady 4 °C for days or weeks on end without power by means of an ingenious energy storage system based only on ice and water. This means it works particularly well with solar panels or in countries with erratic grid electricity, and is ideal for protecting vaccines in remote rural areas.

- Dearman is in commercial trials of a piston engine driven by the phase-change expansion of liquid air or liquid nitrogen for a variety of applications, the first of which is a highly efficient transport refrigeration unit that delivers both cooling and power from a single tank of cryogen. The technology recently won the Innovation Award at the Cooling Awards 2015.

These examples demonstrate that we are able to innovate in these areas, but significant investment in, and championing of, these technologies by business is still necessary if we are to see changes in waste and resource reduction.

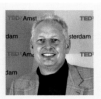

Leo Smit

Insightfully Innovate

The potential of sustainable food packaging

The packaging of food and beverages has undergone a host of innovations over the centuries. Amphorae for holding liquids and dry materials have been found that date back as far as the Neolithic period. Terracotta, ceramics, metal, leather and glass have all been used for storing beverages. Nowadays bottles made of polyethylene terephthalate (PET), invented in 1941, dominate the market for soft drinks. The introduction of the PET bottle (patented in 1973) was driven by the search for a packaging material lighter, and therefore more economical to transport, than glass. Today the focus has shifted from "lightweighting" to sustainability, and the spotlight is on bioplastics – plastics produced from biomass.

The promise of biodegradable plastics attracts considerable attention, on the basis of the belief that decomposition is a natural, and therefore favorable, discharge method. Yet a carefully executed Life Cycle Analysis (LCA)[8] has revealed that, contrary to this view, the composting of bioplastics has a higher environmental impact than other end-of life discharge techniques, such as recycling and even incineration. Moreover, biodegradable plastics cannot easily be left to rot in landfills, as ambient conditions are insufficient to cause the materials to fully decompose; industrial conditions at elevated temperatures are required for this.

If extended to the full usage of packaging materials, LCA shows that less than 10% of total energy usage is attributable to packaging,[9] but that this packaging has a key role to play in ensuring that the food it protects is not wasted. Unconsumed food not only fails to provide people with the nutrition they need; it also produces large amounts of carbon dioxide and methane as it decomposes, and the resources used in production and distribution are lost. Counterintuitively, then, the increased environmental burden of packaging can actually ease the overall burden on the planet by helping ensure that more food remains available for consumption and does not turn straight into waste.

In this light, the concept "sustainable packaging" may be redefined. Packaging is sustainable not simply if the consumption of resources matches the rate of renewal,[10] but if it delivers the most food consumed for the lowest environmental impact.[11]

Packaging materials and technologies that extend shelf life and prevent food wastage will therefore be key to minimizing the environmental impact of the food industry (**Table 1**). Given that some 30–50% of the food produced globally is either lost or wasted, theoretically 9 billion people could be fed if current production levels were to be increased only slightly. The essential requirement is to ensure that all the food produced is actually consumed.

Effective innovations cannot come solely from ingenious scientific innovations, however. Disciplines such as communications and psychology have an important role to play here. Many of the barriers to improving the environmental footprint of the food industry lie in the perceptions, attitudes and behaviors of consumers, who require educating to the true value of food packaging, and to the potential of the wide range of new packaging solutions now available. Food packaging is not a harmful thing in itself: it is essential for ensuring food safety as well as food availability, and many options exist for managing it sustainably.

Table 1 | **Examples of primary packaging technologies to extend shelf life**

Technology	Description	Potential impact on food waste
Multi-layer barrier packaging	Packaging that contains multiple layers to provide the required barriers to moisture, gases and odor. Specific requirements can be met using a combination of polymers, aluminum foil and/or coatings.	Keeping out moisture and oxygen delays product degradation.
Modified atmosphere packaging (MAP)	Gases are added to packaging before it is sealed to control the atmosphere within the pack, and then maintained by a high gas barrier film, e.g., through vacuum packaging. Carbon dioxide is added, alone or with nitrogen and sometimes oxygen, depending on the product (e.g., meat, cheese, fruit and vegetables).	Reduces respiration rates in the product and reduces growth of microorganisms.
Edible coatings	Based on a range of proteins, lipids, polysaccharides and their composites, can be used on fruit, vegetables, meat, confectionery and other products.	Creates a barrier directly around food products (rather than external packaging).
Ethylene scavengers	A range of different technologies that involve chemical reagents added to polymer films or sachets to absorb ethylene. Used for fruit and vegetables.	Removal of ethylene delays ripening and extends the shelf life of fresh produce.
Oxygen scavengers	Substances that remove oxygen from a closed package. They are often in powder form (e.g., rust powder) in a sachet. New technologies include oxygen scavengers in the film itself. Used for sliced processed meat, ready-to-eat meals, beer and bakery products.	Oxygen accelerates degradation of food by causing off-flavor, color change, nutrient loss and microbial attack (bacteria and fungi). Removing oxygen slows the degradation process and extends the shelf life of the food.
Moisture absorbers	Pads made from super-absorbent polymers, which absorb moisture. Used for fresh meat, poultry, and fresh fish.	Maintain conditions that are less favorable for growth or microorganisms.
Aseptic packaging	Packaging that has been sterilized prior to filling with Ultra High Temperature (UHT) treated food. This gives a shelf life of over 6 months without preservatives. Formats include liquid paperboard, pouches and bag-in-box.	High temperatures kill microorganisms, and tight seals on the packaging prevent the entry of microorganisms, gas or moisture that could promote degradation.

Source: Verghese K, Lewis H, Lockrey S et al. The role of packaging in minimizing food waste in the supply chain of the future. Centre for Design, School of Architecture and Design, RMIT University, 2013.

Behavior and attitudes to food

Finally, let us turn out attention to the role of behavioral change and attitudes to food in the developed countries. Retailers across the develop ed world have unique approaches to meeting consumer demands in their respective countries. The United Kingdom will be used as a case study region.

Food waste in the UK is not a new issue: the government-funded Waste and Resources Action Programme has been campaigning on the issue of consumer food for over a decade, but there has been very little change in real terms. History tells us that there is one particularly effective use for food waste that reduces emissions and produces more food: this is, to feed it to pigs. In the UK and across much of Europe, this practice is now illegal, mainly due to fears that it may cause Foot and Mouth Disease.

In the UK, the food retail sector is dominated by large supermarkets that have considerable buying power. To follow consumer preference, they will discard whole crops of food fit for human consumption based on appearance. When we consider our ability to feed the increasing population in the UK and across the globe, we already have enough food, but as a developed society we feel the need to have a buffer of food surplus amounting to around an additional 25% of food consumed. The value of wasted food as a commodity in the UK is so low that it is rarely considered. It is the carbon dioxide and methane emissions from this waste rotting in landfill that have driven change in waste management activities. Politically, it has been easier to tackle the physical management of food waste in the UK rather than the underlying cause of the problem in that nutritious food is discarded by the tonne every minute of every day because is not aesthetically pleasing.

In food outlets and the home in the UK, national and regional governments alike have created a waste management infrastructure that deals with food wastes. However, this approach has not placed further value on food, but rather allowed retailers and families to feel comfortable about wasting food. Significantly more action is required to bring intrinsic value to food and the entire food value chain.

As discussed earlier, while awareness of the problem has increased, not much has actually changed. A study published on August 12, 2015 in the journal *Environmental Research Letters* found that UK households are still throwing away 4.2 million tonnes of avoidable household food and drink annually – the equivalent of six meals every week for the average UK household. According to the research, 80% of food waste was found to be avoidable.12 Much of this waste is triggered at least partly by packaging innovations and labeling requirements. "Best before" dates are often interpreted as "Expired by" dates, which leads to a considerable amount of food being discarded unnecessarily.

It is clear that developed nations such as the UK need to do much more to reduce this waste and actively reuse it within a circular economy. Educating consumers to different behaviors is one factor here, but not the only one. The whole food system must be considered together, else the damaging nature of this waste socially, economically and environmentally will not be addressed.

In the UK, we have excellent knowledge of efficient agricultural practices; we have new clean fuels, biofuel and hydrogen options; we have excellent understanding of communicating behavioral change to both retailers and consumers in order to reduce wastes at the consumption end; and we have good technologies that treat food wastes and produce energy, heat and fertilizers as an output; and yet we fail to implement these in a meaningful way.

As described in section 1, using technologies such as anaerobic digestion on farms can create a systems approach to food production. In the UK, biogas can be used to run adapted farm vehicles, and the excess heat can be piped off to heat barns and other buildings where livestock may be housed, or alternatively used for cooling. Meanwhile the liquor can be used as a fertilizer. By taking a systems approach, those in the farming sector can save money through introducing efficiencies, reducing emissions and waste, and creating a more holistic approach to food production.

The incumbent infrastructure surrounding the food system in the UK, combined with the consumer's desire for "on-demand" products, means that creating a sustainable food system that reflects the needs of future generations as well as our own is a distant dream at present. In the current system, money talks, and it drives down the prices received by farmers and suppliers, creating an environment where the value of food is so low that discarding food is not considered a problem.

In the UK, we have specific behaviors and addictions to certain technologies that mean our ecological footprint for food is much higher than it need be. Our knowledge of advanced agricultural, processing, and storage technologies means that we waste proportionately less in the fields in the UK than is the case in developing countries. However, due to the supply chain of food into the UK and our desire to consume food products that are not available in the UK or else are out of season, our behaviors and attitudes can have a devastating impact on farmers overseas, who rely on UK retailers to purchase their crops.

This was outlined by The Sustainable Food Trust, using Kenya as an example. Kenya is a key supplier of fruit and vegetables to the UK and other European countries, but due to the stringent cosmetic standards of the supermarkets and consumer demand, up to 40 percent of the harvest is thrown away.13 Very recently in the UK, a few supermarkets have tried to move away from this, but it is very little action in what is a massive retail sector. We cannot solve this complicated issue overnight, but engineers are committed to raising awareness and to working with government and industry on this issue. The world does not have infinite resources, and we need to take action now to ensure people today and in the future are able to feed themselves sustainably and with nutritious food.

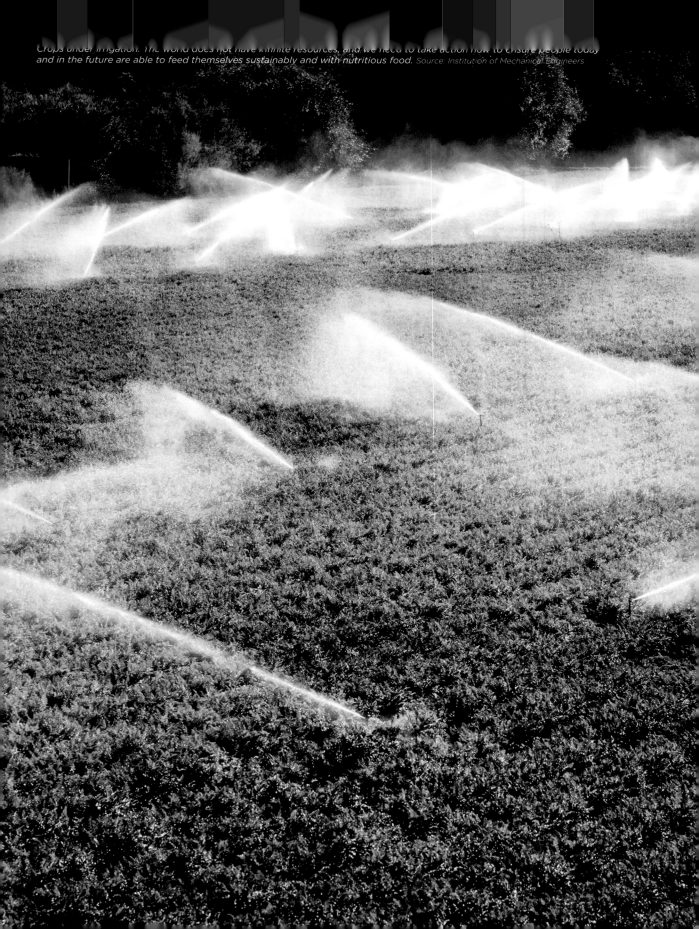

Crops under irrigation. The world does not have infinite resources, and we need to take action now to ensure people today and in the future are able to feed themselves sustainably and with nutritious food. *Source: Institution of Mechanical Engineers*

My personal view

Jenifer Baxter

Engineering out food waste in nutrition

As an engineer, it is relatively easy to see how to solve many of the problems globally associated with food wastage. Effective transportation chains, cooling and consumer management of food will enable it to last longer and to retain its nutritional value, thereby helping to improve health globally. However, these changes do not all involve new technologies, and they are not being implemented in developed countries due to the high financial investment and potential policy changes that would be necessary to create a clean and low-waste food chain.

The low political and financial value placed on waste food in developed countries has led to a situation whereby low income families are seeking support from charity food banks while a waste management infrastructure has evolved that is designed to deal with huge amounts of waste fit for human consumption. The lack of political will to change things for the better has in turn stifled innovation and created a society in which food must be perfectly formed in order to perceived as fit for consumption rather than being seen as nutritious fuel for humans.

In the developing nations, there is an opportunity – if it can be financially supported – to improve the situation and create a sustainable and clean food production environment through the implementation of policies and technologies described in this chapter. Without forward planning for developing and transitioning nations, there will much more food waste globally as populations swell and associated resources are wasted, driving up emissions and contributing to global warming.

We can feed the projected population of 2075 today, but it is necessary to change our attitudes, behaviors and technologies to ensure that everyone in the world, developing and developed, benefits.

Further reading

WRAP, *Synthesis of compositional food waste: sites/files/wrap/hhfdw-synthesis-food-waste-composition-data.pdf.*

Counting the cost of food waste: EU Food Waste Prevention, House of Lords. http://www.publications.parliament.uk/pa/ld201314/ldselect/ldeucom/154/154.pdf

Food Wastage Footprint: Impact on Natural Resources. Food and Agriculture Organization of the United Nations. http://www.fao.org/docrep/018/i3347e/i3347e.pdf

References

1   *Global Food: Waste Not, Want Not. Institution of Mechanical Engineers 2013.*

2   *http://www.un.org/en/development/desa/policy/wesp/wesp_current/2013country_class.pdf .*

3   *Global Food: Waste Not, Want Not. Institution of Mechanical Engineers 2013.*

4   *Global Food: Waste Not, Want Not. Institution of Mechanical Engineers 2013.*

5   *Doing Cold Smarter, University of Birmingham. 2015.*

6   *http://www.johnsoncontrols.com/content/dam/WWW/jci/be/integrated_hvac_systems/hvac_equipment/chiller_products/absorption_single/Absorption_Single_Stage_Application_Guide_PDF.pdf.*

7   *https://www.soilassociation.org/LinkClick.aspx?fileticket=trTYwH9W6Ck%3D&tabid=1862. 20/10/2015.*

8   *Rossi V, Cleeve-Edwards N, Schenker U et al. Life cycle assessment of end-of-life options for two biodegradable packaging materials: Sound application of the European waste hierarchy. Presented at avniR, November 6–7, 2012, Lille.*

9   *Verghese K, Lewis H, Lockrey S et al. The role of packaging in minimizing food waste in the supply chain of the future. Centre for Design, School of Architecture and Design, RMIT University, 2013.*

10 *Robertson GL, Trends in food packaging. fstjournal.org August 24, 2015.*

11 *McEwan Associates. The Value of Flexible Packaging in Extending Shelf Life and Reducing Food Waste. Flexible Packaging Association, 2014.*

12 *http://www.wrap.org.uk/content/household-food-and-drink-waste-uk-2012. Accessed October 20, 2015.*

13 *http://sustainablefoodtrust.org/articles/global-food-waste. Accessed October 20, 2015.*

From Science to Solutions: Effective deployment of evidence-based science for improved nutrition and successful policy-making at international, national and local levels

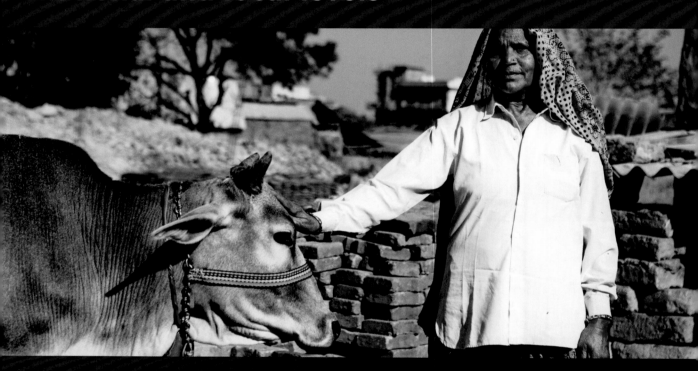

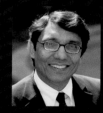

Zulfiqar A Bhutta
Founding Director, Centre of Excellence in Women and Child Health, The Aga Khan University, Karachi, Pakistan; and Co-Director & Director of Research, Center for Global Child Health, The Hospital for Sick Children, Toronto, Canada

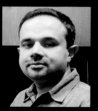

Jai K Das
Assistant Professor, Centre of Excellence in Women and Child Health, The Aga Khan University, Karachi, Pakistan

"Our foremost priority is the removal of poverty, hunger and malnutrition, disease and illiteracy. All social welfare programmes must be implemented efficiently. Agencies involved in the delivery of services should have a strong sense of duty and work in a transparent, corruption-free, time-bound and accountable manner."

Pratibha Patil, 12th President of India (2007–12)

Key messages

- Globally, 159 million children under age 5 are too short for their age (stunted), 50 million do not weigh enough for their height (wasted), and 41 million are overweight.

- Although a great deal of progress is being made in reducing malnutrition, this is still too slow and too uneven, while some forms of malnutrition – namely adult overweight and obesity – are actually increasing.

- A concerted effort from both the nutrition-specific and nutrition-sensitive sectors is required for addressing both kinds of malnutrition synergistically.

- Steps are required to create a more enabling political and financial environment, along with nutrition-friendly systems, to drive sustainable development forward.

The burden of malnutrition

Malnutrition affects all countries of the world and one in three people globally. Nearly half of all countries in the world are currently dealing with more than one type of malnutrition. There are about 795 million people undernourished worldwide (down by 17% over the past decade), of which the vast majority – 780 million – live in the developing regions of the world.[1]

Malnutrition is highly prevalent among women and children. In the year 2014, of the 667 million children in the world under 5 years of age, an estimated 159 million – almost a quarter of the population – was stunted. Moreover, this burden was unevenly distributed, as 90% of the stunted children are from low- and middle-income countries (LMIC)[2] (**Figure 1**). There has been a decrease in the prevalence of stunted children since 1990 (from 39.6% to 23.8%), but it has been highly disparate, as upper-middle-income countries have observed a 77% decrease, while only a 32% decrease has occurred in low-income countries. Wasting affects the lives of 50 million children across the globe, as approximately one in every 13 children in the world is wasted and nearly a third of all wasted children are severely wasted, with a global prevalence in 2014 of 2.4 per cent.[2,3]

At the other extreme, the burden of overweight and obese children is rising, as there were 41 million overweight children in the world in 2014 – about 10 million more than there had been two decades ago, as the prevalence of overweight went up between 1990 and 2014, from 4.8% to 6.1%. This rise has been observed in all regions of the world, and these numbers have doubled in LMIC since 1990 from 7.5 million to 15.5 million.[2] In 2014, almost half of all overweight children under 5 lived in Asia and one quarter in Africa. Africa has witnessed a massive 91% increase since 1990, Asia 22%, and Latin America and the Caribbean 5%.[2] The rate of increase in childhood obesity has been more than 30% higher than that of high-income countries. If the number of obese children keeps rising globally at the current rate, there will be more than 70 million overweight and obese by the year 2025. Without an intervention, these overweight and obese children will probably continue to be obese during adolescence and adulthood and will be more likely to develop non-communicable diseases. The relevance of nutrition during pregnancy and early infancy in defining short-term health and survival has been well established, and the Developmental Origins of Health and Disease (DOHaD) paradigm suggests that the effects of early nutrition and

Figure 1 | **Global prevalence and distribution of stunting**

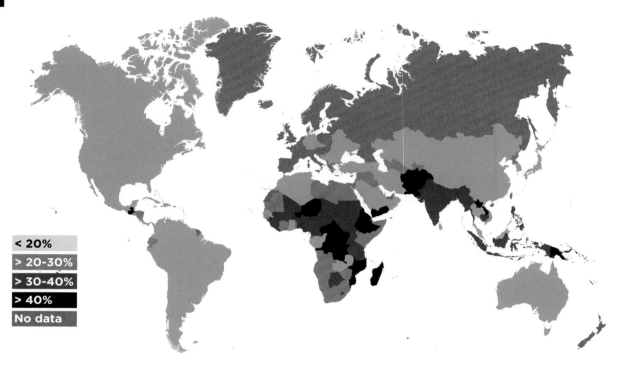

< 20%
> 20-30%
> 30-40%
> 40%
No data

Source: Levels and trends in child malnutrition. UNICEF – WHO – World Bank Group joint child malnutrition estimates.

growth are closely linked to long-term health, including manifestation of chronic disease in adult life (diabetes mellitus, metabolic syndrome).

Although it has decreased over the years, the prevalence of low BMI (<18.5 kg/m²) in adult women in Africa and Asia still remains higher than 10%, while the prevalence of overweight (BMI ≥25 kg/m²) and obesity (BMI ≥30 kg/m²) has been rising in all regions.[4] On the other hand, nearly half of all pregnant women are anemic, and 19% have iron deficiency anemia.[4] Women who are underweight before pregnancy have a 25% higher risk of preterm birth, and a 64% higher risk of having small-for-gestational-age (SGA) babies. In 2010, an estimated 32.4 million infants were born SGA, which is 27% of all births in LMICs; of these, 10.6 million infants were born at term and were low birth weight (LBW).[5] The global prevalence of LBW is 15.5%, which amounts to about 20 million infants born each year, 96.5% of them in developing countries. Vitamin and mineral deficiencies are highly prevalent throughout the developing world, including deficiencies in vitamin A, iron, iodine, zinc and folate.

Nutrition-specific actions

There are tried and tested interventions which can tackle most of the existing burden affecting women and child malnutrition. We undertook a comprehensive review of potential interventions, aiming to assess the evidence of the potential nutritional interventions and to estimate their effect on nutrition-related outcomes of women and children (**Table 1**).

Among the maternal interventions, daily iron supplementation results in a 69% reduction in incidence of anemia, a 20% reduction in incidence of LBW, and an improved mean birth weight. Multiple micronutrient (MMN) supplementation during pregnancy significantly decreases the number of LBW infants (by 14%) and SGA infants (by 13%). By comparison with standard iron and folate use, MMN supplementation results in a significant 11% decrease in the number of LBW and a 13% decrease in SGA babies, and demonstrates comparable effects on rates of anemia and iron deficiency anemia. Balanced protein energy supplementation reduces the incidence of SGA by 32% and risk of stillbirths by 45%.

Table 1 | **Nutrition-specific interventions and impacts**

Intervention	Estimates
Maternal Iron and Iron / Folic acid Supplementation	LBW (RR: 0.81, 95% CI: 0.68–0.97)
	Birth weight (MD: 30.81g, 95% CI: 5.94–55.68)
	Hemoglobin (MD: 8.88 g/l, 95% CI: 6.96–10.80)
	Anemia at term (RR: 0.30, 95% CI: 0.19–0.46),
	Iron deficiency (RR: 0.43, 95% CI: 0.27–0.66)
	Iron deficiency anemia (RR: 0.33, 95% CI: 0.16–0.69)
	Side effects (RR: 2.36, 95% CI: 0.96–5.82)
	Preterm birth (RR: 0.88, 95%CI: 0.77, 1.01)
	Neonatal death (RR: 0.90, 95%CI: 0.68, 1.19)
Maternal Multiple Micronutrient Supplementation	LBW (RR: 0.88, 95%CI: 0.86–0.91)
	SGA (RR: 0.89, 95% CI: 0.83–0.96)
	Stillbirth (RR: 0.92, 95% CI: 0.86–0.99)
Maternal Calcium Supplementation	Pre-eclampsia (RR:0.45, 95% CI: 0.31–0.65)
	Birth weight (MD: 56.40g, 95% CI: 13.55–99.25)
Maternal Balanced Energy Protein Supplementation	SGA (RR: 0.79, 95% CI: 0.69–0.90)
	Stillbirth (RR: 0.60, 95% CI: 0.39–0.94)
	Birth weight (MD:40.96g, 95%CI: 4.66–77.26)
Breastfeeding Promotion	Educational/counseling interventions increased EBF by 43% (9%–87%) at day 1, by 30% (19%–42%) till 1 month, and by 90% (54%, 134%) from 1–6 months
	Significant reductions in rates of no breastfeeding were also observed; 32% (13%, 46%) at day 1, 30% (20%, 38%) 0–1 month, and 18% (11%, 23%) for 1–6 months
Complementary Feeding Promotion	Nutrition education in food secure populations
	Height gain (SMD: 0.35; 95% CI: 0.08–0.62)
	HAZ scores (SMD: 0.22; 95% CI: 0.01–0.43)
	Stunting (RR: 0.70; 95% CI: 0.49–1.01)
	Weight gain (SMD: 0.40; 95% CI: 0.02–0.78)
	Nutrition education in food insecure population
	HAZ (SMD: 0.25; 95% CI: 0.09–0.42)
	Stunting (RR: 0.68; 95% CI: 0.60–0.76)
	WAZ (SMD: 0.26; 95% CI: 0.12–0.41)
	CF provision with or without education in food insecure population
	Height (SMD: 0.31; 95% CI: 0.02–0.6)
	HAZ (SMD: 0.41; 95% CI: 0.08–0.75)
	WAZ (SMD: 0.23; 95% CI: 0.06–0.42)
	Stunting (RR: 0.33; 95% CI: 0.11–1.00)
Vitamin A Supplementation (6 months to 5 years)	All-cause mortality: (RR:0.76, 95% CI: 0.69–0.83)
	Diarrhea related mortality (RR: 0.72, 95% CI: 0.57–0.91)
	Incidence of diarrhea (RR: 0.85, 95%CI:0.82–0.87)
	Incidence of measles (RR:0.50 95%CI: 0.37–0.67)
	Measles related mortality (RR:0.80,95%:0.51–1.24)
	ARI related mortality (RR: 0.78, 95%CI:0.54–1.14)
Zinc Supplementation	Height (6 mo–1 year) (SMD:0.26, 95%CI:0.19, 0.33)
	Weight (6 mo–1 yr) (SMD:0.31, 95%CI:0.25–0.38)
	Incidence of diarrhea (RR:0.87, 95%CI:0.86–0.89]

ARI: *Acute respiratory infections;*
EBF: *Exclusive breastfeeding;*
MD: *Mean difference;*
SMD: *Standard mean difference;*

CF: *Complementary feeding;*
HAZ: *height-for-age z score;*
RR: *Relative risk;*
WAZ: *weight-for-age z score.*

CI: *Confidence interval;*
LBW: *Low birth weight;*
SGA: *small-for-gestational age;*

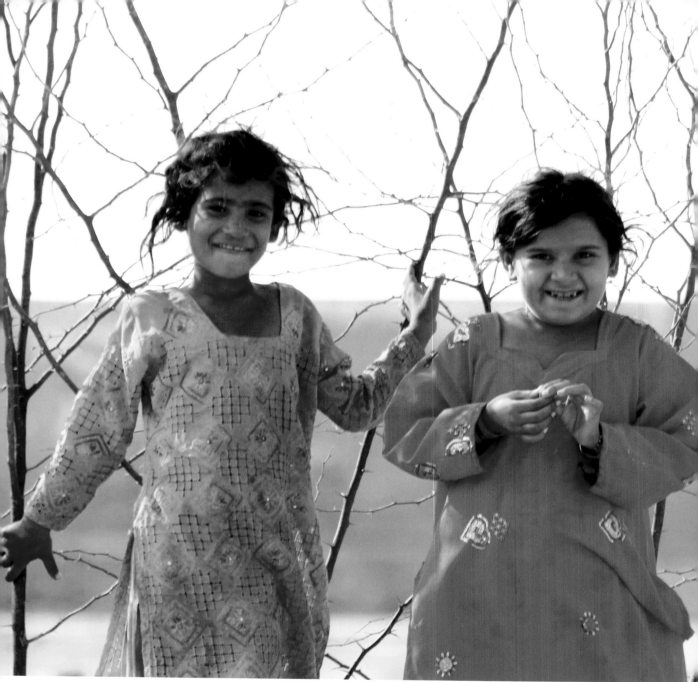

The double burden – within a rural community of Pakistan.
Source: Department of Pediatrics and Child Health, Aga Khan University, Karachi

Among the maternal malaria prevention interventions, antimalarials (when given to pregnant women) increase the mean birth weight significantly, cause a 43% reduction in LBW, and reduce severe antenatal anemia by 38%, while insecticide-treated bed nets in pregnancy reduce LBW by 23% and fetal loss in the first to fourth pregnancy by 33%.

Smoking cessation interventions also reduce LBW by 17% and preterm birth by 14%, accompanied by an increase in birth weight.[6] Recent research has underscored linkages of preconception interventions with improved maternal,

perinatal and neonatal health outcomes, and it has been suggested that several proven interventions recommended during pregnancy may be even more effective if implemented before conception.

Among the neonatal and child interventions, educational/counseling interventions increase exclusive breastfeeding (EBF) rates by 43% at day 1, by 30% till 1 month, and by 90% from 1–6 months, with significant reductions in rates of zero breastfeeding – 32% at day 1, 30% for 0–1 month, and 18% for 1–6 months. Vitamin A supplementation reduces all-cause mortality by 24% and brings about a 14% reduction in the risk of infant mortality at six months; it also reduces diarrhea-related mortality by 28% in children 6–59 months of age and additionally reduces the incidence of diarrhea and measles in this age group. Intermittent iron supplementation in children reduces the risk of anemia by 49% and iron deficiency by 76%; it also significantly improves hemoglobin and ferritin concentration.

Complementary feeding for infants refers to the timely introduction of safe and nutritional foods in addition to breastfeeding, i.e., clean and nutritionally rich additional foods introduced at about six months of infant age. These foods are typically provided to children from 6 to 24 months of age, and multiple complementary nutrition promotion interventions targeted to improve the nutritional status of children have been reviewed and have been shown to be effective.

Multiple micronutrient supplementation during childhood shows small effects on outcomes of growth, including improved length/height and weight, but there is limited evidence for an impact on outcomes such as morbidity and cognitive function. Preventive zinc supplementation in populations at risk of zinc deficiency reduces the incidence of premature delivery, decreases morbidity from childhood diarrhea and acute lower respiratory infections, and increases linear growth and weight gain among infants and young children. Therapeutic zinc supplementation as an adjunct in the treatment of diarrhea has been shown to reduce the duration of acute diarrhea by 0.5 days and that of persistent diarrhea by 0.68 days.[6]

Most of the evidence on preventing obesity in specific settings comes from schools. A recent meta-analysis of multiple studies shows moderately strong evidence of the effectiveness of school-based interventions to address childhood obesity.[7,8] These include professional development for teachers and other staff to train them in implementing health promotion strategies and activities, as well as support for parents in encouraging children to be more active, eat more nutritious foods, and spend less time in screen-based activities at home.

Nutrition-sensitive actions

At a global level, the evidence is clear, and it is largely agreed that nutrition cannot be improved through nutrition-specific interventions alone but requires a broader approach, drawing on sectors which can aid or augment these nutrition-specific actions. This sphere of activity is better known as nutrition-sensitive interventions. Improvements in development outcomes – such as poverty alleviation, food

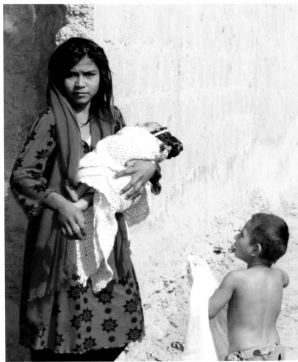

Motherhood at an early age.
Source: Department of Pediatrics and Child Health,
Aga Khan University, Karachi

security, women's education and empowerment, access to improved water and sanitation, social protection, agricultural interventions and improved food supply – are powerful drivers for improved nutrition.[9] Some developing countries, including Vietnam, Brazil, Bangladesh and Nepal, have done really well in combating undernutrition through the combination of nutrition-specific and nutrition-sensitive interventions. Their example may inspire other countries to achieve the same.

Maternal education and empowerment can have a positive influence not only on the health of the mother herself but also on child health, growth and development. Evidence suggests that the risk of stunting decreases significantly among mothers with at least some primary schooling and falls even more sharply among mothers with secondary schooling; paternal education at both primary and secondary level also reduces the risk of stunting.[9] Despite this overall association, wide discrepancies exist between individual countries, as the situation on the ground depends upon the quality of education as well as the quality of relevant data available. Education also helps develop personal capacity and increase earning-power and provides an opportunity to form social connections which can indirectly affect nutrition.

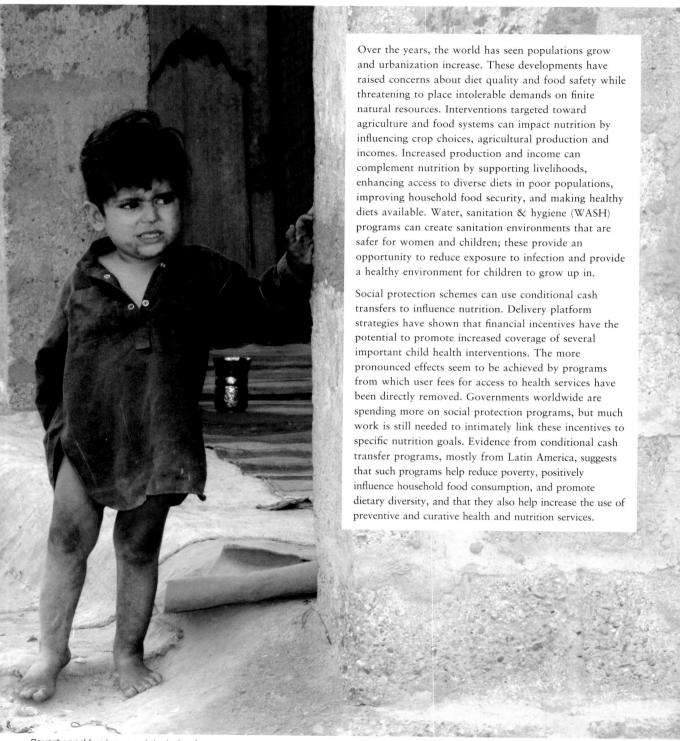

Over the years, the world has seen populations grow and urbanization increase. These developments have raised concerns about diet quality and food safety while threatening to place intolerable demands on finite natural resources. Interventions targeted toward agriculture and food systems can impact nutrition by influencing crop choices, agricultural production and incomes. Increased production and income can complement nutrition by supporting livelihoods, enhancing access to diverse diets in poor populations, improving household food security, and making healthy diets available. Water, sanitation & hygiene (WASH) programs can create sanitation environments that are safer for women and children; these provide an opportunity to reduce exposure to infection and provide a healthy environment for children to grow up in.

Social protection schemes can use conditional cash transfers to influence nutrition. Delivery platform strategies have shown that financial incentives have the potential to promote increased coverage of several important child health interventions. The more pronounced effects seem to be achieved by programs from which user fees for access to health services have been directly removed. Governments worldwide are spending more on social protection programs, but much work is still needed to intimately link these incentives to specific nutrition goals. Evidence from conditional cash transfer programs, mostly from Latin America, suggests that such programs help reduce poverty, positively influence household food consumption, and promote dietary diversity, and that they also help increase the use of preventive and curative health and nutrition services.

Poverty and hygiene are intertwined.
Source: Department of Pediatrics and Child Health, Aga Khan University, Karachi

Turning knowledge into action: What will it take?

Scaling up interventions: Despite consensus on actions to improve nutrition globally, much less is known regarding specific strategies to implement the right mix of nutrition-specific and nutrition-sensitive interventions equitably and at scale. The global coverage of key essential nutrition-specific interventions is low and variable. The median coverage of iron and folic acid supplementation for pregnant women is low, at 29%. Among the supplementation and fortification programs, vitamin A supplementation has the best coverage at 87%, followed by universal salt iodization (57%). Continued breastfeeding has one of the highest levels of coverage at 80%, but coverage is considerably lower for exclusive breastfeeding (35%) for infants under 6 months, and early initiation of breastfeeding within one hour of birth stands at just 51%. Even with this low coverage of essential interventions, wide variations exist between individual countries. This calls for urgent steps to help find ways and means to improve coverage, including reaching out to the poorest of the population through community-based interventions and innovations in financial incentives.

Leadership: The importance of strong political will and a sustained, focused leadership cannot be sufficiently stressed. The government, along with all the national and international organizations and players, needs to operate strategically to steer agreed initiatives at all levels of operation. The political environment should be conducive to nutrition-improving actions and investments in high-impact, cost-effective nutrition interventions. A coherent effort from all sectors (nutrition-specific and nutrition-sensitive) should be geared toward improving the nutritional status of the population, and appropriate policies should be adopted in a wide range of economic and social sectors.

Finances: The current budgets for health are not adequate in many LMICs, and budget specifically for nutrition-related activities is not sufficient at all. An analysis of 14 countries shows allocations to nutrition ranging from 0.06% of the total government budget to 2.90%. Ending malnutrition and striving for progress would require the scaling-up of nutrition financing and capacity to meet the nutrition needs. More governments at all income levels need to make their nutrition budget allocations more transparent, and to direct more financial resources to actions that will reduce malnutrition. Although there are budget allocations to nutrition-sensitive sectors such as agriculture, social protection, water, sanitation & hygiene, and education, this does not translate into a large impact on nutrition, as interventions in these sectors are not geared specifically toward nutrition. Innovation is required to make interventions and budgets more nutrition-sensitive.

Filling data gaps: To monitor progress nationally and internationally, it is essential to have regular, reliable and high-quality data. Of the 12 nutrition-specific interventions recommended by the latest Lancet Series, only four have internationally comparable coverage data, two have data collected on proxy indicators, and six have no internationally comparable data collected on them, while of the data collected on six interventions, only 13 countries collect them all.[3] This missing and poor data presents a significant obstacle to monitoring progress and accountability.

Building capacity and advocacy: A critical mass of nutrition-related or nutrition-trained people is required at all levels from policy makers, implementers, supervisors, healthcare professionals, and community workers, and care should be taken to develop and deploy human resources for nutrition at district level. These workers should have expertise and training in nutrition, and should work full-time on nutrition activities in both nutrition-sensitive and nutrition-specific sectors. Stronger mechanisms are needed to ensure that commitments result in action and give workers the confidence to increase their efforts on nutrition; this involves building better competency, reward, and incentive frameworks for particular parts of the nutrition workforce. There should be greater focus on strengthening behavior change and nutrition awareness activities and on building forms of community leadership, accountability and activism. Influential leaders from government, academia, media, business, and civil society should be encouraged to champion the cause of nutrition.

Researchers and academics: There is a continued need for academics and researchers to develop metrics, methods and tools to track progress of nutrition-related actions and to analyze their effectiveness. They should also evaluate the contextual factors around programs and suggest ways to amend or improve them.

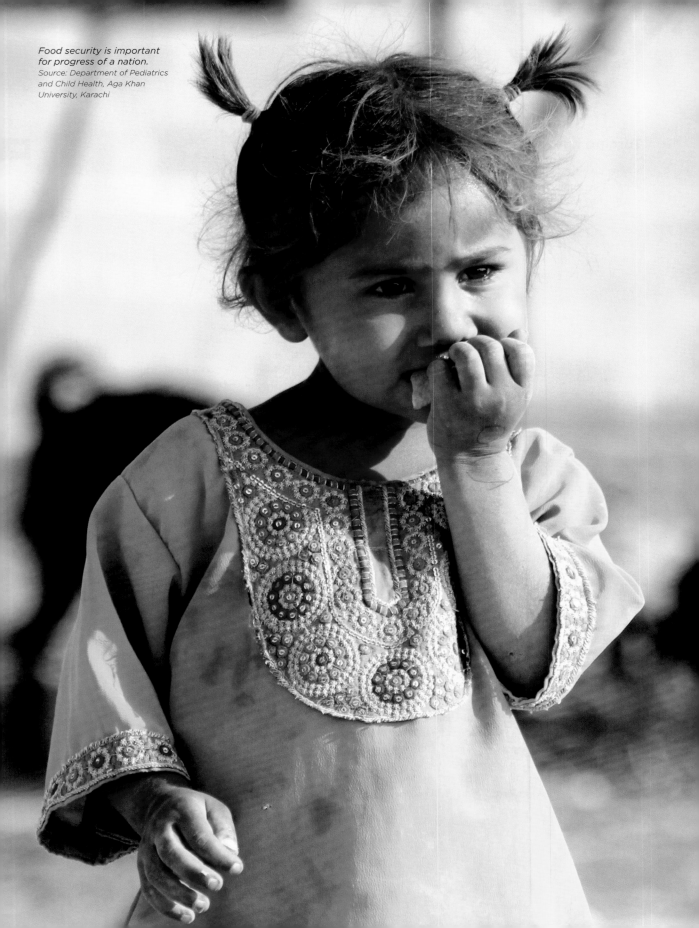

My personal view

Zulfiqar A Bhutta

Improving the nutritional status of the population is intrinsically linked to economic development. It is high time for leaders to recognize this and place nutrition at the front of any development agenda and regard nutritional indicators as development indicators rather than ones that relate solely to health.

There is a virtuous circle of escalating performance between improved nutrition status and sustainable development. Steps are required to create more enabling political environments, healthier food environments, and nutrition-friendly systems.

Further reading

Global Nutrition Report 2015: Actions and Accountability to Advance Nutrition and Sustainable Development

The Lancet Nutrition Series 2013

Levels and trends in child malnutrition. UNICEF – WHO – World Bank Group joint child malnutrition estimates. 2015

WHO e-Library of Evidence for Nutrition Actions (eLENA)

References

1   FAO, IFAD, WFP. *The State of Food Insecurity in the World 2015. Meeting the 2015 international hunger targets: taking stock of uneven progress. Rome, FAO.* available at http://www.fao.org/publications/card/en/c/c2cda20d-ebeb-4467-8a94-038087fe0f6e/. Accessed on 27 September 2015. 2015.

2   IGME. *Levels and trends in child malnutrition. UNICEF – WHO – World Bank Group joint child malnutrition estimates. Key findings of the 2015 edition. Washington DC Sep 2015.* available at http://www.who.int/nutgrowthdb/jme_brochure2015.pdf?ua=1. Accessed on 26 September 2015. 2015.

3   International Food Policy Research Institute. *Global Nutrition Report 2015: Actions and Accountability to Advance Nutrition and Sustainable Development. Washington, DC. 2015.* available at http://ebrary.ifpri.org/utils/getfile/collection/p15738coll2/id/129443/filename/129654.pdf. Accessed on 27 September 2015. 2015.

4   Black RE, Victora CG, Walker SP et al. Maternal and child undernutrition and overweight in low-income and middle-income countries. *Lancet.* 2013;382(9890):427–451.

5   Lee A, Katz J, Blencowe H et al. National and Regional Estimates of Term and Preterm Babies Born Small-for-Gestational-Age in 138 Low-Income and Middle-Income Countries in 2010. *Lancet Global Health.* 2013;1(1):e26–e36.

6   Bhutta ZA, Das JK, Rizvi A et al. Evidence-based interventions for improvement of maternal and child nutrition: what can be done and at what cost? *Lancet.* 2013;382(9890):452–477.

7   Wang Y, Cai L, Wu Y et al. What childhood obesity prevention programmes work? A systematic review and meta-analysis. *Obes Rev.* 2015;16(7):547–565.

8   Waters E, de Silva-Sanigorski A, Hall BJ et al. Interventions for preventing obesity in children. *Cochrane Database Syst Rev.* 2011(12):CD001871.

9   Ruel MT, Alderman H. Nutrition-sensitive interventions and programmes: how can they help to accelerate progress in improving maternal and child nutrition? *Lancet.* 2013;382(9891):536–551.

The Power of People-Centered Nutrition Interventions

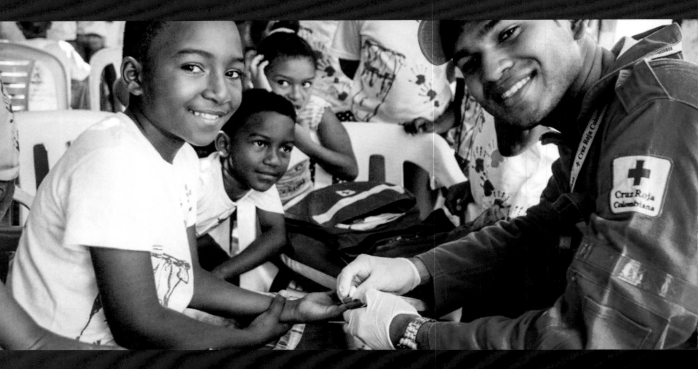

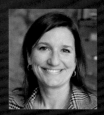

Sera Young
Assistant Professor of
Anthropology, Northwestern
University, Evanston, Illinois,
USA

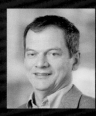

Shawn Baker
Director of Nutrition, Bill &
Melinda Gates Foundation,
Seattle, WA, USA

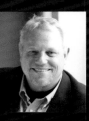

Rolf Klemm
Vice President of Nutrition,
Helen Keller International (HKI)
and Senior Associate in the
Program in Human Nutrition,
Department of International
Health, Johns Hopkins
Bloomberg School of Public
Health, Baltimore, MD, USA

"You can't solve a problem on the same level that it was created on. You have to rise above it to the next level."

Albert Einstein (1879–1955), *German-born theoretical physicist who developed the general theory of relativity.*

Key messages

- Nutrition problems are often more complex than they appear.

- People-centered design can effectively inform nutrition interventions and help ensure that the needs of end-users are better served.

- People-centered design is based on design thinking, which includes end-users in the selection and design of services, and products and behaviors.

- Design thinking is based on a five-step process: understand, define, ideate, make tangible, and iterate.

- Anthropology and allied social sciences can offer analogous methodologies for approaching the people-centered design of nutrition interventions.

- Putting people at the heart of nutrition interventions often requires hard work and creativity, but delivers better results in the long run.

"Meeting people where they are"

In a 2013 interview with *Wired Magazine*, Melinda Gates went on record as saying that people-centered design is in her opinion the single innovation that is changing the most lives in the developing world. She explained people-centered design as: "Meeting people where they are and really taking their needs and feedback into account. When you let people participate in the design process, you find that they often have ingenious ideas about what would really help them. And it's not a onetime thing; it's an iterative process."[1]

Melinda Gates's co-interviewee, the anthropologist and physician Paul Farmer – co-founder of the international social justice and health organization Partners In Health (PIH) and Professor at Harvard University – followed up this observation with an example of how people-centered design works in practice: "In Haiti I would see people sleeping outside the hospital with their donkey saddle under their neck — they'd been waiting there for days. And no one was asking them, 'What are you eating while you're waiting? What is your family eating while you're gone?' We have to design a health delivery system by actually talking to people and asking, 'What would make this service better for you?' As soon as you start asking, you get a flood of answers."

"The first time I went to Haiti and saw Paul in 2003," continued Melinda Gates, "he said, 'How can we expect them to take these pills if they have nothing to eat?' He decided that they needed healthcare workers who could follow patients, and that they had to be people from the community."

In other words, solutions were needed that addressed problems beyond the one that had been identified (in this case, medication adherence). Although this conclusion may sound obvious, the process of understanding what the problems *actually* are, and of developing appropriate solutions – i.e., design thinking – can be quite challenging. In fact, there are far more examples of public health solutions that ignore the end-user than of ones that are built with the end-user in mind. For this very reason, the goal of this chapter is to convey the relevance of people-centered design to nutrition interventions, and to share some strategies for putting people at the heart of nutrition interventions.

199

Design thinking

In its modern incarnation, people-centered design has its roots in technology, with antecedents in cooperative design, which originated in Sweden during the 1970s and gave designers and users an equal share in the design of IT systems. Participatory design and contextual design are also near cousins of cooperative design. Crucially, however, people-centered design as it is applied to nutrition is not technology-driven. As Atul Gawande (professor at the Harvard School of Public Health and also the Department of Surgery at Harvard Medical School) puts it, "People talking to people is still how the world's standards change."[2]

Although its origins are in the engineering world,[3] "design thinking" is a term that has achieved much wider currency in the past decade, thanks to both the business press and popular media.[4] In fact, it is now being discussed in forums as different as software design, personal growth, and clinical trial development.

While specific details of the approach to design thinking may vary, design thinking is basically a process whereby decisions about services, products and behaviors are built on a deep and clear understanding of peoples' context, needs and desires. Crucially, it includes end-users in the selection and design of services, products and behaviors, usually employing an iterative process to do this.

A street scene in India. Design thinking involves meeting people where they are.
Source: Sight and Life

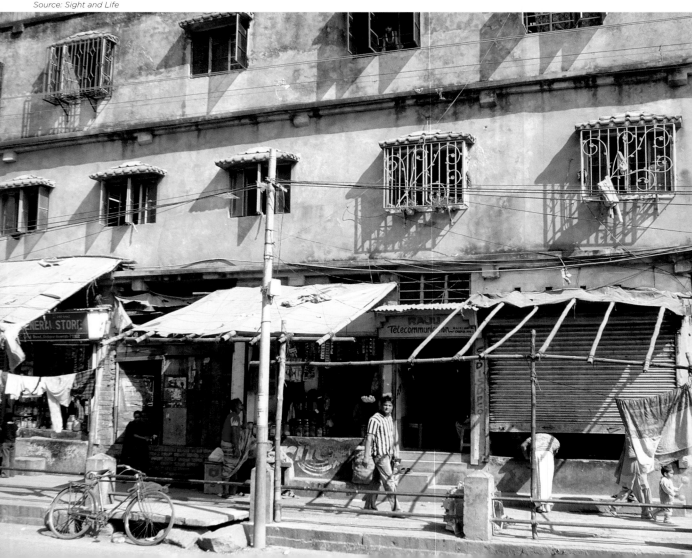

There are five basic steps to design thinking:

Step 1: Understand the issue

Step 2: Define the problem

Step 3: Ideate

Step 4: Make tangible

Step 5: Iterate relentlessly

Although we have not seen the term "design thinking" used widely in public health nutrition, there are many parallels with what social scientists have been doing for decades (see especially Nichter et al., 2004).[5] In what follows, we have mapped these perspectives and data collection techniques onto the above five design thinking steps. It is our hope that this will facilitate nutrition interventions that place people truly at their core.

Step 1: Understand: formative research strategies to understand the issue

"Formative research" is a term used across many disciplines to refer to the use of qualitative and quantitative methods to inform the development of some sort of product, from stump speeches to research surveys. Standard ethnographic techniques have come to be used frequently in formative research.[6]

Qualitative approaches such as ethnographic interviews, participant observation, and focus group discussions are the approaches commonly used to describe what can perhaps best be termed the "lived experiences" of any given phenomenon. Quantitative ethnographic techniques such as surveys, behavioral checklists, and ranking or grouping exercises[7] are also useful formative strategies, but because qualitative approaches are more commonly used, we will focus on these here.

a. The ethnographic interview

Unstructured or semi-structured interviews are a hallmark ethnographic technique. Generally, such interviews are conducted with those who are experiencing the topic at hand (e.g., anemia during pregnancy), as well as those who are somehow connected to the problem (e.g., traditional healers, clinic staff, medicine vendors, family members).

Examples of ways to begin unstructured interviews about infant feeding practices are as simple as: "Tell me about the lack of blood during pregnancy." Indeed, an ethnographic interview need not always be formal; it can even sound like a casual conversation. As interviews become more structured, i.e., guided by a topic list or even a set list of questions, it is important to remember that their purpose is to uncover

important themes or experiences that may not be susceptible to determination *a priori* (i.e., they may not be on the checklist). Thus, the researcher must become skillful at keeping the interview germane to the research question while following novel threads that will allow new findings to emerge. There are no rules about the duration of an interview, but 90 minutes seems to be the point at which fatigue or inconvenience begin to set in.[8]

Ethnographic interviews may occur over multiple encounters, and the rapport between researcher and respondent will probably evolve over time. As the ethnographic researcher establishes rapport among members of the target culture, interviews may become more formal and more structured. Doing this too quickly may result in informants feeling interrogated, however. Alternatively, a structured interview may feel more comfortable before the interviewer and interviewee know each other well. Follow-up conversations may then become more informal, expanding on what was already formally inquired about, with the respondent feeling more at ease and therefore able to provide richer insights.

b. Observation

Observation is another useful ethnographic technique in formative research.[9] Observation may happen at a distance, in the form of sitting, observing, and writing notes on e.g., exchanges at a prenatal clinic, in an open-air market, at a daycare center, or in a family's home.[10] It may also be more participatory, in which the researcher acts as well as observes, e.g., joins breastfeeding support groups. Ethnographic observation can be labor-intensive, but the observations can be extremely valuable for exploring previous confusions or sparking additional lines of inquiry.

c. Visual techniques

Space precludes enumeration of all possible visual techniques for studying nutritional problems, but an overview would be incomplete without the mention of at least one. Photovoice – see following trio of photographs – is a participatory technique in which images relevant to the area of exploration are photographed by participants. These photos are then discussed in one-on-one and group settings.[11] We have successfully used Photovoice to explore how food insecurity impacts infant feeding strategies in Kenya and Uganda.

PhotoVoice is one possible visual technique for "understanding the issue,"
the first step in people-centered nutrition interventions.

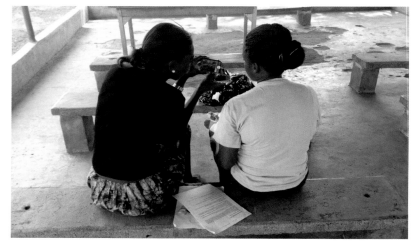

In the first Photovoice encounter, participants are lent cameras. They then take photographs about the topic under discussion over a period of time, e.g., two weeks. In the second phase, pictured here, these photos become the centerpiece of the interview. Here, a mother (sitting on the right, with her infant on her lap) is explaining to a study staff member (left) why she has taken a photo.
Source: Angela Arbach

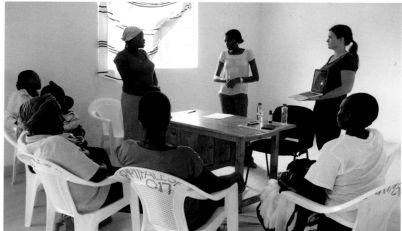

The third phase of the Photovoice activity is a focus group discussion, in which participants select two or three photos that they have taken with a view to talking about these. Here, women are discussing their experiences of how food insecurity impacts the way they feed their infants.
Source: Beryl Oyier

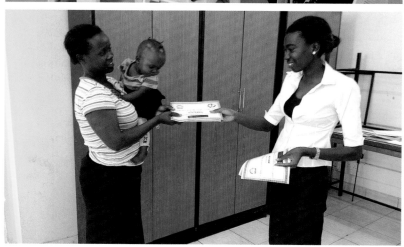

On conclusion of the Photovoice study, a participant receives a certificate of appreciation and a copy of the photos she took for the study.
Source: Angela Arbach

Case Study

Grandmothers promote maternal and child health: the role of Indigenous Knowledge Systems Managers

In virtually all societies, the managers of indigenous knowledge (IK) systems that deal with the development, care and wellbeing of women and children are senior women, or grandmothers. In that function, grandmothers are expected to advise and supervise the younger generations. However, most development programs neither acknowledge their influence nor explicitly involve them in efforts to strengthen existing family and community survival strategies.

There is a need to broaden the concept of indigenous knowledge in development programs: first, to view IK in the context of community and household systems; and second, to consider both beneficial and harmful practices in indigenous knowledge systems related, for example, to health, nutrition or initiation rites.

Methodology to strengthen grandmothers' role as knowledge managers

In community programs, first in Southeast Asia and later in West Africa, the "generic grandmother-inclusive" methodology[12] was developed by The Grandmother Project (an American non-profit NGO) for working with grandmother networks to strengthen their role and knowledge in promoting optimal practices related to maternal and children health and wellbeing. The five key steps in the methodology are:

1 Rapid assessment of grandmothers' role and influence in the household and community related to the issue of interest

2 Public recognition of grandmothers' role in promoting health and development of families and communities

3 Participatory communication/education activities that engage first, grandmother networks, and second, other community members, in discussion of both traditional and modern practices

4 Strengthening the capacity of grandmother leaders and networks to promote improved practices with other grandmothers, in families and in the community-at-large and

5 Ongoing monitoring and documentation for learning.

Through process documentation and evaluation, a number of other positive and unanticipated outcomes of

the grandmother-inclusive methodology were documented among different community groups. Here are examples of changes observed following use of the non-formal education and empowerment approach:

Grandmothers:

- Greater sense of confidence and of empowerment in the community

- Stronger sense of solidarity between grandmothers

- Emergence of grandmother leaders

- Grandmother leaders encourage other grandmothers to consider new ideas

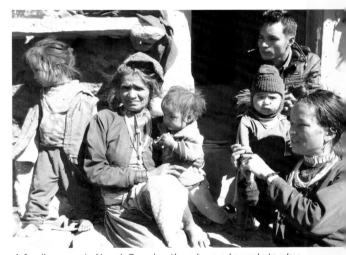

A family group in Nepal. Grandmothers have a key role to play in promoting maternal and child health.
Source: Sight and Life.

Male community leaders:

- Increased respect for grandmothers' advice combining "indigenous" and "modern" knowledge

- Increased public recognition of grandmothers' contribution to women's and children's wellbeing

Household level:

- Positive changes in grandmothers' advice to younger women and men

- Increased confidence of other household members in grandmothers' advice

Continued overleaf

Continued from previous page

- Increased confidence of health/development workers in grandmothers' advice

- Improved communication between mothers-in-law and daughters-in-law.

These experiences illustrate how change can be brought about from within indigenous knowledge systems when key actors in those systems, i.e., the indigenous knowledge managers, are involved in deciding if and how to combine global knowledge with traditional knowledge. The approach described here empowers community actors to make such strategic decisions themselves, while simultaneously strengthening the interrelated roles, relationships, norms and practices within family and community systems.

Source: *IK Notes, http://www.worldbank.org/afr/ik/ default.htm, accessed September 3 2015 (abridged).*

Case Study

Identifying the sociocultural barriers and facilitating factors to nutrition-related behavior change: Formative research for a stunting prevention program in Ntchisi, Malawi

The Scaling Up Nutrition (SUN) Movement has heightened the world's focus on integrated nutrition interventions. In 2013, the Government of Malawi, with support from the World Food Programme and partners, initiated such an intervention in Ntchisi District. Aimed at reducing the prevalence of stunting, the intervention had several components, including the provision of a small-quantity, lipid-based nutrient supplement (SQ-LNS) for children aged 6 to 23 months.

This study aimed to answer the following questions:

- What cultural perceptions and household behaviors exist in relation to childhood illnesses, concepts of healthy growth and development, and food utilization?

- How can an ethnomedical model, which describes a local body of knowledge about a specific illness or group of illnesses, be developed for salient nutrition-related illnesses in this setting?

- What are community members' attitudes toward an SQ-LNS that will be introduced as part of the integrated nutrition intervention in this setting?

Data were collected from February until May 2013 in all seven traditional authorities (geographic areas) of Ntchisi District, which lies in the Central Region of Malawi and is home to approximately 250,000 residents.

Caregivers had positive impressions of the SQ-LNS, and children aged 6 to 23 months were highly accepting of its flavor, a driver of product sharing and overuse that occurred within and between households. Community members suggested that sustained compliance will be more feasible with development of culturally appropriate packaging that includes the sachet language in Chichewa as well as locally developed images and clearer instructions for use. Most people asked for larger quantities of the SQ-LNS, comparing it to the locally produced ready-to-use therapeutic food (RUTF) Chiponde, which is already being used in Ntchisi for the treatment of acute malnutrition and has a weight of 92 g.

When asked directly for their perceptions of the SQ-LNS, 10 caregivers said that the product was a medicine, three that it was a food, and five that it had qualities of both a food and a medicine. They either called the product by its name, referred to it as Chiponde [an area of Malawi], or called it "chakudya," Chichewa for "food." Nine of 12 caregivers indicated that they would pay a nominal price for a sachet of the product if it was introduced through a market-based system, citing their children's health as the reason for this willingness.

The study revealed that the SQ-LNS was accepted as an energy-giving food, but that health education and communications tailored to local understanding of nutrition and health are necessary to ensure its appropriate utilization.

Source: *Kodish S, Aburto N, Hambayi MN et al. Food and Nutrition Bulletin 2015, Vol. 36(2) 138–153 (abridged).*

Step 2: Define the problem using ecological frameworks

Step 2 of the design process is all about defining the problem. The incorporation of an ecological model is a systematic way to ensure that the scope of the understanding outlined in Step 1 is complete.

There are a number of ecological models from which to choose, including the Ecological Model of Food and Nutrition,[13] and the Socio-Ecological Framework.[14,15] Both attempt to identify the multiple social and environmental factors that affect nutritional issues in a simple but holistic schema.

While aspects of society are not nearly as tidily compartmentalized as **Figure 1** might imply, this scheme of relationships is a useful heuristic tool for drawing attention to and organizing the complexities of human nutrition. Some sectors will ultimately be much more important than others, but one must consider the potential role of each at the outset.

Figure 1 | **An ecological model of food and nutrition**

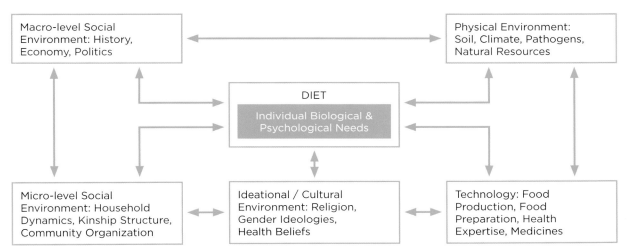

Source: Young SL, Pelto GH. Core Concepts in Nutritional Anthropology. In N. Temple & et al. (eds) Nutritional Health: Strategies for Disease Prevention Totowa, NJ: Humana Press, 2012 pp. 523-537; adapted from Jerome N, Kandel R, Pelto G. An ecological approach to nutritional anthropology. In N. Jerome, R. Kandel, & G.H. Pelto (eds.) Nutritional Anthropology: Contemporary Approaches to Diet and Culture. Pleasantville, NY: Redgrave Publishing, 1980.

Step 3: Ideate: Focus group discussions to generate ideas

Ideation, or brainstorming, is the phase in which new ideas are generated. This phase is perhaps the most difficult to base on examples from prior endeavors in public health nutrition, both because brainstorming sessions are difficult to share, and because new ideas often arrive in an ethereal way. However, focus group discussions are a forum conducive to both generating a number of ideas and receiving feedback about them quickly.

Focus group discussions are an approach to formative research in which the researcher gathers together a group of people (usually 6–8) to discuss a common issue.[16] A facilitator moderates the discussion, keeping participants focused on the topic of interest while promoting dialogue and discussion.

There are a number of advantages to focus group discussions. Given that people commonly work and discuss in groups, focus group discussions can be a very comfortable

mode for sharing ideas. They are also a method for hearing the opinions of many individuals in a very short period of time.[17] Further, the group's responses to other participants' comments are often very informative, and they can be a metric of how resonant that experience is.

However, focus group discussions may be less appropriate for sensitive issues or the discussion of private matters. They can also be uncomfortable for individuals who have differing opinions or experiences than the majority of the group, potentially resulting in an individual remaining quiet. Focus group discussions have been conducted with many vulnerable populations and about many complex subjects. Ultimately their appropriateness must be determined by the research team, and their success relies heavily on the skill of the facilitator. Finally, logistically, they can be difficult to organize.

Step 4: Make tangible: Program implementation pathways to build prototypes

It is much harder to make nutrition interventions tangible through prototyping than it is to, say, create software prototypes. However, a prototype of a nutrition delivery pathway can be built using a Program Implementation Pathway (PIP).

The Program Implementation Pathway is the pathway from an intervention input through programmatic delivery, and household and individual utilization, to its desired impact.[18] One can conceptualize a nutrition intervention as a flow, in which the nutrient(s) and/or the information (e.g., behavior change communication materials) enter into the delivery system and move through a sequence of steps that lasts all the way until the deliverable is consumed or used by the intended beneficiary. As inputs are placed into the stream, they can encounter problems, even in programs that have been very carefully planned.

A bottleneck can be very serious, and may bring an intervention to a complete halt. An obvious example is a break in a vaccine cold chain, in which the vaccine is no longer functional. Everything that follows after the break may be fine, but the intervention itself is a failure. A partial blockage is much more common in nutrition interventions. This can take various forms, including blockages internal to the delivery system as well as blockages in the (household) utilization system. Both the pathways and the barriers and promoters of the "flow" through the pathway can be imagined/trialed/prototyped.

Some common problems in programs in the delivery system that are formally reported in program reports or evaluations, or informally acknowledged by program administrative staff, reflect partial blockages.[19] Examples of delivery system partial blockages include:

i   supplements not being routinely available at delivery points;

ii staff turnover leading to gaps in knowledge about management of the delivery process;

iii frontline workers not understanding the purpose or intent of the program;

iv frontline workers not being well trained in delivering the supplement or not knowing how to give instructions on how to use it; and

v   frontline workers delivering incorrect information in the course of behavior change communication activities.

At the household level, there can also be a number of partial blockages. These include:

i   the intervention failing to reach the households where the need is greatest;

ii for interventions that involve an intermediary to the beneficiary (e.g., infants and young children), caregivers not understanding how to give the supplement or how to prepare and feed the recommended foods;

iii other household members interfering with the actions the caregiver needs to carry out; and

iv caregivers giving the intervention a try but failing to continue it for various reasons.

The concept of Program Implementation Pathway as a tool for program monitoring and evaluation is gaining recognition in nutrition. For example, in a project in Haiti designed to test a preventive versus a curative approach to reducing infant and young child malnutrition,[20] the PIP was used progressively and iteratively over the course of the study.[21,22] It provided the framework for designing both the "process evaluation" after the intervention was fully implemented, and the end-line evaluation to assess the success and comparative impact of the two different models. Other recent examples include in Vietnam the pathways by which the Alive and Thrive campaign impacted infant and young child feeding practices in Vietnam.[23,24]

Step 5: Iterate relentlessly: Evaluative ethnography for iterative redesign

Redesign is core to design thinking; proposed solutions are always re-evaluated. Evaluative ethnography, or research grounded in ethnographic techniques and theories, that is undertaken to inform and improve the translational process from discovery-oriented research to implementation-research, does just this.[25]

We would argue that evaluative ethnographic techniques can, and should, be used throughout the lifespan of the nutrition intervention: before its implementation (see Step 1), during implementation (i.e., as a strategy for process evaluation), and after the intervention has concluded (i.e., as impact evaluation).

Understanding low usage of micronutrient powder in the Kakuma Refugee Camp, Kenya: Findings from a qualitative study

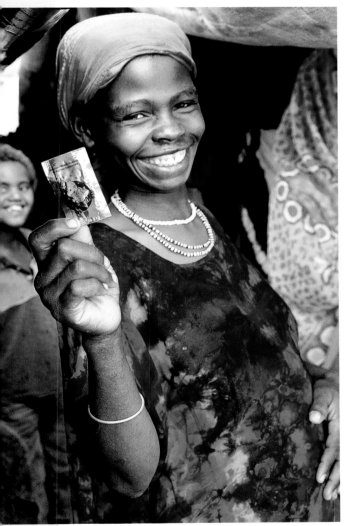

A pregnant woman in Kakuma Refugee Camp, Kenya, with a sachet of the micronutrient powder MixMe™.
Source: Sight and Life

In recent years, home fortification with micronutrients in the form of powders, crushable tablets, and lipid-based spreads has been recognized as a promising approach to prevent micronutrient deficiencies in vulnerable population groups, such as young children who cannot swallow tablets. In particular, the use of micronutrient powder – a mix of vitamins and minerals in powder form that can be added to food just before consumption – has gained popularity since its inception in the late 1990s due to ease of use and low cost.

There has also been abundant scientific evidence from diverse settings demonstrating the efficacy of micronutrient powder in the treatment and prevention of anemia, primarily among young children. In general, micronutrient powder is packaged in single-dose sachets targeted to provide 1 RNI (Recommended Nutrient Intake) of micronutrients per person per day.

In continuing efforts by the United Nations World Food Programme (WFP) and the United Nations High Commissioner for Refugees (UNHCR) to address the high prevalence of undernutrition and micronutrient deficiencies among refugees, a large-scale micronutrient powder program targeting the entire population (approximately 50,000) of the Kakuma Refugee Camp in Kenya was initiated in February 2009. This was enabled by the partnership of WFP and DSM known as "Improving Nutrition – Improving Lives."

The objectives of the micronutrient powder program were to reduce the prevalence of micronutrient malnutrition among the refugees by the 17-month provision of home fortification with micronutrient powder, and to determine the feasibility of distributing micronutrient powder in combination with general food rations in a refugee camp setting. The program provided each individual with a once-a-day micronutrient powder sachet with the brand name MixMe (DSM Nutritional Products Ltd., Kaiseraugst, Switzerland) containing a low dose of iron and 15 other vitamins and minerals for a period of 17 months. One box containing 30 micronutrient powder sachets for each family member was distributed monthly, together with standard food rations.

During the course of the program, uptake of the micronutrient powder at distribution points dropped nearly 70%, from 99% to a low of 30%, and remained at 45% to 52% despite increased social marketing efforts.

A study was therefore initiated to identify factors leading to the low uptake of micronutrient powder through a qualitative inquiry. In-depth interviews were conducted with community leaders, stakeholders, implementing partners, and beneficiaries. Direct observations of food preparation

Continued overleaf

Continued from previous page

and child feeding were conducted. Focus group discussions were employed to examine perceptions and practices of beneficiaries regarding micronutrient powder use.

The study concluded that superficial formative research and lack of interagency coordination had led to insufficient social marketing prior to the program. In addition, community health workers were inadequately trained. This resulted in inadequate communication regarding the health benefits and use of micronutrient powder to the beneficiaries. Reliance on personal experiences with micronutrient powder and issues with its packaging, in part, led to confusion and deleterious

rumors, resulting in decreased uptake of micronutrient powder at distribution points.

From this study it can be concluded that a successful micronutrient powder program requires careful design, with emphasis on conducting thorough formative research, ensuring the involvement and commitment of all stakeholders from the outset, investigating the role of cultural factors, and ensuring provision of sufficient, adequate, and timely information to the beneficiaries.

Source: *Kodish S, Rah JH, Kraemer K et al. Food and Nutrition Bulletin. September 2011. DOI: 10.1177/156482651103200315. Source: PubMed (abridged).*

Conclusion

Melinda Gates and Paul Farmer articulated a truism when pointing out the need to "meet people where they are," but this is not as easy to do as it might at first appear. While it might seem clearly essential to take into consideration the lived

experiences of people when designing proposed improvements, this complex proposition can best be achieved through hard work, creativity, and a commitment to Design Thinking to create and maintain people-centered nutrition interventions.

Our personal view

Sera Young, Shawn Baker and Rolf Klemm

Learning from failures as well as successes

Design thinking encourages us to "fail fast, fail often and fail early." But how exactly should one define failure?

Currently, there are roughly three types of information used to design a nutrition intervention or program. These three types of information pertain to biomedicine (e.g., disease burden, intervention efficacy), context (e.g., social norms, family structure, access behaviors), and delivery systems (e.g., clinic infrastructure, front line workers, private sector). Successful programs are those that are responsive to the constraints and opportunities implicit in each of those three domains. We think that these three

considerations are necessary, but not sufficient, to prevent a program from failing.

We argue for a fourth consideration for nutrition program design, which is meeting the end user's needs. In most cases, mothers (and their children), especially those in low-resource settings, are the target for interventions. But many interventions are not mindful of the burden they place on women, and specifically on their most valuable asset, which is their time. Fetching nutritional supplements from a far-off clinic, sitting through long behavior change sessions, preparing special complementary foods, and even exclusive breastfeeding, all take an extraordinary amount of time from the person who is often the first to wake up and the last to go to sleep each day.

Programs and interventions that are mindful of the end-user and her priorities have the greatest likelihood of success. And as such, we implore that end-user perspectives should be used to modify the intervention or product, right from the earliest stages, so as to create the greatest chances for nutritional success.

Further reading

Young SL, Tuthill E. Ethnography as a tool for formative research and evaluation in public health nutrition: illustrations from the world of infant and young child feeding. In Brett J, Chrzan J (eds) Research Methods for the Anthropological Study of Food and Nutrition. New York: Berghahn Press, 2016.

Chapter 9: "Evaluative Ethnography For Maternal and child nutrition interventions " in http://www.tandfebooks.com/isbn/9781315762319 pp 157–178.

Kolko, J. Design Thinking Comes of Age. In: Harvard Business Review 2015:66–71.

References

1   *The Human Element: Melinda Gates and Paul Farmer on Designing Global; Health. http://www.wired.com/2013/11/2112gatefarmers. Accessed March 1, 2016.*

2   *Gawande A. Slow Ideas: Some innovations spread fast. How do you speed the ones that don't? The New Yorker. Annals of Medicine July 29, 2013 Issue. Accessed March 1, 2016.*

3   *McKim RH. Experiences in Visual Thinking. 2nd ed. Monterey, CA: Brooks/ Cole Publishing Company, 1980.*

4   *Roth B. The Achievement Habit: Stop Wishing, Start Doing, and Take Command of Your Life. HarperBusiness (July 7, 2015).*

5   *Nichter M, Quintero G, Mock J et al. Qualitative Research: Contributions to the Study of Drug Use, Drug Abuse, and Drug Use(r)- Related Interventions. Substance Use & Misuse 2004;39:1907–1969.*

6   *LeCompte MD, Schensul JJ. Designing and Conducting Ethnographic Research. Volume 1 of Ethnographer's Toolkit, Second Edition Series. Rowman Altamira, 2010.*

7   *Bernard HR. Research Methods in Anthropology: Qualitative and Quantitative Approaches. Altamira Press. Fourth revised edition (28 October 2005).*

8   *Spradley JP. The Ethnographic Interview. Belmont CA:Wadsworth Publishing Co Inc 1979.*

9   *Ibid.*

10   *Levy MM, Dellinger RP, Townsend SR et al. The Surviving Sepsis Campaign: results of an international guideline-based performance improvement program targeting severe sepsis. Crit Care Med. 2010;38(2):367–74. doi: 10.1097/CCM.0b013e3181cb0cdc.*

11   *Wang C, Burris MA. Photovoice: concept, methodology, and use for participatory needs assessment. Health Educ Behav. 1997;24(3):369–87.*

12   *Aubel, J. Generic Steps in the Grandmother-Inclusive Methodology. The Grandmother Project, Chevy Chase, Maryland, 2004.*

13   *Jerome NW, Kandel RF, Pelto GH (Eds). Nutritional anthropology: Contemporary approaches to diet and culture. Pleasantville: Redgrave. 1980.*

14   *Centers for Disease Control and Prevention (CDC). The Social-Ecological Model: A Framework for Prevention.http://www.cdc.gov/violenceprevention/ overview/social-ecologicalmodel.html. Accessed March 1, 2016.*

15   *Bronfenbrenner U. Ecological models of human development. In International Encyclopedia of Education, Vol. 3. 2nd Ed. Oxford: Elsevier, 1994.*

16   *Krueger RA, Casey MA. Focus Groups: A Practical Guide for Applied Research. SAGE Publications, Inc; 4th edition (October 15, 2008).*

17   *Ibid.*

18   *Young, S.L. & Pelto, G.H. Core Concepts in Nutritional Anthropology. In N. Temple & et al. (eds) Nutritional Health: Strategies for Disease Prevention, Totowa, NJ: Humana Press, 2012.*

19   *Ibid.*

20   *Ruel, MT, Menon P, Habicht J-P et al. Age-based preventive targeting of food assistance and behavior change and communication for reduction of childhood undernutrition in Haiti: a cluster randomized trial. Lancet 2008;371:588–595.*

21   *Loechl CU, Menon P, Arimond M et al. Using programme theory to assess the feasibility of delivering micronutrient Sprinkles through a food-assisted maternal and child health and nutrition programme in rural Haiti. Matern Child Nutr 2009;5(1):33–48. doi: 10.1111/j.1740-8709.2008.00154.x.*

22   *Menon, P. et al. From research to program design: use of formative research in Haiti to develop a behavior change communication program to prevent malnutrition. Food and Nutrition Bulletin, 2005;26(2):241–242.*

23   *Nguyen, P.H. et al. Program impact pathway analysis of a social franchise model shows potential to improve infant and young child feeding practices in Vietnam. J Nutri 2014;144:627–1636.*

24   *Rawat, R. et al. 2013. Learning how programs achieve their impact: embedding theory- driven process evaluation and other program learning mechanisms in Alive & Thrive. Food and Nutrition Bulletin 2013;34:S212– 225.*

25   *Chapter 9: "Evaluative Ethnography For Maternal and child nutrition interventions " in Ethnographic Research in Maternal and Child Health ed. Dykes F, Flacking R. Taylor & Francis 2015.*

208

The Use of New and Existing Tools and Technologies to Support the Global Nutrition Agenda: The innovation opportunity

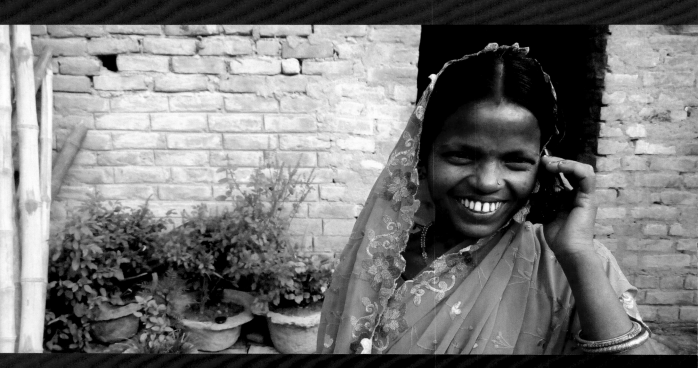

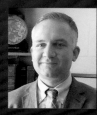

Alain B Labrique
Associate Professor & Director, JHU Global mHealth Initiative

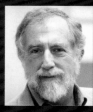

Marc Mitchell
President, D-tree International and Adjunct Lecturer on Global Health, Harvard T.H. Chan School of Public Health

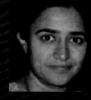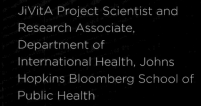

Sucheta Mehra
JiVitA Project Scientist and Research Associate, Department of International Health, Johns Hopkins Bloomberg School of Public Health

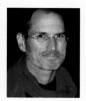

"Creativity is just connecting things."

Steve Jobs (1955–2011), *American information technology entrepreneur and inventor, and co-founder, chairman, and chief executive officer of Apple Inc.*

Key messages

- The pace of information, communication and digital services continues to accelerate globally.

- Governments and NGOs are harnessing this infrastructure to test and scale innovative new solutions.

- The world's ability to capture data on system performance and population health is increasing rapidly.

- The global nutrition community has been at the forefront of many such innovations.

- Further innovation is still needed to achieve Universal Health Coverage.

Since 2013, the International Telecommunications Union (ITU, the United Nations agency charged with tracking the state of information and communications technologies around the globe) has reported that the number of connected mobile devices is nearly equal to the number of human beings on the planet (**Figure 1**). Seemingly saturated by technology, populations around the world have continued to leverage this new connectedness to further accelerate the pace of access to information services such as the Internet.

Only 20 years ago, this might have seemed like a pipe dream to many in the development sector, but today this is recognized as a "leapfrogging" event in the traditional course of development. Across sectors from health through agriculture and education to nutrition, government and non-government actors are harnessing this infrastructure to test and implement innovative solutions. From a health systems perspective, these technologies are helping dissipate obstinate roadblocks to reaching effective coverage of interventions of known efficacy. As we enter a MDG (Millennium Development Goals) era striving toward Universal Health Coverage, the need for further innovation to accelerate progress is clear.

Figure 1 | **The rapid exponential growth in global cellular telephony between 2001 and 2014, culminating in nearly 7 billion subscribers globally, equivalent to the number of people on the planet.**

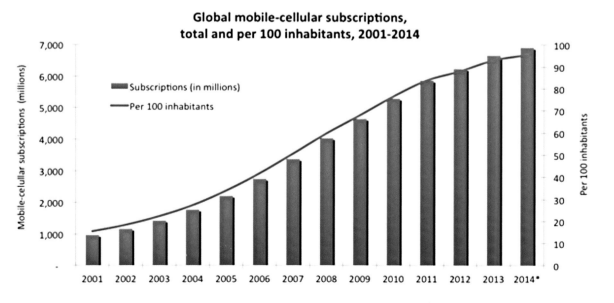

*Note: * Estimate. Source: Mobile subscriptions near the 7-billion mark – Does almost everyone have a phone? https://itunews.itu.int/en/3741-Mobile-subscriptions-near-the-78209billion-markbrDoes-almost-everyone-have-a-phone.note.aspx Accessed August 10, 2015.*

The global nutrition community has been at the forefront of many such innovations – from improving the food supply chain and agricultural performance to tracking population-level nutritional status. Not only is appropriate information now accessible in a timely fashion to more people than ever before; our ability to generate, process and analyze data on system performance and population health is also rapidly accelerating. Through a series of vignettes and examples, we illustrate important trends in how these technologies are being used, at various dimensions of scale, to advance the performance of different components of the nutritional ecosystem, from farm to table – with a focus on low- and middle-income countries (LMICs) around the world.

Improving workforce quality and client engagement

Among the most prevalent use-cases of ICT (Information Communication Technologies) for global nutrition is assisting frontline health workers (FHWs) in the performance of their duties. Especially in LMICs, frontline health workers often serve as the first point of contact with the health system – providing both routine and curative services to the populations they serve.[1] Despite this important role, these armies of workers receive minimal training in short periods of time, with often little post-training support and supervisory follow-up. As such, a commonly noted problem is the adherence to complex, changing treatment guidelines for conditions such as severe acute malnutrition (SAM).

The eNutrition project in Zanzibar (**Figure 2**), a UNICEF Innovation Working Group project implemented by D-Tree International and the Ministry of Health of Zanzibar, used a mobile decision-support tool, providing access to guidelines for outpatient therapeutic care. Responding to the public health crisis of 20–30% of children with severe acute malnutrition dying despite treatment, eNutrition aimed to lower case fatality to below 5%. The pilot study, conducted between 2010 and 2013, was implemented across 12 health centers in two districts and eventually scaled up to the entire island. The eNutrition strategy has demonstrated an ability to improve FHW's diagnostic capacity by 20%, while also relieving the burden of paper-based registration and record-keeping, as reported by system users. A unique facet of this program is a private-sector partnership with a major local Network Operator, Zamtel, who supported the project through reduced airtime and data charges as part of its corporate social responsibility strategy in Zanzibar.

Figure 2 | **Outpatient Therapeutic Care**

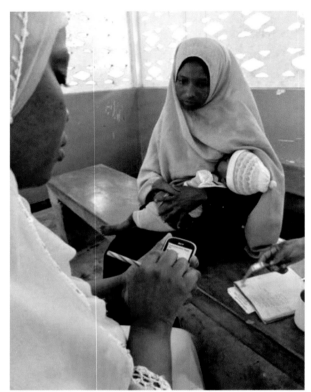

Health worker in Zanzibar using D-Tree's eNutrition software on a mobile device to ensure adherence to Ministry of Health and Social Welfare's guidelines for Outpatient Therapeutic Care.
Source: http://www.africanstrategies4health.org/
uploads/1/3/5/3/13538666/enutrition.pdf Credit: D-tree International

In the villages of Madhya Pradesh, typical of many similar populations across the greater Gangetic floodplains, the problem of recognizing malnutrition at the community level is among the most critical limitations to reducing incidence of severe acute malnutrition. The Real Medicine Foundation in India used the CommCare platform's Growth and Monitoring Promotion (**Figure 3**) features to enable frontline health workers to collect mid-upper arm circumference data over time.[2] Complex anthropometric calculations and trends could be task-shifted to servers processing the data in real-time, freeing up workers to focus on providing treatment or facilitating referrals to care.

The ability to detect moderate alterations in growth trajectories (e.g., faltering or moderate acute malnutrition) is exceedingly difficult to achieve using paper-based ledgers, but relatively straightforward by digital tracking of longitudinal data. Specific cutoffs or slopes of decline can be readily calculated by servers, which automatically alert individual

Chapter 4.3 | The Use of New and Existing Tools and Technologies
to Support the Global Nutrition Agenda: The innovation opportunity

212

workers and supervisors when an intervention is required. Initial measures of system impact found dramatic decreases in data review by a Program Coordinator – from 45 days with the preceding paper-based system to a mere 8 hours with the digital method. The data completeness measured changed from 67% to 84% using the CommCare platform. Interestingly, frontline health workers also reported increases in their levels of social respect, since their data was being immediately "shared with a computer in Delhi (the capital of India)." Parents were reportedly more attentive during counseling sessions where these digital systems were used. The role of mobile technology in this instance seemed to involve improvements in data quality, timeliness of care delivery and faster referrals, but also had an effect on how workers were perceived now that they were connected more integrally to the health systems they represent within communities.

Figure 3 | The CommCare platform

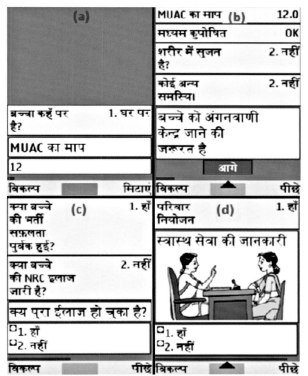

Screenshots of a typical CommCare feature phone screen series a) MUAC value of a child, b) branching questions about moderate malnutrition, triggered by the first response, and c), d) referral and counseling screens.
Source: http://research.microsoft.com/pubs/170446/Medhi-NordiCHI2012-CommCareCasestudy.pdf. Credit: Dimagi/CommCare

Frontline health workers are often overwhelmed by the archaic paper-based systems on which many health systems in low- and middle-income countries rely. In addition to being time-consuming, these systems introduce delays in processing and are prone to transcription errors, as data is summarized at multiple health-system levels. The Liberian Agriculture Upgrading Nutrition and Child Health (LAUNCH) project began in 2010, as a project to improve food security and reduce chronic malnutrition of vulnerable women and children under 5.[3] Focused on the delivery of supplementary food rations, the project employed a Beneficiary Based Commodity Management System to calculate commodity needs for distribution points as well as monitoring stock levels. Shifting to a mobile-phone based registration process significantly reduced beneficiary wait times from 14 to 5 weeks. By leveraging the camera function common to many smartphones, the LAUNCH project was able to transition away from a dysfunctional fingerprint beneficiary system towards one which used client photographs. In addition to system performance improvements, the digital data streams created by this mobile system allowed system-generated data to be used for monitoring and evaluation purposes – for example, using digital timestamps to identify and mitigate bottlenecks in the system.

Globally, a number of programs have used either direct messaging to clients or communication facilitated by frontline health workers using mobile device-based media content (audio, video, or images) to enhance nutrition counseling at the point of care in villages from India to Nigeria. Programs such as USAID's Mobile Alliance for Maternal Action (MAMA)[4] have established messaging "curricula" that cover basic information about pregnancy, child care, health seeking and nutrition from early pregnancy until several years postpartum. In 2015, the MAMA activity was nationalized in South Africa as the Ministry of Health's MomConnect Program,[5] providing free access to pregnant women nationwide. Subscribers receive stage-based messages on their phones at reduced or no cost, depending on the country implementation. Evaluations of this program are presently ongoing to measure behavior changes and health outcomes attributable to these messages.

Digital platforms such as CommCare have been used in multiple settings to assist frontline health workers in counseling clients,[6] leveraging multimedia content (images, local dialects, music) to reinforce knowledge and using quiz-based testing for the health workers themselves. Multimedia use has been shown to increase client engagement,[7] while also raising the credibility of frontline

Chapter 4.3 | The Use of New and Existing Tools and Technologies
to Support the Global Nutrition Agenda: The innovation opportunity

213

health workers through the use of "trusted" audio recordings by health professionals, amplified by the FHWs' subsequent counseling. Within the global Alive & Thrive nutrition program led by FHI360 to improve Infant and Young Child Feeding, University of North Carolina researchers incorporated text and voice messages into a breastfeeding promotion study in rural Nigeria. Women leaders of small microcredit groups (n=4-6) were provided with a single low-cost phone and charged with relaying weekly messages to their members. A randomized trial evaluation of the program showed significant increases in exclusive breastfeeding at 3 and 6 months of life, and a reduction by half of feeding water to <6-month-old infants.[8]

Nutrition workforce capacity-building

Finally, numerous projects are using worker-owned devices to provide access to in-service training programs which strive to reinforce and supplement material delivered during the often expedited face-to-face orientations that frontline health workers receive. The expenses of extracting health workers from their routine activities for training – in terms of productive time lost, travel, and other opportunity costs – can be extremely high.

The CapacityPlus program led by Intrahealth International has been carefully studying the lessons from mobile-based education (referred to as mLearning) which could be applied across the wide range of health verticals.[9] While smartphone penetration is still fairly limited in low- and middle-income countries, innovations in using text messaging and voice to deliver content are needed. Interactive-voice-response (IVR) systems are familiar to many developed-country readers who encounter automated phone menus (e.g., *Press "1" for service, Press "2" for rentals*) in their daily lives.

This strategy has been used successfully by IntraHealth in Senegal and by BBC Media Action's Ananya program in India, to offer in-service "continued education" for frontline health workers. Evaluation of the system in Senegal showed that the interactive-voice-response training was not only feasible and acceptable, but also resulted in greater retention of training material up to 14 months post-exposure. In Bihar, India, Ananya's 190-minute course is delivered to over 200,000 frontline health workers at a cost of ~US$1.50 per worker, issuing them, upon successful completion, a certificate of basic health and nutrition training. The content is available from any mobile phone, no matter how simple, lowering the access threshold to any health worker with a rudimentary device.

Improving agricultural performance

At the other end of the nutritional continuum, innovations in mobile-device enhanced agriculture have set a challenging bar for mNutrition and mHealth entrepreneurs to meet. The OneFarm project in Cuddalore, India reaches over 300,000 smallholder farmers each year with hyper-personalized advisory services. Customized to local micro-climates on their own phones in their local language, OneFarm provides farmers with weather forecasts, crop management advice and soil nutrient guidance, while also alerting them to disease trends and market price fluctuations (**Figure 4**). This program by Ekgaon Technologies aims to reduce unnecessary agri-inputs, increasing profit margins while at the same time improving crop management and productivity. Crop choices and market demands can be better met using such technologies, reducing the market price of vegetables and other staples. Two-year impact assessments have estimated reductions in fertilizer and pesticide use of ~30%, with over 15% increases in crop yields.[11,12] This "digital" agricultural extension approach has been used by numerous innovators, expanding the reach and availability of bespoke, on-demand advice to the small farmers whose crops are essential to geographically localized dietary diversity. In Bangladesh, over 1000 farmers have subscribed to mPower Social Enterprises' Farmer Query System (**Figure 5**) – a system which, like the examples described above for frontline health workers, uses technology to amplify the capacity of local agricultural extension workers.

Figure 4 | **Digital weather reports**

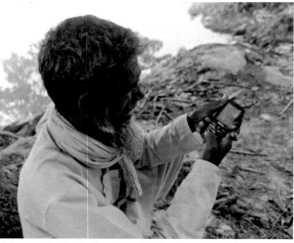

A farmer checks the local weather forecast on a cell phone. Nominal fee-based subscriptions allow messages and alerts to be customized to individual farmers for their specific agricultural zones and crops. Source: Digital Green

Chapter 4.3 | The Use of New and Existing Tools and Technologies
to Support the Global Nutrition Agenda: The innovation opportunity

214

Figure 5 | **Mobile Farming**

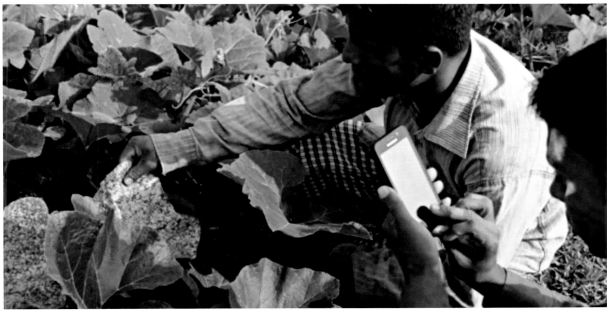

Agricultural extension and farmer support by phone – allows for real-time planting, troubleshooting and sales information to be accessed, as needed, by farmers. Newer phone features, such as high-resolution cameras, allow photos of pests or crop damage to be sent to experts for immediate diagnosis and action recommendations. Pictured here is the Farmer Query System in Bangladesh being used to send crop disease images to a remote expert for diagnosis and treatment recommendations.
Source: Mridul Chowdhury, CEO, mPower Social Enterprises – Farmer Query System, Bangladesh

When approached by farmers with a specific crop issue, such as a pest or disease, agricultural extension workers can capture details using text and images, send these to a remote expert, and receive immediate guidance on remediation of the problem. Initially supported by USAID funding, the project's goal is to migrate to a minimum fee-for-service model, possibly complementing the sparse ranks of Government agricultural extension workers with private-sector experts.

ICT-based solutions to bridge the information gap for small-scale farmers have also developed for livestock management. Often, information gaps caused by illiteracy and poor access to information lead to the use of suboptimal practices that are detrimental to the crop or livestock output. In rural Kenya, the iCow program (**Figure 6**) was created by a Kenyan farmer, supported by the UK Indigo Trust Foundation. This mobile-phone-enabled system allows individual animals to be registered on a central system using simple text messaging.[12] The service then sends reminders to farmers about milking schedules, immunizations and nutrition tips to improve cattle health. By keeping artificial insemination and breeding records, the system also aims to reduce inbreeding and thus sustain overall herd health. As

with the previous D-Tree example, iCow partnered with one of the leading telecommunications providers in Kenya, Safaricom, to provide greater service reach across the country.

Figure 6 | **The iCow application**

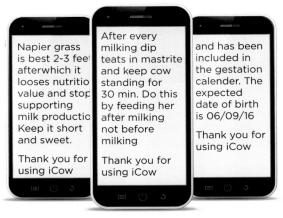

iCow is An award-winning Mobile application being deployed in Kenya in collaboration with national Telecom network operators, to provide text-message access to customized information to small farmers.
Source: http://www.icow.co.ke/images/stories/mobi-images.png

Chapter 4.3 | The Use of New and Existing Tools and Technologies
to Support the Global Nutrition Agenda: The innovation opportunity

215

Another interesting example of information "democratization" with impressive results is the DigitalGreen program by NGO MSSRF (**Figure 7**). With a reach now exceeding 7,600 villages across northern India, from Rajasthan to Odisha, Digital Green engages communities to generate localized video content on best agricultural practices. With a rapidly expanding library of 3,780 videos, the group identifies local farmers adopting best practices, uses them to create training material for their peers, and then facilitates a "mediated video viewing session" with members of that farmer's community and beyond. Communities thus become creators and consumers of "knowledge products" around nutrition and agriculture in the form of digital videos.

A trial of DigitalGreen in Karnataka demonstrated a 7-fold increase in methodology adoption when compared with traditional extension worker methods, at a 10-fold lower cost.[13] Interestingly, these methods have been able to achieve high levels of female participation, upwards of 70% – a potentially exciting result for typically male-dominated, conservative communities. Although primarily focusing on improving agricultural practices, the potential to use this blending of digital content generation, community-based sharing, and mediated change management for other aspects of the nutritional continuum is quite promising – from improving infant and young child feeding to home gardening.

Figure 7 | **Digital tools to support local training**

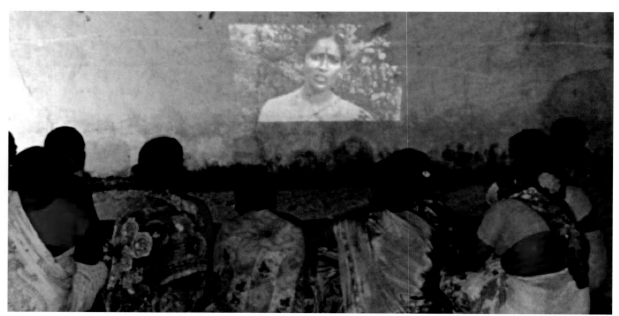

Digital Green and partner NGO workers use simple digital equipment to create highly localized training and information content for peer-to-peer community-based dissemination on farming best practices, using low-cost, battery-powered projectors.
Source: http://blogs.worldbank.org/endpovertyinsouthasia/files/endpovertyinsouthasia/video-shoot-movie.jpg

Technologies for individual self-efficacy

In higher-income countries where smartphone penetration is high, the use of "apps" for daily activities from checking email, news and weather to ordering food and lifestyle management is highly prevalent. The wearable, sensor-based device market has, in the past five years, made substantial strides in providing lower-cost, robust solutions which track energy expenditure, activity intensity and biometric indicators such as heart rate. Some estimates suggest that by 2021 the "wearables" market

will exceed US$15 billion, last measured at ~US$3.5 billion in 2014.[14] As early as 2011, Pew research surveys of US adults suggested that 29% of smartphone users downloaded apps to "track and manage health."[15] Although nascent, there is a growing evidence base testifying to the efficacy of these phone- and sensor-based strategies in improving nutritional outcomes of those who use them. One study by Lin et al[16] found that tailored text messages helped maintain significant weight loss in

Chapter 4.3 | The Use of New and Existing Tools and Technologies
to Support the Global Nutrition Agenda: The innovation opportunity

216

obese African-American adults in urban settings, strongly associated with the degree of engagement with the technology.[17] This emergent field continues to be closely watched by both researchers and industry, with extensive reviews and "state of evidence" reports published with some frequency.[18,19]

Although mobile "apps" will continue to dominate general thinking about technologies for global nutrition, their use for individual nutritional support may be limited by the fact that (a) they cannot yet quantify food and portion choices accurately, beyond the limitations of self-reported information, (b) that many of these software offerings are not tailored to the food composition tables of individual countries, and (c) that there is limited drive or market incentive toward seeking validation for such new technologies against established methods.

The probability remains that technology focusing on individualized nutritional behaviors and choices will, however, make more rapid progress in developed economies than in less developed economies, although the transfer of that technology will be indeed be rapid wherever conditions are appropriate. Among such conditions is one important for the future development of personalized nutrition, and that is mass access to a sophisticated food chain infrastructure (on-line food shopping, electronic elements of retailing, out-of-home dining, loyalty cards, etc.).

One out-spin of personalized nutrition technologies which is immediately applicable to emerging economies is that of dried blood spot technology, which was used to access blood samples remotely in the Food4Me project described in chapter 5.1. This technology allows home- or school-based blood sampling, which is a cheap, easy, highly mobile, postal service independent of freezing or centrifugation and aliquoting. Everywhere in the world, personalized nutrition using e-mobile technology has its challenges, but there is no doubt that the full spectrum of personalized nutrition technologies will eventually penetrate all corners of the globe, albeit at different rates.

Three directions for mNutrition in the future

These above vignettes illustrate, in brief, the breadth of the innovation landscape, from farm to table, that ICT bring to the challenge of improving global nutrition. It is important to keep in mind, however, that these projects and programs vary widely in scale and actual impact. The evidence base around whether these strategies are sustainable, impactful and cost-effective is still emerging. Certain approaches, such as direct-to-client messaging, have scaled at the national level, despite what some might argue to be low levels of evidence of impact.

Direction 1: Institutionalization and scale

Digitizing paper-based systems and processes does improve the quality and speed of information, to drive responsive public health nutrition decision-making. Freeing up health workers from the drudgery of paper-based tracking, reporting and summarizing data – processes that consume limited resources – opens the possibility of improving coverage of nutritional and health interventions of known efficacy.

Systems such as the WHO-led OpenSmartRegister platform are becoming available (OpenSRP, *www.smartregister.org*) to facilitate the digital transition at scale – for enterprise clients like governments and large NGOs. Well-designed, simple digital interfaces which prioritize the user's experience over complex formularies allow population health data to be collected systematically, while complex algorithms on the back-end of the system identify missed visits and high-risk families, and collate statistics and indicators for district- and national-level consumption.

Currently being integrated into frontline health worker workflows by four countries, in technical consultation with the WHO, OpenSRP is designed to integrate with other national-level health management information systems such as DHIS2 and OpenMRS.[20] This example heralds a new chapter in mHealth and mNutrition, where "best-of-breed" strategies are being integrated into an enterprise-grade solution which is designed to be country-owned, but also to break out of the cycle of small "pilot" studies which characterized the early years of this innovation space. Frameworks which illustrate how mHealth strategies "fit" within the broader global agenda for Universal Health Coverage have been proposed, to illustrate how mHealth strategies can, in certain scenarios, contribute to improvements in accountability, supply, demand, quality or costs of health services (**Figure 8**).

For each component part of the health system, we see how shortfalls in reaching levels necessary to support universal health coverage may be improved by the inclusion of single, or concerted mHealth strategies.[21]

217

Figure 8 | A cascading model to prioritize and select integrated mHealth strategies for achieving UHC, drawing from the UNICEF Bottlenecks and Tanahashi frameworks.

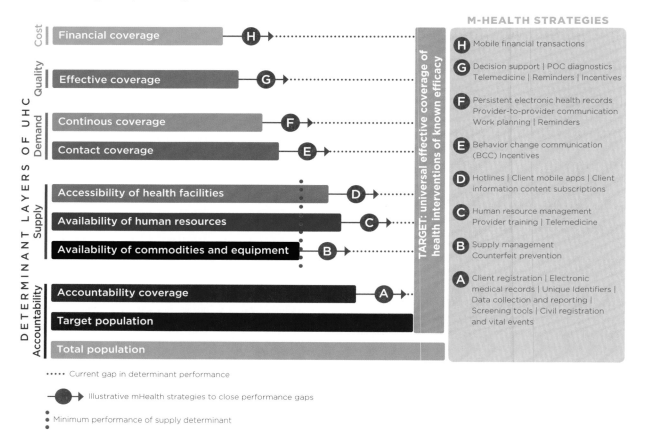

···· Current gap in determinant performance

Illustrative mHealth strategies to close performance gaps

Minimum performance of supply determinant

Source: From Mehl G, Labrique AB. Prioritizing integrated mHealth strategies for universal health coverage. Science 345, 1284 (2014). Reprinted with permission from AAAS.

Chapter 4.3 | The Use of New and Existing Tools and Technologies
to Support the Global Nutrition Agenda: The innovation opportunity

218

Direction 2: Wearable technologies to improve nutritional assessment

Low-cost devices containing tiny chips which measure the direction and intensity of movement, known as accelerometers, have proliferated in high-income settings over the past five years. Linking data on number of steps taken, stairs climbed or hours exercised to diet-logging websites has become a popular method of weight management, often linked to personal mobile devices for graphical visualizations. As the cost of accelerometers continues to drop, it is very likely that widespread use of FitBit®-like devices will also increase in global nutrition research to better quantify energy expenditures. Devices could be provided to research participants or patients under treatment to monitor closely changes in movement and intensity as markers of decline in health.

Similarly, new advances in nano-biotechnology are enabling small-footprint, complex biochemical assays to be developed, powered by mobile computing, to assess a range of conditions from infection to micronutrient deficiency. It is plausible to imagine a not-too-distant frontier where mNutrition innovations brings today's high-performance liquid chromatography (HPLC) and mass spectrometer to the doorstep of the African village, allowing for instantaneous assessment of individual nutritional status at the point of care. Advances in proteomics and metabolomics could be used to inform the direction of these innovations, prioritizing assays which could impact the largest populations – identifying levels of "hidden hunger" faster and with greater reliability than currently possible.

Direction 3: Big Data

One of the least recognized opportunities implicit in most of these technological innovations is the fact that these systems can now generate massive quantities of easily available, analytically ready digital data. In a short span of time, we are moving from a data vacuum where paper records provided unreliable, outdated information to one where frontline workers and populations themselves are generating real-time data, captured by these various systems. Moving from the "annual report" status quo to more frequent looks at health system and nutritional ecosystem performance is a challenging transition. However, from crop yields to dietary diversity, from real-time incidence of stunting or changes in breastfeeding – if the appropriate systems are established to capture these data (provided quality checks, validation and worker training measures are in place), the potential to examine patterns at a much more granular temporal scale than ever before is tremendous.

Beyond this, however, lies the yet-untapped space of using true "big data" analytics – such as machine learning and predictive modeling – and developing heuristics which can sift through terabytes of data to identify patterns or warning signs requiring human attention. Already the commercial private sector has begun to harness such methods to integrate complex multidimensional data streams – e.g., climate, market prices, political instability – with individual behavior models in order to predict consumer behavior. "Machine-learning software predicts what a customer is likely to do in the next five seconds or in the next five weeks. It's pattern recognition at scale," said Ralf Herbrich, European Union director of machine learning at Amazon, in a recent Wall Street Journal interview.[22]

In the near future, the current streams of digital data generated by mobile technologies will rapidly turn into fast-moving rivers of information, ready to be tapped for insight using these advanced methods. Machine learning will facilitate simple analytics, from real-time monitoring and prediction of market prices to detecting patterns of FHW performance, as well as more complex tasks which involve integrating unlinked sources of data such as rainfall or indexes of social inequality. It is quite likely that our ability to extract new insights and actionable "intelligence" will increase as exponentially as cell phone ownership in remote villages of Asia and Africa.

My personal view

Alain B Labrique

The low cost and probably minimal risk of sharing information about optimal health and nutrition practices have tipped the scales in favor of implementation in many countries, where program investment has moved faster than the pace of evidence supporting these strategies.

Caution around information supersaturation has been raised in the global mHealth conversation, as populations rapidly become "spammed" by commercial and public health messaging directly to their devices. Ultimately, this may diminish the possible positive impacts these strategies currently enjoy in emerging markets.

Across this busy landscape of mInnovation, however, few strategies are being identified as impactful – with clear, robust evidence of their impact having been measured. Continued measurement and reporting of results will therefore be critical in making the case for continued mHealth and mNutrition scale-up and integration, and for harnessing of the full potential of these developments.

Further reading

African Strategies for Health mHealth Database, Focus on Nutrition: http://www.africanstrategies4health.org/mhealth-database.html?appSession=482174534684344, 2015 (n=26 projects listed).

Higgs ES, Goldberg AB, Labrique AB et al. Understanding the role of mHealth and other media interventions for behavior change to enhance child survival and development in low- and middle-income countries: an evidence review. J Health Commun. 2014;19 Suppl 1:164–89. doi: 10.1080/10810730.2014.929763.

Labrique AB, A Dangour. Nutrition Innovation and Technology. In: Eggersdorfer M, Kraemer K, Ruel M et al (eds). The Road to Good Nutrition: A global perspective. Karger. Kaiseraugst, Switzerland. 2015.

Mitchell M. Imagine a world. http://www.d-tree.org/imagine/imagine-a-world/ Vision statement for DTREE International. 2015.

mHealth Impact Model – a monitoring and evaluation framework to assess technology for development innovations across various sectors: http://www.gsma.com/mobilefordevelopment/mhealth-for-mnch-impact-model, 2015.

Mehl G, Vasudevan L, L Gonsalves et al. Harnessing mHealth in low-resource settings to overcome health system constraints and achieve universal access to health. In: Marsch LA, Lord SE, Dallery J, editors. Transforming Behavioral Healthcare with Technology: The State of the Science. Oxford University Press; 2014.

Mehl G, Labrique AB. Prioritizing integrated mHealth strategies for universal health coverage. Science 2014;345(6202):1284–7. doi: 10.1126/science.1258926.

Labrique AB, Vasudevan L, Kochi E et al. Articulating mHealth Strategies as Health System Strengthening Tools – Twelve Common Applications and a Visual Framework. Global Health Science and Practice 2013; 1(2):160–171.

References

1 Agarwal S, Perry HB, Long LA et al. Evidence on the feasibility and effective use of mHealth strategies by frontline health workers in developing countries: a systematic review. Tropical Medicine & International Health 2015;20(8):1003–1014.

2 http://research.microsoft.com/pubs/170446/Medhi-NordiCHI2012-CommCareCasestudy.pdf

3 mHealth Compendium Vol4. LAUNCH Project. http://www.africanstrategies4health.org/uploads/1/3/5/3/13538666/launch.pdf

4 http://www.mobilemamaalliance.org/. Accessed October 9, 2015.

5 http://www.africanstrategies4health.org/uploads/1/3/5/3/13538666/momconnect.pdf

6 http://www.dimagi.com/wp-content/uploads/2015/02/CommCare-Evidence-Base-March-2015.pdf.

7 Treatman D, Bhavsar M, Kumar V et al. Mobile phones for community health workers of Bihar empower adolescent girls. WHO South-East Asia J Public Health 2012;1(2):224–226.

8 http://www.africanstrategies4health.org/uploads/1/3/5/3/13538666/alive_and_thrive.pdf.

9 http://www.capacityplus.org/files/resources/ivr-system-refresher-training-senegal.pdf.

10 https://www.changemakers.com/serve2gether/entries/onefarm. Accessed October 9, 2015.

11 http://www.digitalgreen.org/press/. Accessed October 9, 2015.

12 http://www.theguardian.com/world/2012/aug/26/africa-innovations-transform-continent.

13 Gandhi R, Veeraraghavan R, Toyama K et al. Digital Green: Participatory Video and Mediated Instruction for Agricultural Extension. Inf Tech & Intl Dev. 5(1):1–15. 2009. http://itidjournal.org/index.php/itid/article/view/322/145.

14 http://www.prnewswire.com/news-releases/smart-sports-and-fitness-wearables-market-to-hit-149-billion-by-2021-528461241.html.

15 http://www.pewinternet.org/2011/11/02/part-iv-what-types-of-apps-are-adults-downloading/.

16 Lin M, Mahmooth Z, Dedhia N et al.Tailored, interactive text messages for enhancing weight loss among African American adults: the TRIMM randomized controlled trial. Am J Med. 2015 Aug;128(8):896-904. doi: 10.1016/j.amjmed.2015.03.013. Epub 2015 Mar 31.

17 http://www.ncbi.nlm.nih.gov/pubmed/25840035.

18 http://www.ncbi.nlm.nih.gov/pubmed/26965099.

19 http://www.ncbi.nlm.nih.gov/pubmed/26965100.

20 http://www.who.int/life-course/topics/AGH01-THRIVE.pdf.

21 Mehl G, Labrique AB. Prioritizing integrated mHealth strategies for universal health coverage. Science 2014;345:1284.

22 http://blogs.wsj.com/digits/2015/08/26/amazon-com-offers-machine-learning-platform-hires-scientists/.

Convergent Innovation for Addressing Malnutrition: Scaling up cross-sector solutions from the social economy

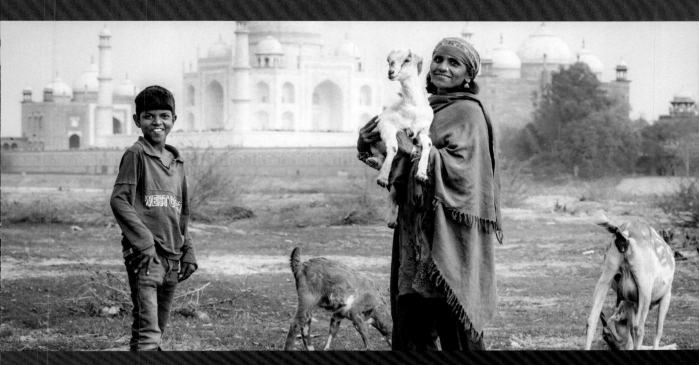

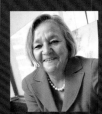

Laurette Dubé
James McGill Professor of consumer and lifestyle psychology and marketing, Desautels Faculty of Management, McGill University, Montreal, Quebec, Canada, and founding chair and scientific director of the McGill Centre for the Convergence of Health and Economics

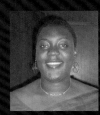

T Nana Mokoah Ackatia-Armah
Postdoctoral Fellow, McGill Center for the Convergence of Health and Economics (MCCHE), Desautels Faculty of Management, McGill University, Montreal, Quebec, Canada

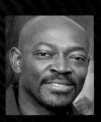

Nii Antiaye Addy
Assistant Professor (Research), Desautels Faculty of Management, McGill Center for the Convergence of Health and Economics, McGill University, Montreal, Quebec, Canada

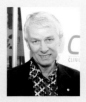

"Each year, several million children either die or suffer irreparable developmental defects because of vitamin A deficiency. Countless others are harmed by malnutrition and starvation. Yet many of these deaths would be preventable if we addressed them head on and used the tools that exist to stop them."

Sir Richard John Roberts, *recipient (together with Phillip Allen Sharp) of the 1993 Nobel Prize in Physiology or Medicine for the discovery of introns in eukaryotic DNA and the mechanism of gene-splicing.*

Key messages

- Business principles of innovation, entrepreneurship, and financing have been increasingly adopted in addressing malnutrition.

- Enterprises and financing schemes of various types have been formed, spanning the social economy, business, and public sectors to simultaneously create social and economic value and increase the impact of efforts to address malnutrition.

- The next challenge in scaling up current efforts is to place nutrition at the core of commercial food innovation, while fostering the social and institutional innovation needed to create an enabling environment for behavioral change and societal transformation.

- Convergent Innovation (CI) is a pragmatic, solution-oriented framework to help decision-makers incorporate the social objectives of nutrition into the economic mission of business, while ensuring that economic viability is better integrated into organizations focused on social benefit.

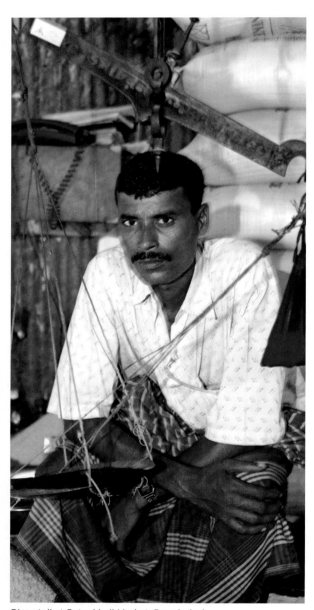

Rice stall at Patuakhali Market, Bangladesh.
Source: Mike Bloem

Chapter 4.4 | Convergent Innovation for Addressing Malnutrition:
Scaling up cross-sector solutions from the social economy

222

Using market-based approaches to address malnutrition

Globally, the adoption of market-based approaches to address social problems, including malnutrition, has gained popularity since the 1990s. For example, the Global Alliance for Improved Nutrition (GAIN, 2014) points out that: "it is crucial to harness the power of business – their technology, their marketing skills and insight into consumer behavior and their reach – for the public good."[1] Also in communities worldwide, the Ashoka network, which provides support for social entrepreneurs transforming the food chain, highlights lessons from business in stating that: "the citizen sector has discovered what the business sector learned long ago: there is nothing as powerful as a new idea in the hands of a first-class entrepreneur."[2] Thus, leadership in addressing malnutrition, once the purview of the public and social sectors (e.g., governments, international agencies and non-profits), is now engaging with business in cross-sector alliances.

Business principles are being integrated into nutrition solutions, with hybrid types of organizations in the *social economy* transcending the traditional bipolar focus on creating either social benefit or commercial value. Accordingly, concepts such as "social" and "inclusive" businesses, "social entrepreneurship," "social finance," and "development impact bonds" are increasingly encountered in the discourse around market-based approaches to address malnutrition.

Despite this new trend, bottlenecks remain in the attempt to transcend the boundaries of social economy organizations so as to more fully harness the capabilities and resources of the private sector in scaling up nutrition. This is especially the case when it comes to mainstreaming nutrition into core commercial activities.[3] Indeed, food businesses have been blamed for significantly contributing to obesity, diabetes and other diet-related diseases.[4] For example, business-driven advancements in technology for producing ultra-processed food, while profitable, have encouraged the consumption of calorie-rich ultra-processed foods, which has led to global overweight and obesity.[5] The Bulletin of the World Health Organization (2015) noted that in a study of 69 countries (24 of them high-income, 27 middle-income and 18 low-income), increased calorie intake was enough to explain concurrent increases in body weight linked with obesity in 45 countries between 1971 and 2010.[6]

Yet, with consumers acquiring most of their food through commercial sources (even in emerging economies)[7] there is a pressing need for efforts that simultaneously transform both the food supply chain *and* consumer behavior. This can be achieved through convergence between commercial and social objectives, in single and collective action by organizations across the social economy, government, and business. This is what Dube et al[8] have called "*Convergent Innovation*" (CI).

Drawing upon Convergent Innovation, this chapter provides a framework for guiding decision-makers across sectors of society to act individually and collectively to scale up current efforts that adopt business approaches to address malnutrition. The rest of the chapter proceeds as follows: first, to illustrate questions that decision-makers face, we draw upon a case of the Ghana Nutrition Improvement Project – a private-public-partnership (PPP) that is exploring business and financial models to scale up its development and marketing of a complementary food supplement to address malnutrition. Next, to elaborate on current efforts creating social and economic value, we use an interactive approach developed by social economy experts Quarter et al. (2009)[9] and Mook et al. (2015)[10] to characterize organizations in the nutrition space, based on (i) the orientation of their mission (i.e., social, commercial), and (ii) their sources of funding (i.e., government, market, civil society).

This approach differs from conventional categorization into private, public, and social/plural/third sectors, which, while useful for classifications, does not convey the complexity of how organizations blend sectoral elements. Given our interest in market-oriented solutions for nutrition, we focus on solutions spanning the social economy and private sectors. We elaborate on organizational types that depend on substantial government funding (i.e., *local development enterprises [LDEs]*, which include *social enterprises*) and those that do not (i.e., *social economy businesses [SEBs]*, which include *social businesses*). Illustrating some of the approaches being adopted, we present eKutir, an India-based social business leveraging information and communication technology to address multiple facets of smallholder farmer poverty, and Wholesome Wave, a US social enterprise creating partnership-based programs to enable underserved consumers to make healthier food choices. With financing being a key challenge across the board, we then discuss *social financing* within the framework used. To guide partnerships scaling up innovations in cases such as the ones we describe, we present the *Convergent Innovation* framework for engaging diverse types of organizations to act individually and collectively in simultaneously creating social and commercial value to address malnutrition and transform society. A fundamental idea behind Convergent Innovation is that deep insight into human behavior – in both food supply and demand – is needed to bring about societal transformation. We conclude with a consideration of the possibilities for the coming years and decades.

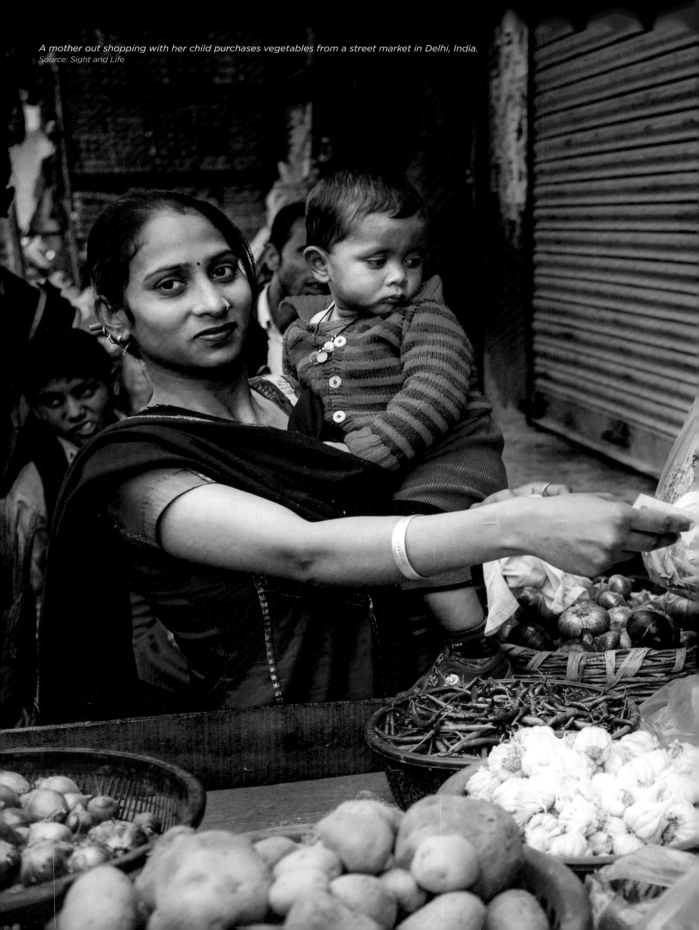

A mother out shopping with her child purchases vegetables from a street market in Delhi, India.
Source: Sight and Life

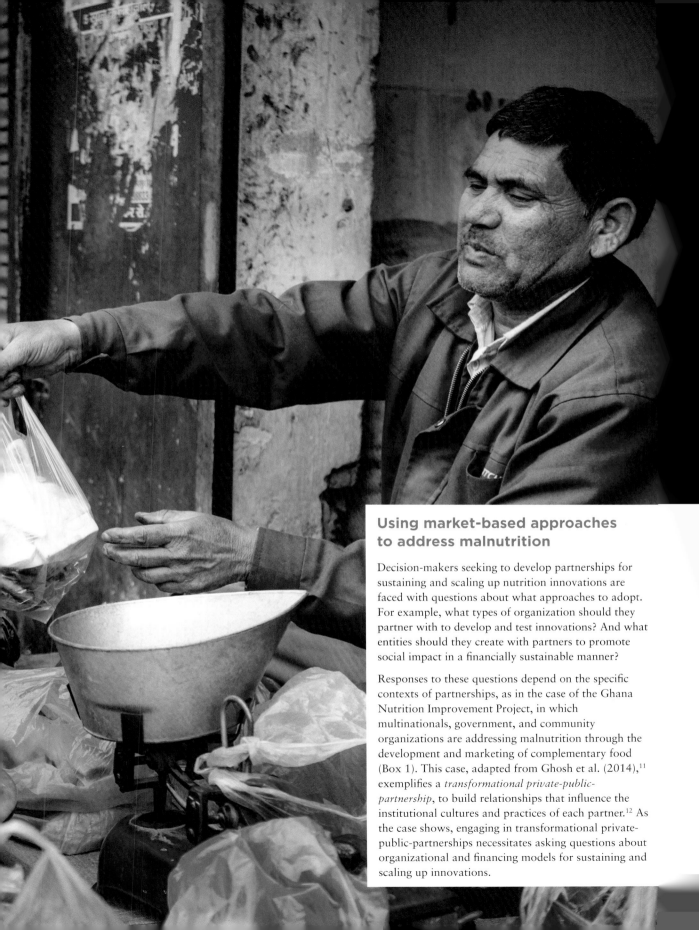

Using market-based approaches to address malnutrition

Decision-makers seeking to develop partnerships for sustaining and scaling up nutrition innovations are faced with questions about what approaches to adopt. For example, what types of organization should they partner with to develop and test innovations? And what entities should they create with partners to promote social impact in a financially sustainable manner?

Responses to these questions depend on the specific contexts of partnerships, as in the case of the Ghana Nutrition Improvement Project, in which multinationals, government, and community organizations are addressing malnutrition through the development and marketing of complementary food (Box 1). This case, adapted from Ghosh et al. (2014),[11] exemplifies a *transformational private-public-partnership*, to build relationships that influence the institutional cultures and practices of each partner.[12] As the case shows, engaging in transformational private-public-partnerships necessitates asking questions about organizational and financing models for sustaining and scaling up innovations.

Box 1 | A private-public-partnership addressing malnutrition in Ghana

The Ghana Nutrition Improvement Project (GNIP) was launched in 2010 to address the poor quality of complementary foods (CFs) by (i) producing a low-cost complementary food supplement, KOKO Plus™, to be added to fermented maize porridge, koko (a typical complementary food consumed by Ghanaian infants and young children); and (ii) testing social entrepreneurship and social business models in the distribution and delivery of the product, for scaling up the initiative.

The Ghana Nutrition Improvement Project is led by a tripartite public-private-partnership consisting of the following, who lead on topics briefly outlined:

- University of Ghana: Research & development (R&D) based on in-depth understanding of local needs; testing potential for KOKO Plus™, facilitating collaboration with government agencies, such as Ghana Health Service

- Nevin Scrimshaw International Nutrition Foundation (INF): Research & development testing

- Ajinomoto Inc. (multinational food company): Local production, together with Yedent Agro Processing Venture Ltd, a local for-profit food producer, employing expertise in food technology and amino acid nutrition.

Figure 1 | Ghana Nutrition Improvement Project partners

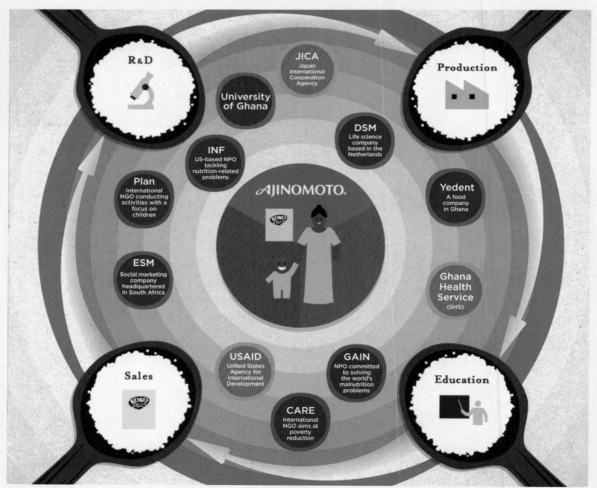

Chapter 4.4 | Convergent Innovation for Addressing Malnutrition:
Scaling up cross-sector solutions from the social economy

226

Other partners are bilateral and multilateral development agencies, and global and national/local organizations from the public, private, and social sectors (**Figure 1**), who, beyond R&D and production, are also engaged in education for demand creation, through communicating the importance of nutrition to local mothers; and in developing an innovative distribution model for sales.

The Ghana Nutrition Improvement Project aims for an "inclusive business" approach by employing (i) 2,000 women entrepreneurs to sell the supplement, (ii) workers at the factory, and (iii) suppliers of the main ingredients. The Project has been exploring business and financing models to implement for sustaining and scaling up the initiative.

In a study, Ghosh et al (2014) note that for sustainability there is a need to manage investments and expectations about returns by the private sector partners, within the context of addressing public sector requirements and societal need for improved access to good nutrition. They also note the need to address questions about business models that could be potentially adopted to sustain and scale the production, distribution, and delivery of products such as KOKO Plus™.

Hybrids creating social and commercial value

Sustaining and scaling efforts such as the Ghana Nutrition Improvement Project requires that decision-makers across sectors – for example, social and commercial entrepreneurs exploring what strategic partnerships to develop; investors seeking returns, while having a social impact; and policy-makers and legislators deliberating on how to create enabling environments – be consistently abreast of innovative approaches being adopted. Departing from traditional conceptualizations, we adopt the interactive approach used by social economy experts Quarter et al. (2009) and Mook et al. (2015) to highlight diverse types of organizations interacting with each other across the fluid boundaries of the social economy, public, and private sectors, creating social and economic value (**Figure 2**). Mook et al. (2015) define the social economy as bridging "the many different types of self-governing organizations whose focus is fulfilling social objectives and, in balance, whose social objectives assume priority over their economic purposes."

The interactive approach facilitates an understanding of emerging types of organizations that decision-makers, initially embedded within different sectors, create to develop and scale up nutrition innovations. As our case studies show, government agencies may initially enter into partnerships with businesses and civil society as separate entities, but then create hybrid organizations that also evolve over time.

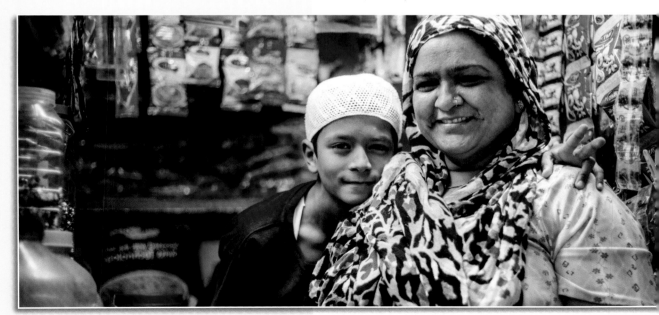

Obese mother with son in her snack stall at Karnataka, India.
Source: Mike Bloem

Chapter 4.4 | Convergent Innovation for Addressing Malnutrition:
Scaling up cross-sector solutions from the social economy

227

Figure 2 | **The social economy in interaction
with the public and private sectors**

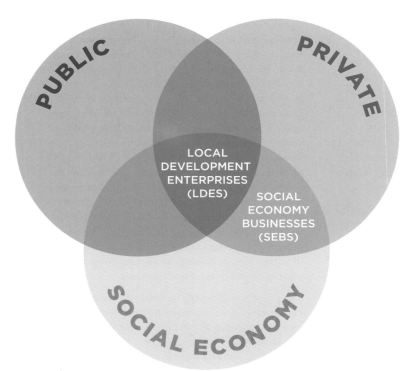

Given our interest in market-oriented solutions for nutrition, among the multiple types of organizations we focus on those spanning the social economy and private sectors. We differentiate between those that depend on substantial government funding, *local development enterprises*, and those that do not, *social economy businesses*. We note that in reality the distinctions are subtle, and organizations may evolve from one type to another, as illustrated by the open boundaries of **Figure 2**. **Table 1** summarizes the orientations and examples of the two types.

In addressing the issue of economic viability and financing that is especially critical for sustaining and scaling up nutrition, we elaborate on *social businesses* as examples of SEBs and *social enterprises* exemplifying local development enterprises. In the section on social financing, we also elaborate on *development financial institutions* (DFIs), which are likewise local development enterprises.

Table 1 | **Social economy organizations spanning the private
sector (adapted from Quarter et al., 2009 and Mook et al., 2015)**

Component	Social Economy Businesses (SEBs)	Local Development Enterprises (LDEs)
Orientation/Mission	Public at large (e.g., non-profits) Members (e.g., coops)	Community (usually defined geographically, or around a common interest)
Sources of Funding	Revenue from market, clients, members	Mixture of government, market, and donors
Examples	Cooperatives Non-profit organizations Social businesses Low-profit limited liability companies (L3Cs) Benefit corporations	Community development corporations (CDCs) Social enterprises Community development financial institutions Business improvement districts Workforce development organizations Workforce enterprises for marginal social groups Performing arts organizations Rural infrastructure development organizations Affordable home ownership organizations

Chapter 4.4 | Convergent Innovation for Addressing Malnutrition:
Scaling up cross-sector solutions from the social economy

228

Straddling the social economy and the private sector

Straddling the social and private sectors, social economy businesses are organizations that have a social mission but earn all or most of their revenues from commercial activities. These include *co-operatives*, some *non-profits*, and *social businesses*. New types of social economy business are also emerging. For example, *benefit corporations*, which have been expanding in the US and other parts of the world since 2007, are a type of for-profit corporate entity (i.e., treated the same as for-profit for tax purposes), with legally defined goals, including that of having a positive impact on society and the environment, in addition to the goal of making a profit. Additionally, *low-profit limited liability companies* are socially-oriented limited liability companies in some US states. Low-profit limited liability companies were inaugurated in 2008 to lower investment risk for private foundations that are looking to invest portions of their program-related investments, which are made to generate specific program outcomes, rather than for commercial returns.

Among social economy businesses, social businesses in particular have been playing a key role in addressing malnutrition globally. Social businesses are legal entities within the private sector (i.e., belonging to either shareholders or private owners), although they have strong social objectives as part of their mission (we note that some commentators classify them differently, placing them squarely in the private sector – which is illustrative of the fluidity

between the boundaries in Figure 2. Social economy experts Quarter et al. [2009] describe the distinctions as "splitting hairs"). Nobel Laureate Muhammad Yunus (2010)[13] defines social business as a "self-sustaining company that sells goods or services and repays its owners' investments, but whose primary purpose is to serve society and improve the lot of the poor." Although investors in social businesses are expected to receive their investment back, dividends and capital appreciation are not expected. The Grameen family of companies are well-noted examples of social businesses. Particularly relevant in the context of nutrition is Grameen Danone, a partnership between Grameen and Danone, the French multinational, that offers an affordable and easily available yoghurt, produced locally and distributed by local women entrepreneurs, to fulfil the nutritional needs of Bangladeshi children (Quarter et al., 2009).

Profit-oriented businesses owned by the poor, and thereby bringing them benefits, can also be social businesses. Related to this, a concept promoted by the World Business Council for Sustainable Development and the United Nations Development Programme is "inclusive business," which involves the poor in the corporate value chains – either as employees, entrepreneurs, suppliers, distributors, franchisees, retailers or customers, or else as sources of innovation.

While social businesses have shown some success at developing innovations to address malnutrition, they also face challenges in scaling up. Even as hybrids created from partnerships, they need to engage in further partnerships for increasing impact, as the case of eKutir in India shows (Box 2).

Chapter 4.4 | Convergent Innovation for Addressing Malnutrition:
Scaling up cross-sector solutions from the social economy

229

Box 2 | Social business creating partnerships: eKutir in India

eKutir is an India-based social business that has been providing a range of services to rural farmers and consumers with the aim of positively impacting nutrition since 2009. Viewing agriculture and rural development from an enterprise paradigm, its initiatives are premised on the understanding that deep insight into human behavior is needed in order to bring about change.

We focus here on eKutir's agricultural yield initiative and its healthy food access retail initiative, VeggieKart. For improving farmer yields, eKutir partnered with Grameen Intel Social Business in initiating a pilot study, which revealed dysfunction in the traditional agricultural value chain. Poor, often illiterate farmers, in addition to laboring

in the fields, were required to undertake various activities, ranging from assessing the state of the soil through accessing credit and market information and identifying purchasers to organizing transport for produce. eKutir developed an initiative to identify, select and train village-level micro-entrepreneurs, who utilize participatory methodology to understand the needs of farmers, and use contextualized ICT tools to provide services such as soil testing and nutrient management, helping to reduce production costs and improve productivity and yields with the objective of sustaining farmers' incomes.

With improved yields, eKutir also tackled demand-side challenges in another initiative, VeggieKart. It established a collaboration to provide market linkages by connecting farmers (mostly women) directly to the variety of consumers across different income groups, providing price variability through different retail outlets, and increasing accessibility to healthy produce in order to address malnutrition. **Figure 3** shows the relatively higher value being received by farmers growing potatoes, in the case of VeggieKart 59%, as compared with 41% traditionally. With green vegetables, the case of VeggieKart is 61%, as compared with 27% traditionally.

To acquire financing, eKutir is collaborating with corporate-sector partners such as MGM Agri Ventures, an agriculture investment firm, for retailing VeggieKart; and with ONE Acre Venture, a crowdfunding platform connecting investors to people at the Base of the Pyramid, including farmers, farming communities, and rural households. eKutir also has partnerships with local governments, notably for improving the livelihoods of women famers, so as to empower them.

Moving forward, Krishna Mishra, eKutir's founder, indicates that eKutir will continue to develop partnerships to scale up the impact of their work in India and globally.

Figure 3 | **Improvement in food value chain with eKutir intervention**

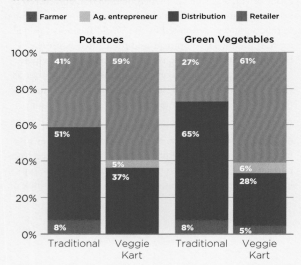

Source: Suvankar Mishra, Executive Director, eKutir Social Business Group – http://www.ekutirsb.com.

Straddling the social economy, private, and public sectors

Another set of organizations playing a key role in bringing innovations to scale are local development enterprises, which differ from social economy businesses in relying substantially on government funding (e.g., grants and contracts, particularly during early stages), beyond civil society (e.g., community-supported arrangements) and market sources. Local development enterprises include social enterprises. As with other types of organization in the fluid local development enterprise space, social enterprises

are oriented towards the economic and social development of communities (often geographically specified). They are also driven by diverse sets of values, including a mission to serve underdeveloped communities. The forms of social enterprises vary depending on their specific goals, as well as on the policy and legal environments within which they are created. For example, in the case presented below (Box 3), Wholesome Wave was established in the USA as a non-profit social enterprise partnering with local farmers' markets to increase access to healthier foods for underserved communities that receive government benefits.

Box 3 | Non-profit social enterprise: Wholesome Wave

Wholesome Wave is a US-based non-profit organization with strong linkages between food supply and demand: small and mid-sized farmers. The organization targets underserved communities to motivate healthier food choices, thereby improving nutrition and health outcomes. Wholesome Wave collaborates with more than 80 community-based partners, government, and businesses, with its programs having expanded from three states in 2007 to 33 states and Washington, DC in 2015, and is currently being implemented in over 500 farmers' markets, food hubs, and food retail outlets such as schools, restaurants, hospitals, and community health centers throughout the USA.

Wholesome Wave programs include:

- National Nutrition Incentive Network, which changes the consumption behavior of low-income households from unhealthy to healthier diets by providing double the monetary incentive to consumers who spend their Supplemental Nutrition Assistance Program (SNAP) benefits on fresh fruits and vegetables at farmers' markets and other retail outlets; and advocates at city, state, and federal levels for policies that generate additional opportunities for small and mid-sized farm businesses.

- Fruit and Vegetable Prescription Program, which provides

families affected by diet-related diseases with a prescription for fruits and vegetables, to be spent at participating farmers' markets and retail outlets. From 2010 to 2014, there have been 1,131 overweight/obese patients enrolled in the Fruit and Vegetable Prescription Program, and 5,655 low-income families impacted, with numbers expected to grow as the program expands to more states.

- Healthy Food Commerce Investments, which improves the supply chain for local food by working with food hubs to structure investments, and enter large wholesale markets in collaboration with businesses, government entities, investors, and customers (**Figure 4**).

Very significantly, Wholesome Wave's advocacy has affected US federal policy, specifically the US Farm Bill that includes funding for nutrition incentives at US$20 million per year, for five years, increasing funding for the Farmers' Market and the Healthy Food Financing Initiative, among other incentives. Wholesome Wave's success has further attracted additional funding. In 2015 it obtained a US$3.77 million grant from United States Department of Agriculture to support the increase of affordable access to fruits and vegetables for more than 110,000 SNAP consumers, thereby further positively impacting food security and nutrition.

Figure 4 | **Wholesome Wave model for its Healthy Food Commerce Investments**

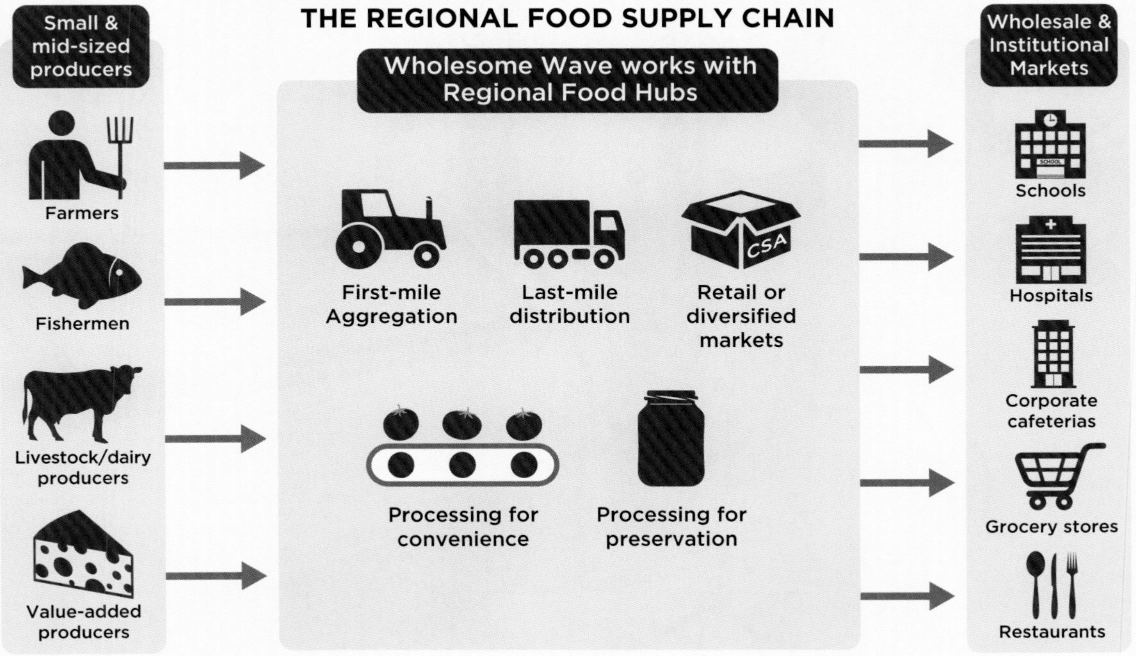

Source: Wholesome Wave - http://www.wholesomewave.org

Chapter 4.4 | Convergent Innovation for Addressing Malnutrition:
Scaling up cross-sector solutions from the social economy

231

Social financing

While the case of Wholesome Wave shows the possibilities for scaling up using public resources, given cuts in such funding, market-based and community financing remain crucial. Yet accessing such sources continues to be one of the biggest challenges faced in addressing malnutrition, due to the low return on such investments. For example, as compared with unhealthy processed foods or technology-based enterprises, initiatives targeting nutrition (particularly those by organizations in local food systems [e.g., in primary production, fresh/whole foods]) tend to take time and have lower growth potential, so that with traditional equity investors looking for anywhere between a 20% and a 100% return on investment, venture capital and financing for scaling up nutrition innovations is hard to come by.[15]

Local development enterprises that focus on financing, such as *development finance institutions*, potentially play a key role in addressing challenges to bringing innovations to scale in various parts of the world. Development finance institutions – which include banks (e.g., for agriculture and rural development), credit unions, loan funds, and venture capital funds that target development, as well as microfinance institutions, microenterprise development loan funds, and community development corporations – are

oriented towards the economic and social development of communities. Development finance institutions are able to pool resources from government, from civil society (e.g., crowdfunding), and from exchanging services in the marketplace for attaining some financial independence.

At a global level, such pooling of resources is emerging as an important source of funding for scaling up impact. For example, *Development Impact Bonds* are emerging as a means of socially and commercially oriented investing, in which savings realized by government (for instance, due to reductions in healthcare costs attributable to improved nutrition) are recouped by investors. Noting that investors may be better attracted where pooled funds are backed by global financial institutions, the Global Alliance for Improved Nutrition (GAIN) has partnered with the International Finance Corporation (IFC) and other financial institutions to provide access to various types of financing (e.g., grant, debt, equity) and expertise, and to share risk and generate additional financial resources by leveraging capital from investors for nutrition-related innovation.[16] These "nutrition-themed investment funds" include social investment funds (e.g., Root Capital), impact investments (e.g., LGT Venture Philanthropy), and other forms of patient debt/equity investors (e.g., Acumen Fund).

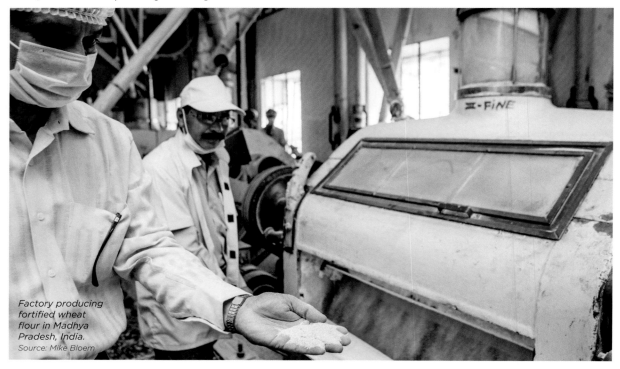

Factory producing fortified wheat flour in Madhya Pradesh, India.
Source: Mike Bloem

Chapter 4.4 | Convergent Innovation for Addressing Malnutrition:
Scaling up cross-sector solutions from the social economy

232

Convergent Innovation for scaling up cross-sector nutrition efforts

Despite advances made by social businesses, social enterprises, development finance institutions, and other types of organization spanning the social economy, the public sector, and the private sector in bridging tensions between socially and commercially oriented objectives for addressing malnutrition, more remains to be done. A next step for scaling up efforts is to make the social objectives of nutrition more central to for-profit organizations, while business approaches are further integrated into socially oriented organizations.

One pragmatic way of doing so is through convergent innovation partnerships. Until now, food innovation efforts have mostly been designed and managed as distinct domains (i.e., agricultural inputs, farming, food processing, community development, healthcare, media, etc.), by different sectors (i.e., government, commercial, civil society) and at different levels (i.e., local, city, state, country, global). For instance, while governmental and non-profit efforts typically focus on economic access to food that people need for subsistence and health, the success of businesses is rooted in a flow of food innovations that consumers want and are willing and able to pay for. Further, nothing on the food-supply side is possible unless farmers and others in the value chain are willing and able to produce. Convergent innovation finds the "sweet spot" for convergence in agriculture, wealth, and health in "one world," scaling the efforts of social economy hybrids that span sectors (**Figure 5**).

Convergent Innovation is a concept to guide decision-makers in initiating and developing partnerships to bring about behavioral change and societal transformation through accelerating successful go-to-market strategies for appealing and nutritious food innovations in a manner that is both financially and environmentally sustainable, while improving diets for society overall. Convergent Innovation harnesses the power of business and jointly targets economic growth and human development, enabled by the engagement of private enterprise, cross-sector collective action, and digital technologies (**Figure 6**).

Figure 5 | **The Convergent Innovation sweet spot for scaling up nutrition efforts**

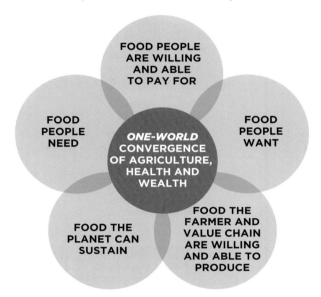

PUBLIC | SOCIAL ECONOMY | PRIVATE

FOOD PEOPLE ARE WILLING AND ABLE TO PAY FOR

FOOD PEOPLE NEED

ONE-WORLD CONVERGENCE OF AGRICULTURE, HEALTH AND WEALTH

FOOD PEOPLE WANT

FOOD THE PLANET CAN SUSTAIN

FOOD THE FARMER AND VALUE CHAIN ARE WILLING AND ABLE TO PRODUCE

To realize desired goals, Convergent Innovation comprises three pillars that the case studies in this chapter showed: technological innovation (e.g., novel agriculture inputs and food processing, applications for tracking nutrition behavior and healthcare), social innovation (e.g., changes to the value chain, organizational forms, and financial models), and institutional innovation (e.g., changes to informal norms and formal policy, consumer choice and market architecture design). As the developers of Convergent Innovation point out, it is important to note that each innovation pillar reinforces the other, since the absence of one pillar would limit the realization of the full potential of other pillars (Jha et al., 2014).[17]

Chapter 4.4 | Convergent Innovation for Addressing Malnutrition:
Scaling up cross-sector solutions from the social economy

233

Figure 6 | **The Convergent Innovation Framework**

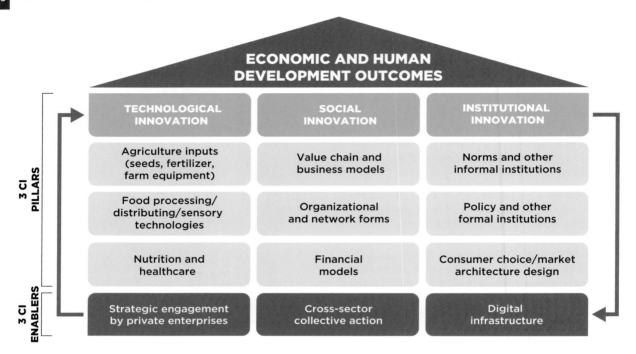

Convergent Innovation is deployed through collaborative platforms, convening partners from academia, the social economy, private and public sectors across education, health and other domains, with the highest aspiration to "change the world through food." These partnerships progressively transform institutions, such that Convergent Innovation becomes the new standard in a commercially successful and healthy food system.

We have developed the Convergent Innovation concept and methods, taking pulses (e.g., dried peas, lentils, chickpeas) as the first proof of concept, with a Global Pulse Innovation Platform launched as part of the official 2016 International Year of Pulses declaration. National Pulse Innovation Platforms are to be launched in 2016 in Canada and India, with the goal of sparking a world movement that will collectively pool ideas and resources, and engage in supply- and demand-side action for years to come.

The development and deployment of Convergent Innovation (CI) has benefited from the support of the International Development Research Centre (IDRC) and the Social Sciences and Humanities Research Council (SSHRC) of Canada.

Chapter 4.4 | Convergent Innovation for Addressing Malnutrition:
Scaling up cross-sector solutions from the social economy

234

My personal view

Laurette Dubé

Market-oriented approaches for addressing malnutrition are necessary in the face of scarce financial resources. Yet simply adopting market-based financing approaches is not enough for scaling up innovations, particularly in nutrition. There is a need to engage all sectors in bringing about behavioral change and societal transformation.

Convergent Innovation provides a framework to guide decision-makers in initiating and developing partnerships to bring about necessary micro-level change and macro-level transformation for addressing malnutrition.

Moving forward, I foresee the diffusion of approaches and financing models that are being used by social businesses such as eKutir in India, social enterprises such as Wholesome Wave in the USA, global development finance institutions' development of "nutrition-themed investment funds," and other emerging approaches and models, particularly those based on deep insights into human behavior. It is my hope that efforts deployed by social, public, and commercial sectors of society will improve human and economic development outcomes to a greater extent than has been possible thus far, with convergent innovation facilitating such transformation, taking a "One World" perspective in addressing both undernutrition and overnutrition in an economically sustainable manner.

Further reading

Jha SK, McDermott J, Bacon Gat al. *Convergent Innovation for Affordable Nutrition, Health and Healthcare: The Global Pulse Roadmap, Ann N Y Acad Sci 2014;1331(1):142-156* – http:// onlinelibrary.wiley.com/ doi/10.1111/nyas.12543/full

Mook L, Whitman A, Quarter J et al. *Understanding the Social Economy of the United States. Toronto, ON: University of Toronto Press, 2015.*

Walker, C., & Schofield, D. *Attracting Investment Capital to Nutrition Interventions. 2014* – http:// micronutrientforum.org/wp-content/uploads/2014/12/0355. pdf & Nutrition-Themed Investment Funds: http://www. gainhealth.org/knowledge-centre/project/nutrition-themedinvestment-funds

Young, C. *Food, Farms, Fish and Finance: Practical impact investment strategies to seed and sustain local food systems. 2015* - http://www.mcconnellfoundation.ca/en/resources/ report/food-farms-fish-and-finance-practical-impact-investment-strategi

Jha SK, Pinsonneault A, Dubé L. *The Evolution of an ICT Platform-enabled Ecosystem for Poverty Alleviation: The Case of eKutir. Management Information Science Quarterly (MISQ) (in press)* – http://www.misq.org/skin/frontend/ default/misq/pdf/Abstracts/13555_RN_SI.pdf

References

1   http://www.gainhealth.org/knowledge-centre/annual-report-2014/.

2   https://www.ashoka.org/social_entrepreneur.

3   Dubé, L. Scaling Up Multistakeholder Partnerships for Non-Communicable Disease Prevention and Control: Threading the Needle between Conflict and Convergence of Interests, Strategic Brief submitted December 16th, 2013 to (PAHO), Pan American Health Organization.

4   Swinburn BA, Sacks G, Hall KD et al. The global obesity pandemic: shaped by global drivers and local environments. Lancet. 2011;378(9793):804–14. doi: 10.1016/S0140-6736(11)60813-1.

5   Popki BM, Adair LS, Ng SW . NOW AND THEN: The Global Nutrition Transition: The Pandemic of Obesity in Developing Countries. Nutrition Reviews 2012;70(1):3–21. doi:10.1111/j.1753-4887.2011.00456.

6   http://www.who.int/bulletin/releases/NFM0715/en/.

7   Tschirley D, Reardon T, Dolislager M et al. The Rise of a Middle Class in East and Southern Africa: Implications for food system transformation. Journal of International Development, J Int Dev 2015;27:628–646. Published online in Wiley Online Library (wileyonlinelibrary.com) DOI:10.1002/ jid.3107.

8   Dubé L, Jha SK, Faber A et al. Convergent innovation for sustainable economic growth and affordable universal healthcare: Innovating the way we innovate, Ann N Y Acad Sci 2014;1331(1):119–141.

9   Quarter J, Mook L, Armstrong A. Understanding the Social Economy: A Canadian Perspective. Toronto, Buffalo, London: University of Toronto Press, 2009

10   Mook L, Whitman A, Quarter J et al. Understanding the Social Economy of the United States. Toronto, ON: University of Toronto Press, 2015.

11   Ghosh S, Tano-Debrah K, Aaron GJ et al. (2014). Improving complementary feeding in Ghana: reaching the vulnerable through innovative business – the case of KOKO Plus. Ann N Y Acad Sci 2014;1331(1):76–89.

12   Kraak VI, Harrigan PB, Lawrence M et al. Balancing the benefits and risks of public-private partnerships to address the global double burden of malnutrition. Public Health Nutrition. 2012;15(03):503–17. doi: doi:10.1017/ S1368980011002060.

13   Yunus M, Bertrand M, Lehmann-Ortega L. Building Social Business Models: Lessons from the Grameen Experience. Long Range Planning 2010;43(2–3):308–325.

14   http://www.wholesomewave.org/about-us/.

15   http://mcconnellfoundation.ca/en/resources/report/food-farms-fish-andfinance-practical-impact-investment-strategi.

16   http://www.gainhealth.org/knowledge-centre/project/nutrition-themedinvestment-funds

17   Jha SK, McDermott J, Bacon G et al. (2014). Convergent Innovation for Affordable Nutrition, Health and Healthcare: The Global Pulse Roadmap, Annals of the New York Academy of Sciences 2014;1331(1):142–156.

Personalized Nutrition: Paving the way to better population health

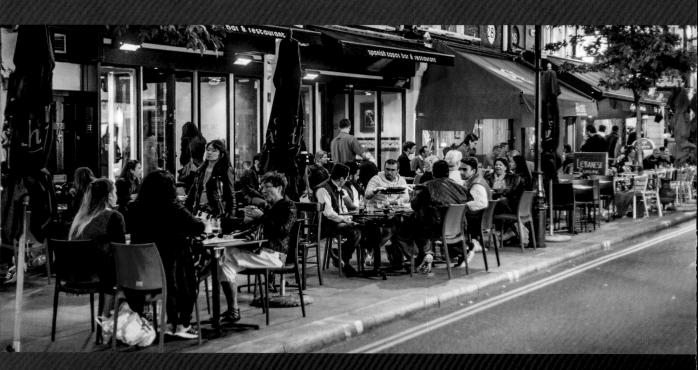

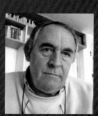

Michael Gibney
Professor of Food and
Health, University College
Dublin, Ireland

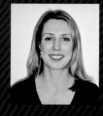

Marianne Walsh
Research Fellow, University
College Dublin, Ireland

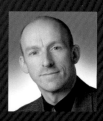

Jo Goosens
Director Bio-Sense,
Belgium, on behalf of the
Food4Me Consortium

"Life is the sum of all your choices."

Albert Camus *(1913–60), French philosopher, author and journalist; winner of the 1957 Nobel Prize for Literature.*

Key messages

- One of our biggest current challenges is how to change eating and behavior patterns so as to produce better health in any given individual.

- The sequencing of the human genome led to a widespread belief that personalized medicine was imminent and soon gave rise to the term "personalized nutrition."

- The essence of personalized nutrition is to "assist individuals in achieving a lasting dietary behavior change that is beneficial for health."

- In a study entitled Food4me, consumers perceived the health benefits of personalized nutrition as outweighing the perceived risks.

- Personalized nutrition will represent an opportunity to achieve optimal health and will support self-realization, both within the realm of health and beyond it.

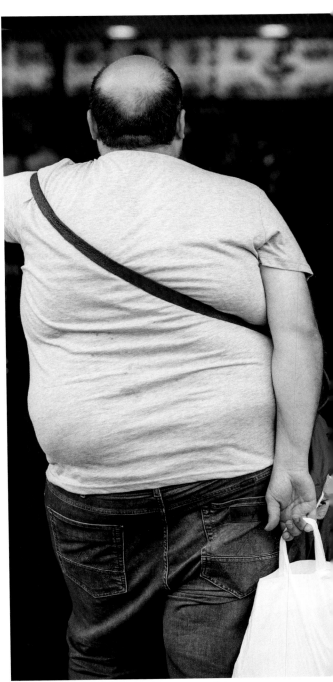

One billion people go to bed hungry every night, while half a billion of the world's citizens are obese.
Source: Mike Bloem

One billion people go to bed hungry every night, while half a billion of the world's citizens are obese. In the developed world, a sedentary and affluent lifestyle in a society with immediate access to affordable food is the main driver of obesity. In developing economies, urbanization is the lead cause of obesity. Traditionally, public health nutrition education programs have followed a "one-size-fits-all" approach. In today's digital age, this will change both in developing and developed countries as emerging information technologies come to dominate many traditional areas of communication. Nutrition education is no exception, and there is no reason not to believe that public health nutrition will be transformed to meet the unique needs of each individual citizen.

From 2011 to 2015, Food 4me, a European Union Seventh Framework project, explored the opportunities and challenges of personalized nutrition in addressing this increasingly concerning problem. Coordinated by University College Dublin and 26 partners across the EU, this project considered what might both help and hinder the development of personalized nutrition for all. The findings of Food 4me were published by the European Food Information Council in March 2015. They explore the concept of personalized nutrition from a scientific, technological, consumer, behavioral and business perspective.

Origins of the concept of personalized nutrition

Roger J Williams (1893–1988) was an American biochemist who named the B-vitamin folic acid and discovered another B-vitamin, pantothenic acid. In 1950, in an article entitled "Concept of genetotrophic disease," Williams wrote thus: *"A genetotrophic disease is one which occurs if a diet fails to provide sufficient supply of one or more nutrients required at high levels because of the characteristic genetic pattern of the individual concerned. This concept, based upon results in genetics and biochemistry, is new in medical thought and is believed to be the basis for many diseases, the causation of which is now obscure. Individual patients are far from standardized specimens, and medical problems should consistently be considered in terms of the genetically diverse patients, rather than in terms of an absolute normal."*

Thus the concept of genetically-based personalized health was first envisaged over six decades ago. It was to remain dormant for over half a century, however. The sequencing of the human genome changed those dynamics and led to a widespread belief that personalized medicine, in which therapeutic strategies would be targeted at patients on a genetic basis, was imminent. Soon, the term "personalized nutrition" began to emerge, accompanied by a belief that the nutritional management of diet-related chronic disease could be considerably improved on the basis of an individual's genomic data. In 2003 – about the time of the release of the human genome – the Institute for the Future at Palo Alto issued a report on personalized nutrition which concluded as follows: "Analysis of the data shows that about one third of American adults are likely to make at least some decisions based on a knowledge of personalized nutrition by 2010. This will create an opportunity for a substantial transformation of the food and nutrition industry in the United States and elsewhere – especially for producers and packagers of foods, retailers, pharmacies, managers of magazines and health reports and health insurance." Clearly, this prediction failed to materialize.

Against the background of such expectations of the potential of personalized nutrition, the European Commission's Directorate-General for Research issued a call in 2009 for proposals to explore this area. The Food4Me consortium was developed in response, and submitted its proposal in 2010. The submission was successful, and the consortium began its program in April 2011, to run until March 2015. The project aimed to explore all elements of personalized nutrition, using a multidisciplinary approach. It delivered the most comprehensive analysis ever of personalized nutrition, taking full account of both the opportunities and the challenges of this exciting new concept.

Definition of personalized nutrition

The essence of personalized nutrition is not to change existing nutritional guidelines, nor to personalize food products, nor indeed to turn food into medicine, but rather to "assist individuals in achieving a lasting dietary behavior change that is beneficial for health." Personalized nutrition can therefore be beneficial to everyone, whether they have already been diagnosed as at risk or they are perfectly healthy. It is an approach that helps everyone to reach the health condition to which they individually aspire.

Personalized nutrition makes healthy dietary suggestions more relevant to the daily life of the individual. Suggested changes to dietary patterns are therefore more effective and lasting. Food4me identified the need for combining the following approaches in order to achieve this.

1 A detailed knowledge of an individual's food choices and resultant nutrient intake has to be established, using internet-based tools.

2 Based on that analysis, the individual needs to receive coaching on how to improve his or her nutrient profile by making better prevailing personal food choices.

3 The use of dried blood spot technology (through special

paper cards delivered in the post to each volunteer) allowed researchers to probe blood profiles so as to enhance the dietary analysis data in terms of understanding each volunteer's unique nutritional profile.

4 Cheek swab samples were returned to the researchers to ascertain the genetic profile of each individual.

A six-month intervention study with over 1500 volunteers, carried out as part of Food4Me, showed this principle to be both feasible and effective. The mere fact that an individual receives dietary recommendations on a personal basis is enough to positively affect his or her dietary behavior. The effectiveness is higher, however, if the advice can be further personalized by providing detailed coaching on how each individual can modify his or her existing food choices so as to improve his/her own nutritional profile. Adding further information (such as blood-based biomarkers or genetic profiling) might result in even greater effectiveness, but this will require further research. The study also showed that it is feasible to deliver personalized dietary advice via an entirely internet-based interface, and that this approach provides a generally representative sample.

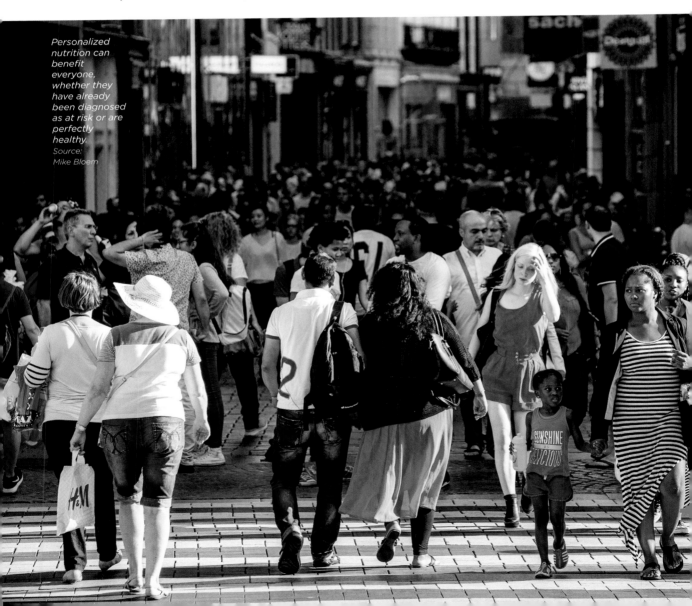

Personalized nutrition can benefit everyone, whether they have already been diagnosed as at risk or are perfectly healthy.
Source:
Mike Bloem

239

The scientific basis for personalized nutrition:
Advice and lessons learned from a proof of principle study

Primary research questions:

Does **personalization of dietary advice** assist and / or motivate participants to eat a healthier diet in comparison with non-personalized, conventional healthy eating guidelines?

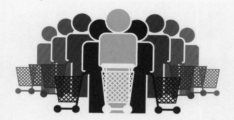

Is **personalization based on individualized phenotypic** or **genotypic information** more effective in motivating participants to make healthy changes, than personalization based on diet alone?

Secondary research questions:

Does **more frequent feedback help participants to improve** their compliance and motivate them to follow a healthier diet and lifestyle in comparison with those receiving less frequent feedback?

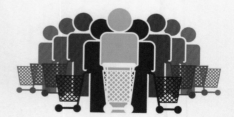

Recruitment flow chart

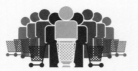

Register online

Interested individuals registered their details on the Food4Me website: **http://www.food4me.org/**

Age, sex, internet access, pregnancy, food intolerances and allergies

1st screening questionnaire

2nd screening questionnaire

Demographic, health, anthropometric and dietary information

Food Frequency Questionnaire (FFQ) to estimate habitual dietary intakes

Screening FFQ

Enrolment into study

Excluded those who were pregnant, lactating, following a prescribed diet or having a food allergy or intolerance or not having access to the internet

Participants completed the online FFQ, took anthropometric measurements, started wearing PA monitors and sent buccal swabs and dry blood spot cards to the research team

Baseline FFQ DNA and blood sample

Month 3 FFQ and provide blood sample

Participants in the *high intensity* group also completed the FFQ, anthropometric and PA at Month 1 and Month 2

Participants were provided with a personalized report (based on diet, phenotype and genotype) regardless of their intervention arm

Month 6 FFQ and provide blood sample

241

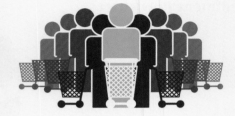

Is personalization based on phenotype or genotype more effective than personalization based on diet alone?

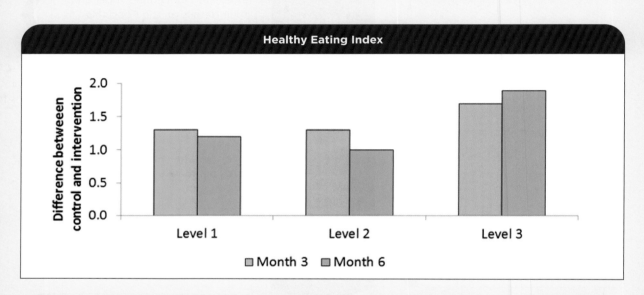

Healthy Eating Index

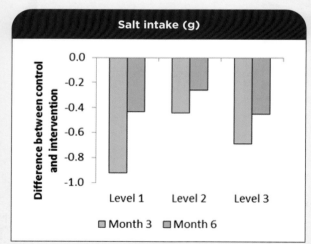

Salt intake (g)

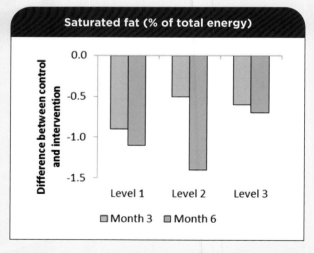

Saturated fat (% of total energy)

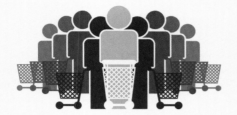

Will the **effect of PN advice on body weight change differ between individuals** with different starting body weights?

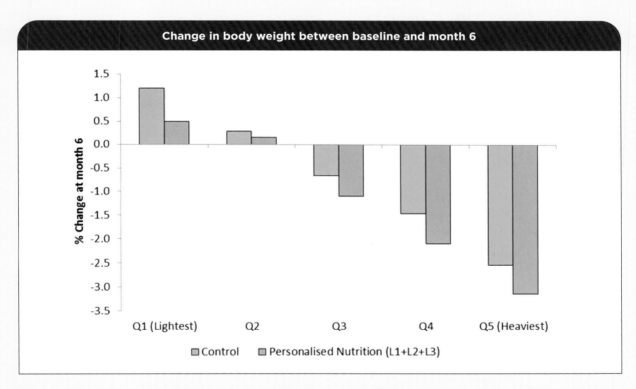

Change in body weight between baseline and month 6

% Change at month 6

☐ Control   ☐ Personalised Nutrition (L1+L2+L3)

The graph above indicates the change in body weight between baseline and month 6 according to the body weight of individuals at baseline (lightest weight [Q1] to heaviest weight [Q5]). Individuals who were underweight gained over 1% of their body weight, compared with individuals who were overweight or obese, who lost up to 3.5% of their body weight.

Adapted from Food4Me White Paper (2015) Accessed May 2015:
http://www.food4me.org/news/226-food4me-white-paper-onpersonalised-nutrition-paving-a-way-to-better-populationhealth.

About Food4Me

At the outset, Food4Me recognized that personalized nutrition would operate on three levels, each of which could either stand-alone or else be combined:

- Personalized dietary analysis

- Personalized phenotype analysis

- Personalized genotype analysis.

The design of the proof-of-principle study presented some novel challenges to the consortium, particularly the recruitment of subjects into a study where all contact between researchers and subjects was via the internet or the postal services. A standard operating procedure of some 900 pages was constructed to ensure consistency in a detailed protocol across each of the seven participating centers (Dublin, Reading, Warsaw, Athens, Pamplona, Munich and Maastricht).

Two centers started ahead of all the rest and, based on their experience, modifications to the standard operating procedure were made, and an intense training program was initiated. The proof-of-principle study kicked off in June 2012 and ended in March 2014. All objectives, milestones and deliverables were achieved which, given the scale and novelty of the study, remains a credit to all involved.

Food4Me recognized that without a detailed understanding of consumer attitudes to personalized nutrition, any insight in this field would fall well short of ideal. Thus a very significant part of the work program was devoted to probing the opinions of EU consumers. An extensive focus group study was carried out in nine participating centers, leading to the development of a questionnaire that would then be administered to 1,000 subjects in each of these centers. In addition, about 700 of those who actually participated in the proof-of-principle study undertook this same questionnaire. The consortium also probed the legal and ethical aspects of delivering personalized nutrition, as well as scoping existing and emerging technologies that individuals can use to learn about their health and lifestyle.

The outcome is an extremely valuable database, which can now be mined to address the many complex questions that will be asked regarding consumer attitudes to personalized nutrition. Allied to an understanding of consumer attitudes to personalized nutrition is the need to understand the viability of any personalized nutrition enterprise, whether driven by social or by private entrepreneurship. Across a series of workshops with stakeholders drawn from a wide range of interested sectors, a number of scenarios were developed which will help shape our thinking about the viable alternatives for the creation of a sustainable personalized nutrition offering.

Consumer responses to personalized nutrition

Consumer responses to the concept of personalized nutrition were found to be surprisingly positive. The perceived health benefits and the self-efficacy in managing personalized nutrition were seen to significantly outweigh any perceived risks.

Consumers share strikingly common views as to the criteria for an acceptable personalized nutrition service. These are:

- Person-to-person contact (either by email, phone or Skype, or else face to face)

- Direct access to an expert advisor who is perceived to have a professional background

- Regular follow-up on the advice given

- Advice covering not just nutrition but also physical activity and lifestyle recommendations.

Consumer attitudes vary much more widely when it comes to who should pay – the individual or public healthcare. They also disagree about what kind of arguments they find most persuasive – scientific explanations on the one hand, or experience-based evidence on the other. Some consumers may prefer group coaching over individual coaching, and some will favor a radical change of diet over a gradual adaptation. There is also greater reservation vis-à-vis genetic profiling than vis-à-vis blood analyses.

Consumers perceive risks especially related to privacy, personal data safety and potential misuse, either by authorities or companies, or as a result of hacking. It is possible that such risks are more keenly perceived when using the internet as an interface, as was the case in Food4Me.

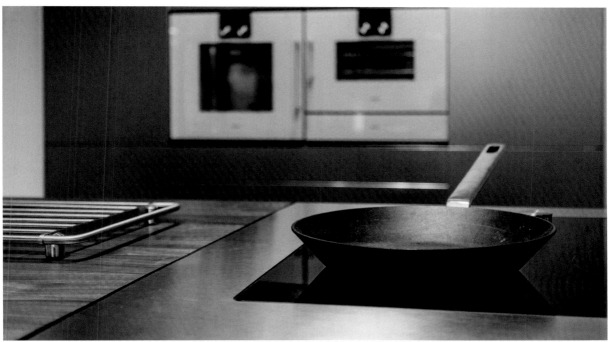

*Self-measurement will be important in personalized nutrition,
as most people want to be more independent and in control.*
Source: Mike Bloem

The role of technology in personalized nutrition

Food4me also looked into the wide range of novel
technologies that play an important role in enabling
personalized nutrition. From the diagnostic phase (monitoring
and assessing a person's nutrition and health status) to
generating dietary advice and making it practically applicable
in daily life, technologies are essential for personalized nutrition.
While individual genotyping is most often referred to in
personalized nutrition, the growing number of diagnostic tools
that help to assess the detailed physical and metabolic profile
of an individual are probably more important and relevant.

Food4Me explored the usefulness and reliability of some of
these technologies. For example, dry blood spot sampling was
used in the intervention study and was shown to be a very
reliable and alternative sampling and measurement tool for a
wide range of biomarkers from blood. Moreover, with proper
video instructions, consumers were perfectly capable of taking
their own blood samples, thus avoiding having to visit a doctor.

Self-measurement will be important in personalized nutrition,
as most people want to be more independent and in control.
Food4Me has shown that self-measurement of body
parameters, physical activity and dietary intake is perfectly
feasible when integrated into their lives – for example, by
means of on-line food frequency questionnaires or wearable
physical activity monitors. Novel technologies for wearable
and on-line monitoring devices are emerging every day and
will eventually allow us to measure a wide range of physical
parameters, from glucose levels to vitamin status and from
blood pressure to sleep quality.

Technical solutions are equally important to enable the
coaching and follow-up of dietary behavior or to measure the
progress of a person's nutritional status against the objectives
set. Using the internet and mobile communications, consumers
could have a choice of direct interfaces in any situation to
support appropriate food choices. These can come in a variety
of forms – from apps such as on-line shopping assistants to
appliances such as intelligent fridges and 3D food printers, or
in the form of complete services such as home-delivered
catering. This is how consumers will mostly experience the
practical use of personalized nutrition. What they will not see
is how these services rely on complex algorithms that convert a
variety of information streams into a set of nutritional
recommendations and, further, into food and meal plans that
fit personal preferences. In this respect, Food4me successfully
demonstrated the feasibility of such an integrated approach
and its delivery through an on-line dietary advice system.

Making personalized nutrition available to society at large

Much more effort will of course be needed before personalized nutrition can benefit society at large. While the volunteers in Food4Me demonstrated that the concept is useful for everyone, it will be a formidable challenge to introduce it to those who are most in need of a better diet, and who are often least interested in changing their dietary behavior.

Food4me explored what supportive business model concepts might possibly emerge in the future. Because dietary behavior and matters of nutrition and health are deeply rooted in societal issues, introducing personalized nutrition will inevitably involve significant societal changes. The timing is right for these changes, as our society urgently needs to take measures to tackle its growing health and nutrition problems.

Given the size and urgency of the problems and the fact that everyone should have the right to benefit from better health through personalized nutrition, a government-led initiative seems the most logical way of making personalized nutrition available to society at large. However, such a development is considered unlikely because governments are inherently reluctant to change such complex systems as public healthcare and also because of the sheer complexity of centrally organizing a personalized nutrition offering.

Personalized nutrition involves a wide range of actors, from diagnostic labs to producers of monitoring devices and app developers, and from advice algorithm developers to big data storage and analysis services. There will be an equally diverse constellation of users, most of them operating as intermediaries between the personalized nutrition service provider and the consumer/patient. These will range from dieticians, nutritionists and doctors, through hospitals, nursing homes, schools and day-care centers, to fitness centers, wellness institutions, retailers, caterers and restaurants, as well as health insurers and employers.

Personalized nutrition providers will thus become new and important integrating actors in society. Private initiatives are therefore the most likely way to drive the introduction of personalized nutrition services, probably with some form of societal support, preferably in the form of public/private partnerships.

Future business models are thus likely to involve networked structures with distributed profit centers that will work in close relationship with communities and other societal actors.

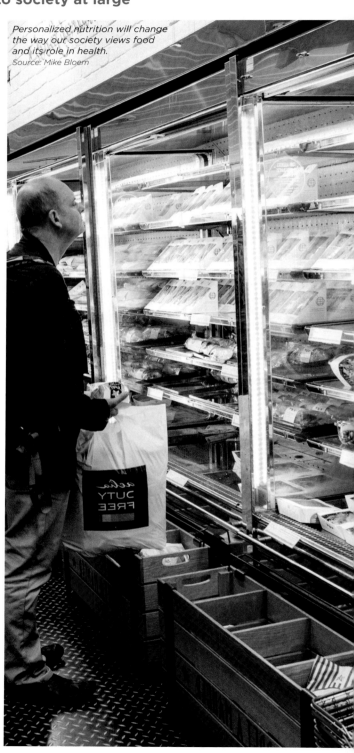

Personalized nutrition will change the way our society views food and its role in health.
Source: Mike Bloem

Legal and ethical considerations

In the light of the profound impact it will have on society, the introduction of personalized nutrition also raises important legal and ethical concerns. These too were examined in depth by the Food4Me project.

As personalized nutrition is making "nutrition-related" health the explicit responsibility of the individual, it will change the way our society views food and its role in health. This will affect the solidarity principle on which health insurance has until now been based. This will happen because personalized nutrition will lift this "veil of ignorance" when it comes to nutrition-related health issues.

The introduction of personalized nutrition brings to the fore concerns about personal freedom (especially if some people prefer not to be informed about individual health risks). It also raises questions about fairness in the system, particularly as concerns those deemed to be at higher risk.

There is also an issue over social inequality and injustice, since not everyone will be able either to understand or to react appropriately to the advice (or even to afford to follow it), while at the same time others might willfully and knowingly ignore this advice and refuse to change any behaviors.

These are complex issues. Significant changes to public healthcare and health insurance systems will therefore be required in order to maintain a balance between the interests of the individual and the common good.

On top of this, the present legal frameworks on food and health afford very little scope for providing this approach to personalized nutritional. Significant changes will be needed when it comes to regulating privacy (personal data access rights and data storage security). This holds true especially for mobile- and internet-based interfaces.

Similar steps being are taken right now towards personalized medicine, and these may also help us find a clearer distinction between nutrition-related health and uncontrollable health risks and the possible new roles that different actors will have as these definitions change.

Personalized nutrition in developed and less developed economies

Chapter 4.3 of this book highlights some of the challenges of technology transfer in the field of personalized nutrition. The Food4Me project focused on a collection of samples and data in affluent EU states. However, all of those technologies – personalized nutrition analysis, personalized anthropometric analysis and personalized genomics – are transferrable to less developed economies. In particular, dried blood spot technologies, as used in Food4Me, offer a rapid, inexpensive, low-technology and mass-distributive solution for blood collection which can be subsequently used for routine blood analysis or more advanced metabolomics analysis using the "hyphenated" (GC/LC/MC and NMR) technologies.

The developments in "Nutrition-workforce capacity building" as outlined in Chapter 4.3 provide the initial input into the building-blocks of personalized nutrition. Digitized personal data can be entered into such systems to help explore personalized nutrition using simple food consumption study methods. Most importantly, this technology can deliver photographic images of food servings, which have much greater communicative potential than linguistically based approaches. Ultimately, e-health in all its aspects will be like the smartphone: ubiquitous and adaptable.

Developing a more positive attitude toward diet and health

It seems possible that, at some point in the future, the move towards personalized nutrition in our society will fundamentally change people's perception of food and its role in health.

With each individual accepting his or her own responsibility for health, and effective use of the technologies that allow us to monitor this and make it happen, our society will gain a growing sense of being in control, and will develop an altogether more positive attitude toward diet and health.

For the majority, it will be enough to have the reassurance that potential health risks are under control. By these means, health will be turned into a manageable asset. For a growing percentage of the population, however, personalized nutrition will represent an opportunity to achieve optimal health. The concept of "health" itself will therefore evolve from one centered on achieving basic health goals to one involving the attainment of a much higher level of knowledge, understanding and self-awareness. Personalized nutrition will support self-realization, both within the realm of health and beyond it.

Food4Me partners

1	University College Dublin	14	Wageningen University
2	Ulster University	15	LEI-Wageningen University Research
3	Maastricht University	16	Philips Netherlands
4	Newcastle University	17	Technical University Munich
5	University of Oslo	18	NuGO-A Association
6	University of Navarra	18	Keller and Heckman
7	Lund University	20	Philips UK
8	University of Reading	21	Vitas
9	Crème GlobalSoftware Ltd.	22	HLK
10	European Food Information Council	23	Porto University
11	National Food and Nutrition Institute, Warsaw	24	Bio-Sense
12	TNO Quality of Life	25	DSM Nutritional Products Ltd
13	Harokopio University, Athens	26	University of Bradford

www.food4me.org

Project Coordinator
Professor Mike Gibney, Director, Institute of
Food and Health, University College Dublin, Ireland

Project Manager
Dr Marianne Walsh, Institute of Food and Health,
University College Dublin, Ireland
www.ucd.ie

Communications
European Food Information Council (EUFIC), Belgium
eufic@eufic.org | www.eufic.org

*Food4me – "Personalized nutrition: An integrated analysis
of opportunities and challenges" received funding from the
European Union's Seventh Framework Program for
research, technological development and demonstration
(Grant agreement no. 265494).*

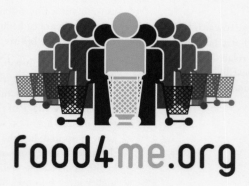

My personal view

Michael Gibney

Food4Me has demonstrated that the internet-based delivery of personalized dietary analysis and advice is not only feasible but also highly attractive to consumers. It has additionally shown that, in the light of the increasing age profile of the internet- and social-media-savvy consumer, the emergence of personalized nutrition is a given. Popular smartphone apps will come and go, but they will – at least for the foreseeable future – lack the complexity of the IT technology seen in Food4Me.

Beyond the simple 20-minute session a consumer might spend on the internet to attain a personalized dietary analysis and nutritional coaching, the next phase will be to integrate that service with smart kitchens, with retailers, and with works canteens. In the white goods industry, there is intense interest in bringing technologies directly into the home kitchen so as to enable consumers to optimize home cooking in order to attain improved nutrient profiling.

This is one step away from linking the home kitchen to the electronic dimension of supermarket purchasing and another step away from the selection of foods at works canteens. The integration of all this data will happen, and the consumer of the future will be able to plan and manage a week's menu so as to optimize gastronomic aspects, price and nutritional wellbeing. As Edwin Land, the MIT professor who pioneered Polaroid photography, said: "The present is the past, biting into the future."

Further reading

Food4Me White Paper (2015) Accessed May 2015: http:// www.food4me.org/news/226-food4me-white-paper-onpersonalised-nutrition-paving-a-way-to-better-populationhealth.

Nordstrom K et al. Values at stake: autonomy, responsibility, and trustworthiness in relation to genetic testing and personalized nutrition advice. Genes Nutr 2013;4:365–72.

Poinhos R, van der Lans IA, Rankin Aet al. Psychological Determinants of Consumer Acceptance of Personalized Nutrition in 9 European Countries. PLoS One. 2014;21:9(10).

Providing Access to Nutrient-Rich Diets for Vulnerable Groups in Low- & Middle-Income Settings

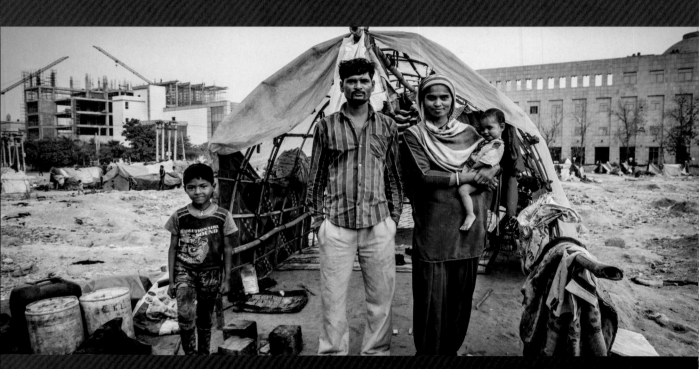

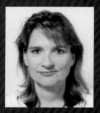

Saskia de Pee
Nutrition Division, World Food Programme, Rome, Italy. Friedman School of Nutrition Science and Policy, Tufts University, Boston, MA, USA

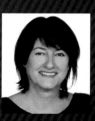

Regina Moench-Pfanner
ibn360, Singapore, Board Member of Rice Bowl Index

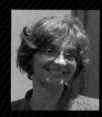

Lynnda Kiess
Nutrition Division, World Food Programme, Rome, Italy

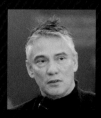

Martin W Bloem
Nutrition Division, World Food Programme, Rome, Italy. Friedman School of Nutrition Science and Policy, Tufts University, Boston, MA, USA. Johns Hopkins School of Public Health, Baltimore, MD, USA

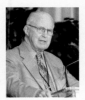

"The first essential component of social justice is adequate food for all mankind. Food is the moral right of all who are born into this world."

Norman Borlaug, American biologist, humanitarian and Nobel laureate, known as "the father of the Green Revolution."

Key messages

- Meeting nutrient requirements is a prerequisite for preventing undernutrition. Ensuring adequate nutrient intake and preventing disease requires direct multi-stakeholder efforts that also address the underlying causes of undernutrition.

- Nutrient requirements are frequently not met due to the limited availability and affordability of an adequately diverse diet that includes plant-source, animal-source, and fortified foods.

- The fortification of foods started almost 100 years ago, and fortification will continue to be an important way of ensuring adequate intake of nutrients such as iodine, iron, folic acid, vitamin A, vitamin B_{12}, and other vitamins.

- Foods fortified for the general population – such as flour, salt, sugar and vegetable oil – "piggy-back" on already existing distribution systems and consumption practices. Special nutritious foods, by contrast, are designed to meet the requirements of specific groups, who need to be encouraged to consume the individual product (e.g., micronutrient powders or fortified complementary foods).

- While a wealth of evidence already exists about the need to meet nutrient requirements and how to do so, more information should be collected on the magnitude of the impact of a combination of nutrition-specific and nutrition-sensitive interventions in a particular context and at a particular cost.

Key terms

Biofortification:
The process by which the nutritional quality of food crops is improved through biological means such as conventional plant breeding.

Dietary diversity:
The number of different foods or food groups consumed over a given reference period. The greater the dietary diversity, the greater the likelihood of meeting nutrient intake recommendations.

Food fortification:
The process of adding micronutrients to foods, during or after processing.

Nutrition-specific interventions and programs:[i]
Interventions or programs that address the immediate determinants of fetal and child nutrition and development –

adequate food and nutrient intake, feeding, caregiving and parenting practices, and low burden of infectious diseases.

Nutrition-sensitive interventions and programs:[ii]
Interventions or programs that address the underlying determinants of fetal and child nutrition and development – food security; adequate caregiving resources at the maternal, household and community levels; and access to health services and a safe and hygienic environment – and incorporate specific nutrition goals and actions. Nutrition-sensitive programs can serve as delivery platforms for nutrition-specific interventions, potentially increasing their scale, coverage and effectiveness.

Supplementation:
The provision of nutrients either via a food or as a tablet, capsule, syrup, or powder to boost the nutrient content of the diet.

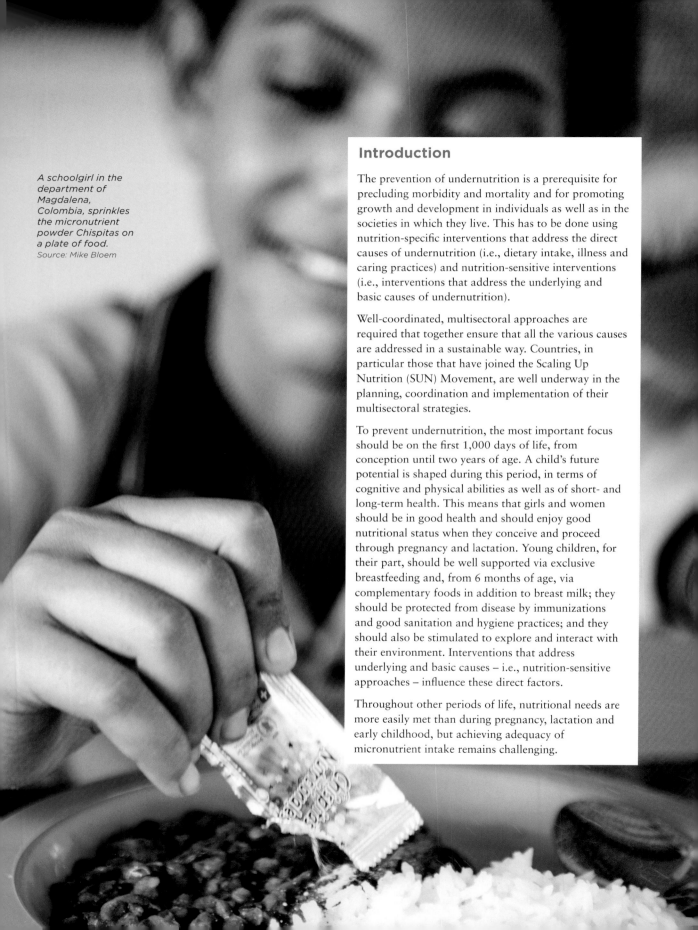

A schoolgirl in the department of Magdalena, Colombia, sprinkles the micronutrient powder Chispitas on a plate of food.
Source: Mike Bloem

Introduction

The prevention of undernutrition is a prerequisite for precluding morbidity and mortality and for promoting growth and development in individuals as well as in the societies in which they live. This has to be done using nutrition-specific interventions that address the direct causes of undernutrition (i.e., dietary intake, illness and caring practices) and nutrition-sensitive interventions (i.e., interventions that address the underlying and basic causes of undernutrition).

Well-coordinated, multisectoral approaches are required that together ensure that all the various causes are addressed in a sustainable way. Countries, in particular those that have joined the Scaling Up Nutrition (SUN) Movement, are well underway in the planning, coordination and implementation of their multisectoral strategies.

To prevent undernutrition, the most important focus should be on the first 1,000 days of life, from conception until two years of age. A child's future potential is shaped during this period, in terms of cognitive and physical abilities as well as of short- and long-term health. This means that girls and women should be in good health and should enjoy good nutritional status when they conceive and proceed through pregnancy and lactation. Young children, for their part, should be well supported via exclusive breastfeeding and, from 6 months of age, via complementary foods in addition to breast milk; they should be protected from disease by immunizations and good sanitation and hygiene practices; and they should also be stimulated to explore and interact with their environment. Interventions that address underlying and basic causes – i.e., nutrition-sensitive approaches – influence these direct factors.

Throughout other periods of life, nutritional needs are more easily met than during pregnancy, lactation and early childhood, but achieving adequacy of micronutrient intake remains challenging.

Strategies to prevent micronutrient deficiencies

To prevent undernutrition, the diet needs to provide all the nutrients required for growth, development and good health. Ideally, people's nutrient requirements will be met by eating locally available foods. However, in the case of some nutrients, it can be difficult to meet requirements from a diet based on local foods. This is particularly true of iodine, which is leeched out of many soils, making seafood the only good natural source of this essential micronutrient. Also for some other nutrients, meeting the requirements of different subgroups of the general population is a challenge. For example, where the average intake of folic acid is low, there is an increased risk of babies being born with neural tube defects (spina bifida), and nutritional anemia is more prevalent where people consume a predominantly plant-based diet, because certain essential nutrients, particularly iron, are not easily absorbed from these diets.

The fortification of commonly consumed foods started some 100 years ago in Europe and North America, and remains an important strategy in those countries and elsewhere for preventing deficiencies in specific micronutrients. For example, to prevent iodine deficiency, many countries have now introduced iodized salt, and for some areas where this is not (yet) possible, supplements are being used. Foods such as flour are fortified with folic acid, to prevent neural tube defects, with iron to prevent anemia and other consequences of iron deficiency, and with B-vitamins. Foods containing fat, such as milk and margarine, are fortified with vitamin A to prevent morbidity and xerophthalmia. To prevent neural tube defects, folate/folic acid intake around conception has to be adequate. However, taking supplements in anticipation of a planned pregnancy is not practiced in a large proportion of pregnancies, due to a lack of knowledge of, or access to, supplements. Fortification of commonly consumed foods, such as flour, is therefore the preferred strategy for protecting most pregnancies, whether planned or unplanned.

It is important to note that dietary diversity, fortification (industrial or domestic), biofortification and supplementation are complementary strategies for meeting nutrient requirements. Supplementation is usually targeted at specific groups with high needs, in particular young children (e.g., vitamin A capsules) or groups not touched by strategies that reach the majority of the population – for example, because of an isolated geographical location.

Industrial fortification reaches people who consume processed, packaged, foods. It can be applied to foods that are consumed by the general population, such as wheat flour, breakfast cereals, vegetable oil, margarine and sugar, and to foods for specific target groups, including infant porridges and special drinks or snacks for pregnant and breastfeeding women.

Biofortification refers to breeding crops with increased concentrations of 1–3 specific vitamins or minerals, which can be achieved either by conventional breeding or else by genetic modification. While industrial fortification can add a greater number of vitamins and minerals to a food consumed widely and regularly by consumers who access processed foods, biofortification has the potential to reach consumers who consume foods that are not processed, or only minimally so.

253

History of food fortification

Food fortification has contributed to the reduction of micronutrient deficiencies in North America, Europe and South America since its introduction approximately a century ago. Over the past two decades, Asia and Africa have also begun to adopt food fortification in order to improve the daily intake of micronutrients that are not provided in adequate quantities by the local diet.

In the early 1920s, as the causes of certain clinical problems were being discovered and vitamins were being isolated and their chemical structured identified, fortification was introduced as a means of eliminating the consequences of specific nutrient deficiencies, e.g., goiter (due to iodine deficiency) and xerophthalmia (due to vitamin A deficiency). Salt iodization was introduced in Switzerland as early as 1923, and in the USA in 1930; vitamin A fortification of margarine in Denmark in the 1930s, and of milk in the UK and USA in 1923; and Denmark also added vitamin D to margarine.

From the 1940s onwards, fortification of flour and cereal products commenced, which typically included iron, folic acid and some of the B-vitamins (especially thiamin, riboflavin and niacin). Meanwhile, the fortification of salt, margarine and milk continued, and vitamin A fortification of sugar was later introduced in Latin America. Also, industrial efforts were initiated to voluntarily fortify porridges and breakfast cereals targeted at young children and the general population. Concurrently, regulatory agencies developed guidelines and regulations on appropriate fortification levels as well as on messages and marketing communications for consumers.

Food consumption surveys show that fortified foods are an important source of micronutrients among consumers in high-income countries such as the USA, Costa Rica and the Netherlands. Some consumers consciously choose fortified products, whereas others are less aware that the processed foods they consume may be fortified. While some consumers speculate that food fortification might result in an excess intake of specific nutrients, there are no cases of toxicity documented in the literature. In fact, because the levels added are very low compared with the levels at which toxicity can occur, it is virtually impossible to eat foods such as breakfast cereals or margarine in quantities that would cause toxicity due to their fortification.

However, it is important to inform consumers about fortification, i.e., why it is done, and which foods are fortified: especially among populations who are not familiar with fortification, hearing that "something has been added to the food" may be misinterpreted as something that might be harmful, which could result in them not consuming the particular food.

The History of Fortification

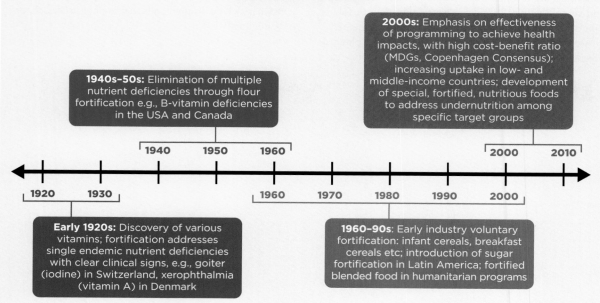

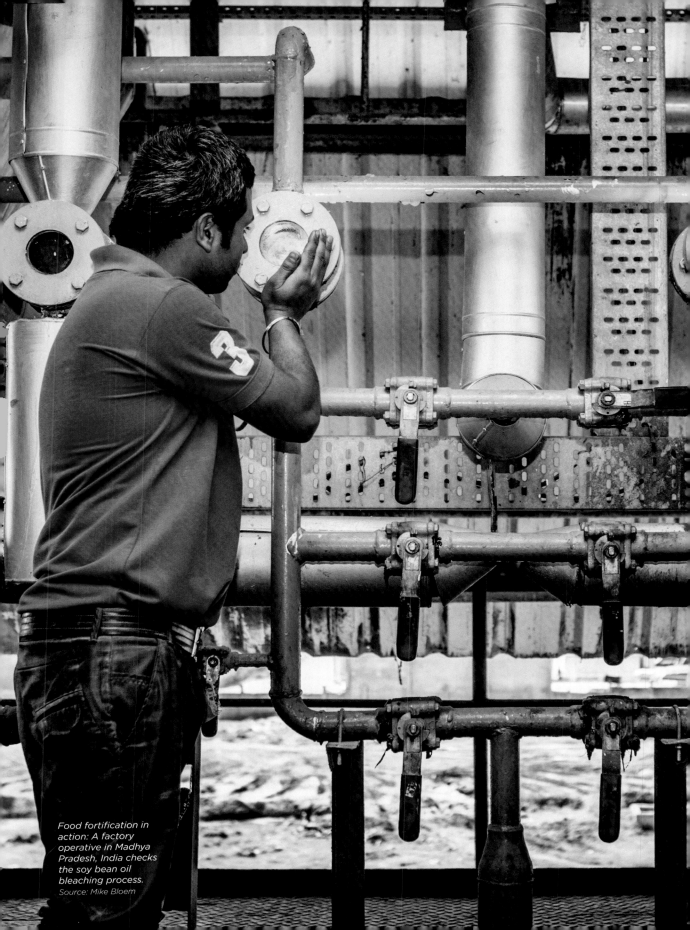

Food fortification in action: A factory operative in Madhya Pradesh, India checks the soy bean oil bleaching process.
Source: Mike Bloem

Nutrient requirements during the first 1,000 days

The diet, including foods, drinks, breast milk and any complements/supplements, needs to provide the nutrients the body requires to be healthy, to be physically active, and to grow. A recommended nutrient intake (RNI) has been established for normal, healthy people of both sexes of different ages, physiological states and activity levels, including young children, pregnant women and others. When that intake is consistently achieved, and the individual is free from disease (which increases the need for nutrients and interferes with their utilization in the body), the individual can be free from undernutrition.

During early childhood, the need for essential nutrients, such as iron, zinc, and essential fatty acids, is very high due to growth, and it may be further increased by the effect of frequent illness, while the energy requirement for physical activity is relatively low due to small body size. For this reason, the diet of young children needs to be far more nutrient-dense than that of adults. Per 100 kcal of food, a 6–8 month-old breastfed infant needs more than four times as much zinc and nine times as much iron as an adult male. However, when an infant is fed a watery porridge, the nutrient density of that meal is much lower than that of the adult male's diet.

Furthermore, it is postulated that the nutrient requirements of young children growing up in an environment where the prevalence of stunting is high exceed the RNI for normal, healthy children. This is for the following reasons:

a   In these settings, the prevalence of infection is high, which reduces appetite, hampers nutrient absorption and utilization, and increases nutrient requirements

b   Children may have been born small for gestational age, due to which they have lower nutrient stores and a higher need for catch-up growth

c   They may be breastfed by mothers who suffer nutrient deficiencies themselves.

How much higher than the RNI their needs are, is unknown, but it is reasonable to assume that they are somewhere between the RNI and the needs of children with moderate acute malnutrition (MAM). For the latter, higher intakes have been recommended in a background paper for the preparation of a WHO meeting on MAM, and these are widely accepted among experts in undernutrition.

Meeting nutrient requirements during the first 1,000 days

In order to determine feasible ways to better meet the nutrient requirements of young children as well as of pregnant and breastfeeding women, and also to ascertain which groups of the population should be targeted, situation analysis is required. Such an analysis should include results from linear programming tools, which are increasingly being used to assess the feasibility of designing adequately nutritious diets – based on the nutrient content and cost of available foods, and the purchasing power of different socioeconomic groups of the population. Good examples of such linear programming tools are the Cost of the Diet tool, developed by Save the Children UK, and Optifood, for which a beta-version is currently being piloted.

Such analyses consistently show that meeting nutrient intake recommendations from a largely plant-based diet is very difficult, as diets that would meet all nutritional recommendations in the absence of fortified foods require very frequent intake of substantial amounts of animal-source foods, such as milk, fish and liver. These foods are often difficult to access, for several reasons. Firstly, their cost limits the amount that can be purchased, especially when we also consider that other family members will also wish to consume some. Secondly, markets where these foods are sold may not be held on more than 1–2 days per week, which limits the number of days on which these foods can be obtained and consumed, as they would require cold storage for safe consumption, and this is not accessible to many households. And thirdly, preparing and feeding nutritious meals for young children 3–4 times per day takes considerable time, which is a constraint for many caretakers who struggle daily to make ends meet.

In addition, diets with the required amounts of animal-source foods are more expensive than diets that include fortified foods. Thus, local foods – including vegetables, fruits and animal-source foods – are essential for meeting nutrient requirements, but achieving adequacy is not easy for specific groups such as young children and pregnant and breastfeeding women, as it is beyond the financial means and practical scope of many households. For some nutrients, such as iron, zinc, iodine and calcium, inadequacies are very likely.

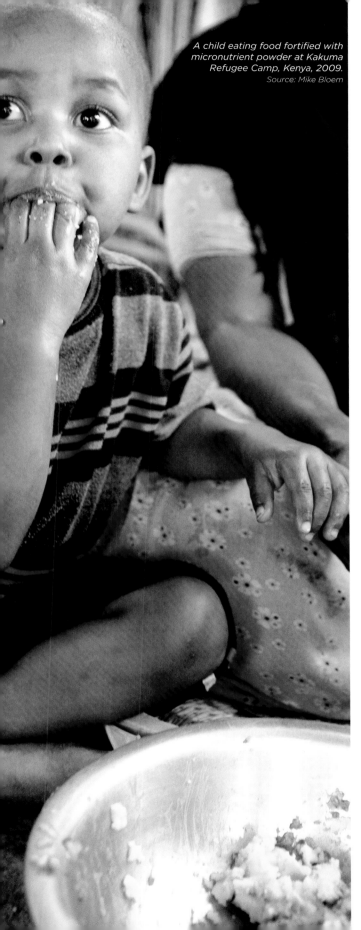

A child eating food fortified with micronutrient powder at Kakuma Refugee Camp, Kenya, 2009.
Source: Mike Bloem

Ways to fill the nutrient gap in a diet

As meeting the RNI is a prerequisite for preventing undernutrition, the consumption of local foods should be optimized and, where necessary for certain groups, complemented by specific foods that provide nutrients that are not supplied in adequate amounts by the local diet.

Ways to optimize consumption of local foods include behavior change communication (BCC), whose object is to raise awareness of the importance of a diverse diet and of ways of feeding nutritious foods to young children. For low-income households, a cash transfer may additionally be required. However, as mentioned above, for specific nutrients, requirements are very difficult to meet, especially between 6–23 months of age and during pregnancy and early lactation, without the inclusion of some fortified food(s) or supplement(s).

For specific groups, such as young children, special nutritious foods have been formulated that are fortified and safe, and which provide a comprehensive set of nutrients, including SUPER CEREAL *plus*, which is a type of infant cereal (see **Table 1**), Ready-to-Use Supplementary Food (RUSF), Lipid-based Nutrient Supplements, medium or small quantity (LNS-MQ, LNS-SQ), and Micronutrient Powder (MNP).

Complementing the diet with such a special food should be done in a way that supports breastfeeding, respects local dietary habits, and promotes a healthy, diverse diet based on locally available and affordable foods. For example, the home diet can be fortified by adding MNP or small-quantity LNS, depending on the likely dietary deficits, or else a fortified infant cereal can be used to prepare 1–3 servings of porridge per day, to which local ingredients and spices can be added.

Approaches to prevent undernutrition can focus on the prevention of wasting, stunting and micronutrient deficiencies. As such, special nutritious foods can be included in programs for the prevention of an increase of wasting during emergencies and periods of severe food insecurity, such as lean seasons, as well as for the prevention of undernutrition during the first 1,000 days of life. In case of the latter, the target group may be reached as part of emergency and recovery programming, when the prevention of wasting is also a major focus, or as part of social protection programming which focuses on the most vulnerable, including during relatively stable periods.

Table 1 | **Composition of SUPER CEREAL *Plus* for complementary feeding**[1,2,3,4]

		Nutrient / 100 g	% RNI in 50 g				Nutrient / 100 g	% RNI in 50 g
Energy	kcal	400	32		Vitamin K	mcg	30	100
Protein	g	16	88		Pantothenic acid	mg	3.6	100
Carbohydrate	g	64			Biotin	mcg	12	100
Fat	g	10	25		Calcium	mg	800	100
Vitamin A	IU	2640	100		Copper	mg	0.44	100
Thiamin	mg	0.6	100		Iodine	mcg	90	35
Riboflavin	mg	0.8	100		Iron	mg	23	62
Niacin	mg	8	100		Magnesium	mg	108	100
Vitamin B$_6$	mg	0.6	100		Manganese	mg	1.2	100
Vitamin B$_{12}$	mcg	1.4	100		Phosphorus	mg	940	171
Vitamin C	mg	60	100		Potassium	mg	773	55
Vitamin D	IU	400	100		Selenium	mcg	15	45
Vitamin E (α-tocopherol)	mg	10	100		Zinc	mg	17	100
Folate, total	mcg	160	100					

Complementary approaches are required to prevent undernutrition

A focus on meeting nutrient intake recommendations should be accompanied by interventions that prevent illness, the other direct cause of undernutrition, as illness increases nutrient requirements and affects nutrient absorption and utilization.

Inadequate caring practices are also a direct cause of undernutrition. Comprehensive social behavior change communication to support appropriate breastfeeding and complementary feeding practices, including the frequency and composition of meals, feeding during illness, food safety, and appropriate use of special food commodities, is essential.

Ensuring adequate nutrient intake, preventing illness and promoting good caring practices requires simultaneous, but different, interventions that reach the same individuals. For example, food systems, including food producers, food processors and markets, should make nutritious foods available; health systems need to provide preventive and curative health services and may distribute supplements or provide nutrition education; safe drinking water and sanitary facilities should be available to all households; antenatal care providers should ensure that pregnant women are assisted in initiating exclusive breastfeeding, while employers and society at large should enable the continuation of exclusive and sustained breastfeeding; the public sector should educate consumers as to healthy food choices; regulators need to work with the food industry to ensure appropriate marketing strategies, and so on.

As these examples show, a multitude of services is required, and these are often implemented by different ministries and/or actors. This is why multisectoral collaboration – which is the essence of the Scaling Up Nutrition (SUN) Movement – is extremely important. In such a collaboration, each partner should contribute in accordance with its own strengths and abilities, as well as its coverage of the target population.

Furthermore, program monitoring and surveillance activities need to assess the coverage of interventions, the adoption of promoted practices, and the patterns of food expenditure, in order to ascertain what is going well and to identify what requires extra effort. For example, the World Health Assembly target is for countries to achieve at least 50% exclusive breastfeeding among children aged 0–5 months. However, according to the 2015 Global Nutrition Report, only 41% of countries with data available are on track to achieve that goal. This means that many children are not exclusively breastfed during the first six months of life. Substantial effort should be put into increasing exclusive breastfeeding and ensuring that children's nutrient needs are being met. Here, multisectoral collaboration is essential in order to agree a common goal and develop solutions for different situations and population sub-groups.

Preventing undernutrition by closing the nutrient gap: options, costs and impact

As explained above, meeting nutrient requirements is a prerequisite for the prevention of undernutrition, and special nutritious foods can be used to fill a potential nutrient gap. This approach is basically the same as food fortification. The only difference is that instead of fortifying foods that are already commonly consumed by a large proportion of the population (such as flour, salt or vegetable oil), individual foods are designed to meet the needs of specific target groups, such as young children, pregnant women, or children with acute malnutrition, and they may receive these foods either through normal marketing channels or else through specific channels, such as the health sector or a social safety net system.

With a clear rationale for providing special nutritious foods for the prevention of undernutrition in circumstances where the risk of undernutrition is high, the main question is how to achieve the greatest impact at the lowest cost, while also maximizing the use of locally grown foods. Although prevention studies under harsh circumstances are rare for ethical and practical reasons, evidence of impact is accumulating. For example, a study in Haiti found that blanket provision of fortified blended food to young children, based on age, was more effective in preventing wasting and underweight than the treatment of individual children with wasting. Studies in Niger during subsequent years, in each of which a different food was provided as a complement to the diet, found lower incidences of wasting, morbidity and mortality with blanket provision of RUTF (ready-to-use therapeutic food), RUSF (ready-to-use supplementary food) and medium-quantity LNS.

Another recent study in Niger found that the incidence of acute malnutrition was comparable among groups that received RUSF or SUPER CEREAL *plus*, (see Table 1) as compared to cash, whereas the cost was approximately four times higher for cash compared to the special nutritious food (roughly 12 vs 48 US$/mo). The incidence was approximately two times lower in groups that received both cash and special nutritious foods as compared to groups that received cash only or special food only, while they received less cash to include the special food. This shows that an income transfer improves a household's access to food and care, which can improve the nutritional status and health of young children; but it also demonstrates that a special nutritious food in this context more cost-effectively improved children's nutritional status and health. Thus, a special nutritious food supports a child's nutritional status directly, whereas household assistance in the form of cash supports vulnerable households and may also have an impact on young children,

depending on how the cash may be used, including whether nutrient-rich foods can be purchased.

The cost of filling the nutrient gap can be estimated in many ways, depending on the approach selected. For example, the Cost of the Diet software calculates the cost of meeting all nutrient requirements of specific individuals based on food prices in a specific location. In the case of Indonesia, the cost- and nutrient-optimized choice of foods for a 12–23-month-old child was US$43–82 per annum, depending on the market price at the various locations. SUPER CEREAL *plus*, (see Table 1), as purchased directly from manufacturers, would cost approx. US$ 20 per annum for 50 grams per day (approx. 200 kcal) for a 12–23-month-old child, while 50 grams per day of LNS-MQ (approx. 260 kcal) purchased directly from the manufacturer would cost around US$ 45 per annum. Each of these would still need to be transported and distributed, and their total costs should be added to the costs of the other foods for the child that are purchased by the family. These estimates align with the cost of complementary feeding of children between 6 and 23 months of age, which have been estimated for the Scaling Up Nutrition Movement at US$ 40–80 for 18 months (i.e., US$ 27–53 per annum).

Findings for the prevention of stunting with complementary feeding interventions have been more modest than those for wasting. This is probably due to several factors:

a The extent to which nutrient requirements were met, which depends on the actual need (which may be increased by illness), and the total intake (which depends on the composition of the supplements, their consumption, and the rest of the diet). It is important to note that interventions to treat or prevent wasting typically provide a larger complement to the daily diet than do interventions to prevent stunting. Studies have used very different complementary foods and were conducted among different populations and contexts, which makes it harder to determine their "overall" impact.

b Period and length of intervention. As stunting accumulates between conception and two years of age, nutrient requirements must be met across this entire period. So the following are key aspects:

i   the duration of the intervention, i.e., the portion of the first 1,000 days during which nutrient requirements are met; and

ii the nutritional deficit that was already present when the intervention commenced.

Furthermore, when interpreting results of studies or

systematic reviews on the impact of nutrition interventions on the prevention of stunting, it is important to keep in mind that, whereas stunting is a good indicator for assessing the prevalence of undernutrition at population level, it should not be the sole indicator for assessing the impact of a nutrition intervention. The reason is that some of the developmental consequences associated with stunting are primarily caused by the co-occurrence of other nutrient deficiencies, some of which have no impact on linear growth (e.g., iron, vitamin B_{12}, essential fatty acids) but rather on other critical health and developmental outcomes. Thus, improving the diet with special nutritious foods is likely to reduce micronutrient deficiencies before – or in some cases even without – improving linear growth. Also, micronutrient stores can be replenished quite easily (although it may not be possible to undo all the consequences of earlier deficits), while catching up on a linear growth deficit takes more time. Thus, the effects on micronutrient deficiencies and functional consequences, such as morbidity and cognitive development, are also important indicators for assessing the impact of nutrition interventions.

In other words, when interventions aimed at improving nutrient intake do not achieve the expected reduction in stunting, this probably means that the requirements were higher than anticipated; that intake was not improved sufficiently for all essential nutrients (which may also be related to substitution for foods that would have otherwise been consumed [i.e., net increase is less than expected]); that the intervention was not sustained over a long enough period of time; or that illness hampered the body's utilization of foods and nutrients consumed. However, if the formulation of the fortified foods has been comprehensive (e.g., WFP's SUPER CEREAL *plus* foods with composition as per GAIN guidance for complementary foods, MNP according to HF-TAG guidance, SQ-LNS as per iLiNS composition), there will very probably have been benefits, such as reduced micronutrient deficiencies, which ameliorate other adverse outcomes – for example, iron and essential fatty acids are essential for brain development and hence cognitive function.

Thus, nutrient intake requirements should be met, and evidence is required on the extent to which undernutrition is prevented by a combination of nutrition-specific and nutrition-sensitive approaches in specific contexts, among specific target groups, and at a specific cost.

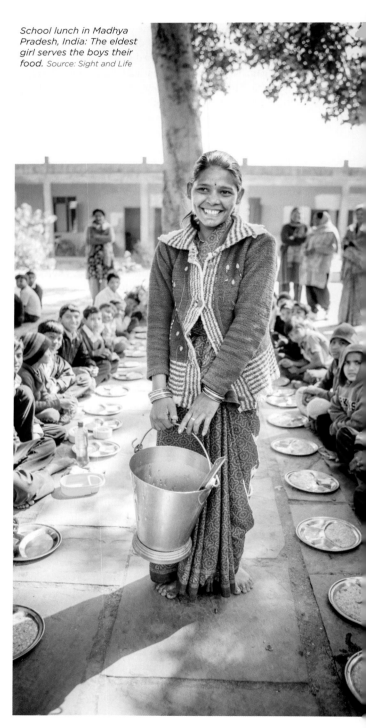

School lunch in Madhya Pradesh, India: The eldest girl serves the boys their food. Source: Sight and Life

Implementing strategies to fill the nutrient gap and prevent undernutrition

Where the incidence of low birth weight and the prevalence of stunting are high, nutrient intake recommendations are very probably not being met, and the diet may need to be complemented with special nutritious foods, which should be made available for self-purchasing, at a commercial or subsidized price, and distributed for free to the poorest who need them the most but would otherwise be unable to access them. Governments and partners are increasingly using vouchers to create demand and stimulate the market availability of nutritious foods, which also provides access to self-purchasing consumers.

It is important to note that using special nutritious products to complement the local diet of specific target groups, who have high needs and limited access due to constraints on availability and affordability, is not a matter of replacing local foods with processed foods. Instead, local foods are complemented. When local foods such as maize and soy are processed into safe, nutritious, fortified foods, such as SUPER CEREAL *plus*, (see Table 1), the availability of, and access to, nutritious foods for specific groups is further increased, and local food producers and processors, including their family members, can also benefit.

Furthermore, the first 450 days – i.e., from conception until 6 months of age, when complementary feeding starts – are more important than was previously recognized. Therefore, meeting nutrient intake recommendations for pregnant and breastfeeding women and women of reproductive age, in particular adolescents, is also essential to prevent children from already having acquired a nutritional deficit when they enter the complementary feeding period. For these reasons, efforts should be increased to reach adolescent girls and pregnant and lactating women with nutrition-specific interventions, as well as other services, including health, e.g., antenatal and obstetric care, family planning, and education.

In addition, exclusive breastfeeding in the first six months of life is critical, and is not fully achieved in many settings.

Finally, the implementation of multisectoral responses that address the underlying and basic causes of undernutrition, alongside interventions that address the direct causes, is essential. It is important to note that addressing underlying and basic causes can impact nutrition through an effect on the direct causes, i.e., dietary intake and/or illness, which in turn affect nutritional status. Nutrition-sensitive interventions should therefore outline the pathways via which the direct causes will be impacted, and should monitor the extent to which this occurs. Intermediate outcome indicators for both nutrition-specific and nutrition-sensitive interventions should include the change of dietary intake (e.g., dietary diversity, nutrient intake, consumption of plant-source, animal-source and fortified foods, breastfeeding) and of illness (incidence, duration and severity).

Social entrepreneurship in South Africa

Social entrepreneurship in South Africa is emerging as a blend of for-profit and not-for-profit approaches, which balances the value and trustworthiness of social organizations with the efficiencies and profit motive of business. The concept of social entrepreneurship introduces a profit motive to the running of an organization, but that profit must be re-invested back into the organization.

Some examples:

• The Oasis Association in South Africa, which generates income through its recycling activities and provides safe, structured employment for people with intellectual disabilities.

• Spark Schools, which helps improve the caliber of teachers by providing teacher training.

• Sizanani Mzanzi (Zulu for "Help each other South Africa"), which is a social business founded by *Sight and Life* and DSM, and which sells nutritious products produced by DSM using microfranchising.

Organizations that start out with a social entrepreneurial bent think differently about how they deliver their services, focusing on sustainability, quality of service, efficiency, and accountability.

Adapted from: http://pressoffice.mg.co.za/gibs/ PressRelease.php?StoryID=261102 and http://www. sightandlife.org/fileadmin/data/Magazine/2015/29_1_2015/ Microfanchise_program_South_Africa.pdf.

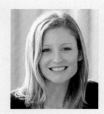

Kristina Spiegel

**Deputy Manager, SUN
Business Network**

The SUN Business Network

Increasing access to nutrient-rich diets for vulnerable groups in low- and middle-income settings – critical to achievement of the ambitious 2030 Agenda – must include engagement of the private sector, which today is largely responsible for the production, distribution and marketing of food. Including the private sector in increasing access to nutritious diets acknowledges how people live and offers the potential to impact nutrition more sustainably and at greater scale.

There are 57 countries that are actively engaged in the SUN Movement – an initiative which unites all stakeholders, including business, in a collective effort to improve nutrition. The SUN Business Network's role is to engage companies, in partnership with the public and civil society, to create value through developing and producing nutritious products, fostering demand for more nutritious foods, and delivering nutritious products and services to vulnerable populations at scale. Ensuring that the private sector is effectively engaged in nutrition strategies at global, national and local levels will facilitate the alignment of critical actions that are required to improve nutrition, leveraging traditional humanitarian and development assistance with private-sector resources and expertise.

The network has seen rapidly growing engagement, with more than 250 companies having signed up to the SUN Business Network (SBN) global platform. This number is significantly increasing with each country that organizes a national SBN platform, with over 200 companies making commitments to nutrition at country level. Supporting national governments and civil society to collaborate with business has emerged as a key request from SUN Countries within the Movement. The network has responded by supporting 11 SUN countries to establish national SBNs, to date, and will look to support a further 15 over the next year. These national networks are identifying entry points for business to support national nutrition strategies, and are developing action plans with business to address the barriers to greater investment.

As countries step up action to build nutritious agricultural food systems, improve the availability and affordability of nutritious foods and strengthen underlying health systems, private enterprise – whether multinationals, national companies or SMEs – can be the source of many valuable innovations. These include new products and technologies, new financing mechanisms, and new distribution models that provide better access to affordable, safe and nutritious foods.

In partnership with the private sector, we can increase access to, and availability of, nutritious foods. To do this, we must:

- Together with all other actors, focus on creating consumer awareness and thus demand for more nutritious foods, making nutritious food available at large scale, affordable, and aspirational.

- Ensure that, along with a focus on the "do no harm" principle, the nutrition community also develops a clearer articulation of the potential and opportunities working with the private sector.

- Emphasize the role of small and medium-sized enterprises (SMEs) as foundational to increasing access to nutritious food and products at country level (providing SME support through technology transfer, technical assistance, and partnership brokering).

- Acknowledge the risks to business to take action on nutrition and understand that positive engagement requires the right mix of policies, standards and legislation.

- Build the evidence base through a more rigorous research agenda to fill evidence gaps and determine what interventions have the greatest positive effect on nutrition outcomes, including market-based interventions.

Business has a fundamental role to play in delivering nutrition, and there is a business case to be made for the private sector to invest in nutrition. While this analysis is now widely accepted by governments and the development community, detailed evidence around the most impactful interventions with business and commercial models needs to be significantly strengthened. It is time to move beyond the rhetoric to the kind of business engagement required to end malnutrition in all its forms.

Conclusion

There is a very strong case for improving the availability of, and access to, nutritious foods, especially among vulnerable populations with a high prevalence or incidence of undernutrition (stunting, micronutrient deficiencies and/or wasting) in order to ensure that nutrient needs are better met and to reduce the risk of undernutrition and its immediate and long-term consequences. For specific target groups with high needs and limited access to adequately nutritious foods, some complement in the form of a fortified food is often required to ensure that nutrient intake requirements are met, whereas adolescents and pregnant women also benefit from foods that are fortified for the general population. Interventions to ensure adequate dietary intake should focus on:

a   Ensuring availability of, and access to, nutritious foods that meet the needs of specific target groups, for example by using vouchers for fresh plant- and animal-source foods and specific fortified foods where these are already on the market, or by distributing them directly where they are not (yet) available.

b   Complementing the diet with special nutritious foods should be done where necessary in a way that supports breastfeeding, respects local dietary habits and promotes a healthy, diverse diet based on foods that are accessible to households.

c   Ensuring that other needs – such as disease prevention, WASH interventions, livelihood assistance, and support for gender-sensitive food production – are also in place, through collaboration with stakeholders who are well positioned to implement these interventions.

d   Partnerships and multisectoral collaboration, e.g., through the SUN Movement and coordination with national governments and via in-country coordination mechanisms, particularly on nutrition, linking food and health systems, and social protection.

WFP: from food aid to food assistance

The World Food Programme (WFP) is the food assistance agency of the United Nations.

Food assistance is one of the many instruments that can help to promote food security which is defined as access by all people at all times to the food needed for an active and healthy life.

WFP works towards eradicating hunger and poverty. The core policies and strategies that govern WFP's activities are to provide food assistance:

• to save lives in refugee and other emergency situations;

• to improve the nutrition and quality of life of the most vulnerable people at critical times in their lives; and

• to help build assets and promote the self-reliance of poor people and communities, particularly through labor-intensive public works programmes.

WFP plays a major role in the continuum that runs from emergency relief to development, including disaster prevention, preparedness and mitigation.

WFP works on ensuring access to food in many different ways, including distribution of food, electronic vouchers and/or cash; providing technical assistance to governments in implementing school feeding and social safety nets; working with smallholder farmers to ensure good-quality produce and access to markets; and helping local manufacturers of nutritious foods to develop capacity. The term "food assistance" has therefore replaced "food aid," in order to better describe the scope of WFP's work.

My personal view
Saskia de Pee

At this moment when nutrition is receiving a lot of attention, it is essential to join forces across disciplines and deliver good results on the prevention of undernutrition.

While it is recognized that both nutrition-specific and nutrition-sensitive strategies are necessary, and that implementing these requires multisectoral collaboration, it is vital that individual stakeholders should focus on what they are good at and coordinate their efforts with those of others in order to ensure that the target group is exposed to the full palette of interventions. In doing so, agencies should build on their strengths and apply them where they fit the context.

For example, where access to clean water and sanitation facilities is limited, this is an important contributor to undernutrition, and ameliorating the situation should be a high priority. Where, by contrast, hygiene and sanitation are already good and people buy most of their foods, instead of producing these themselves, the main priority should be to work with actors along the food value chain to ensure the availability and affordability of nutritious foods. Understanding context and performing a thorough situation analysis are essential for designing and implementing effective strategies for preventing undernutrition.

Further reading

Alive & Thrive. Why stunting matters. Technical brief – Insight 2. 2014. http://aliveandthrive.org/resources/technical-brief-insight-2-why-stunting-matters-english-and-vietnamese/.

Baldi G, Martini E, Catharina M et al. "Cost of the Diet" tool (CoD): First results from Indonesia and applications for policy discussion on food and nutrition security. Food Nutr Bull 2013; 34: S35–42.

Black RE, Victora CG, Walker SP et al. Maternal and child undernutrition and overweight in low-income and middle-income countries. Lancet 2013; 382: 427–51.

Christian P, Shaikh S, Shamim AA et al. Effect of fortified complementary food supplementation on child growth in rural Bangladesh: a cluster-randomized trial. Int J Epidemiol 2015; doi: 10.1093/ije/dyv155.

De Pee S, Grais R, Fenn B et al. Prevention of acute malnutrition: Distribution of special nutritious foods and cash, and addressing underlying causes – what to recommend when, where, for whom and how. Food Nutr Bull 2015; 36: S24–9.

Dewey, KG. The challenge of meeting nutrient needs of infants and young children during the period of complementary feeding: an evolutionary perspective. J Nutr 2013; 143: 2050–2054.

Dror DK, Allen LH. The importance of milk and other animal-source foods for children in low-income countries. Food Nutr Bull 2011; 32: 227–43.

Golden, MH. Proposed recommended nutrient densities for moderately malnourished children. Food Nutr Bull 2009: 30: S267.

Moench-Pfanner R, Laillou A, Berger J. Introduction: Large-scale fortification, an important nutrition-specific intervention. Food Nutr Bull 2012;33:S255–9

Semba RD. The historical evolution of thought regarding multiple micronutrient nutrition. J Nutr 2012; 142:143S–56S

Endnotes

i   Adapted from Ruel MT, Alderman H, and the Maternal and Child Nutrition Study Group. Nutrition-sensitive interventions and programmes: how can they help to accelerate progress in improving maternal and child nutrition? Page 66. The Lancet. 2013.

ii Ibid.

1   This formulation is suitable for the complementary feeding of children aged 6–23 months, based on its contribution to meeting nutrient intake recommendations. Main ingredients: maize (58%), soy (20%), milk powder (8%), sugar (9%), oil (3%), vitamin and mineral premix (2%).

2   The amounts proposed are based on the RNI for 7–11 month-old infants, which is the target nutrient content at the time of consumption. When setting specifications, nutrient losses during processing and storage will have to be taken into consideration, as well as measurement variability.

3   Note that a breastfed child aged 6–8 months should get approximately 420 kcal/d from breastmilk. An amount of 200 kcal from complementary food would add the remaining energy needs.

4   Nutrients for which the nutrient content target is not set at 100% of the RNI, and the rationale:

   - Energy, protein, carbohydrate, fat: because the food complements breast milk and the macronutrient content of its main ingredients

   - Iodine: because of the likely use of iodized salt for preparing the porridge;

   - Iron: because the RNI assumes lower bioavailability then iron fortificants with good bioavailability

   - Phosphorus: because of higher RNI for 12–23 month-old children and the need for the ratio Ca:P to be between 0.8–1.2

   - Selenium: only native content of main ingredients has been stipulated because of risk of toxicity when selenium from micronutrient premix is not homogenously distributed within the product.

Ensuring Good Nutrition for Vulnerable Population Groups such as Elderly and Hospitalized Individuals in Affluent Societies

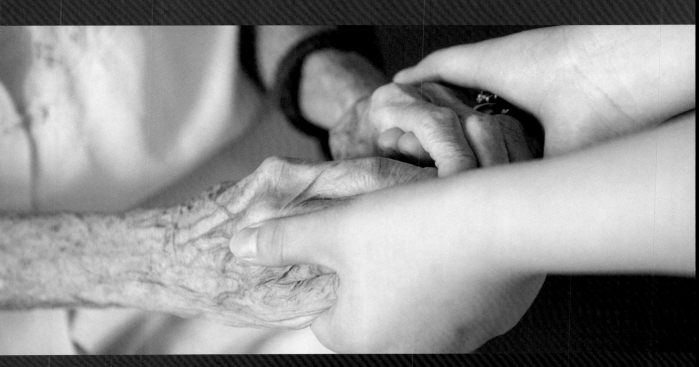

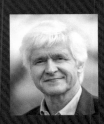

Peter Weber
Professor of Nutrition at the University of Stuttgart-Hohenheim, Germany; Corporate Science Fellow for Human Nutrition & Health, DSM, Kaiseraugst, Switzerland

"Explicit de coquina quae est optima medicina."
("Food is the best medicine.")

From The Form of Cury, *a 1390 collection of cookery books believed to have been compiled by the master chef of King Richard II of England (ruled 1377–1399)*

Key messages

- Micronutrient deficiencies are well established in the developing world, but a growing body of evidence indicates that they exist in the developed world too.

- Life expectancy for populations around the world continues to grow, but the last decade of life is often compromised by the burden of partially preventable health issues.

- Healthy ageing is essential if the elderly are to remain independent and play an integral role in society

- Micronutrient deficiencies and insufficiencies within vulnerable populations in the developed world have serious health and economic consequences.

- The same level of attention that is currently given to overnutrition should be given to undernutrition and appropriate changes made to public health policies and programs.

The Lady with the Lamp

"Every careful observer of the sick will agree in this that thousands of patients are annually starved in the midst of plenty, from want of attention to the ways which alone make it possible for them to take food. This want of attention is as remarkable in those who urge upon the sick to do what is quite impossible to them, as in the sick themselves who will not make the effort to do what is perfectly possible to them. For instance, to the large majority of very weak patients it is quite impossible to take any solid food before 11 A.M., nor then, if their strength is still further exhausted by fasting till that hour. For weak patients have generally feverish nights and, in the morning, dry mouths; and, if they could eat with those dry mouths, it would be the worse for them."[1]

So wrote Florence Nightingale, the founder of modern nursing, in 1898. The words of "The Lady with the Lamp", who began to revolutionize nursing through her management of British field hospitals during the Crimean War of 1853–56, have a troublingly topical ring.

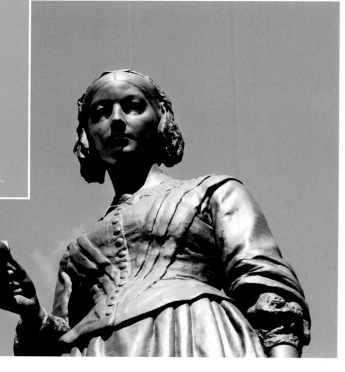

Florence Nightingale, the Lady with the Lamp.

Chapter 5.3 | Ensuring Good Nutrition for Vulnerable Population
Groups such as Elderly and Hospitalized Individuals in Affluent Societies

266

Even in the developed world, an increasing number of people consume nutrient-poor food on a regular basis. Recent surveys in Western countries consistently indicate inadequate intake of nutrients such as vitamins and minerals, compared to recommendations.[2] Especially at risk are elderly people in institutions such as hospitals and nursing homes, whose access to good nutrition is frequently compromised by a multiplicity of factors. These include a phenomenon known as the "anorexia of ageing," which can be aggravated by the negative effects of nutrient-drug interactions. As the average age of

populations in affluent societies increases, this is becoming a growing problem, creating unnecessary human suffering while at the same time driving up the overall costs of medical and residential care.[3] Solutions exist, in terms of nutrition science on the one hand and care management systems on the other, but a significant effort is required to translate this potential into effective public health policies and programs that will support long-term national and global health, economic productivity and stability, and societal resilience.

Figure 1 | **Global vitamin D map**

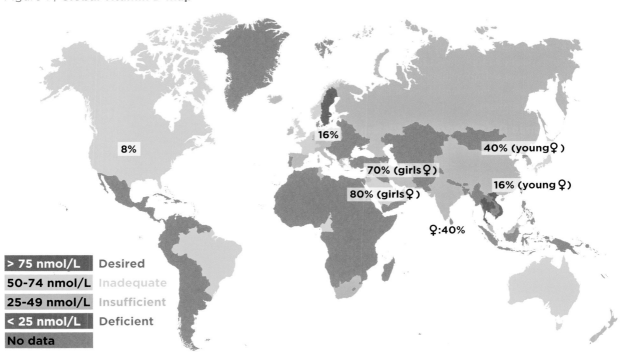

Source: International Osteoporosis Foundation, http://www.iofbonehealth.org/facts-and-statistics/vitamin-d-studies-map.

The return of vitamin D deficiency diseases

According to the International Osteoporosis Foundation's (IOF) latest figures, approximately 88% of the world's population does not have an optimal vitamin D status.[4] This lack is leading to the return of a number of diseases that characterized the Victorian era, such as tuberculosis, scarlet fever and rickets. The lame and sickly child Tiny Tim, for instance, from Charles Dickens's 1843 novella *A Christmas Carol*, has recently been diagnosed as suffering from both TB and rickets.[5]

As cholecalciferol (vitamin D3), vitamin D is synthesized in the skin by the action of ultraviolet light on 7-dehydrocholesterol; it is also present in a small number of foods, most notably fatty cold saltwater fish such as sardines and mackerel. The return of the bone deficiency disease rickets among young people has been associated with lack of exposure to sunlight – a trend attributable partly to an excess of sedentary indoor activities among this age group and partly to the extensive use of UV sun screens to protect against sunburn.

Table 1 | **Vitamin D deficiency/insufficiency**

Area of operation of vitamin D	Consequences of deficiency/insufficiency
Musculo-skeletal system	• Falls and fractures
Immune system	• Infections • Allergies • Tumors
Endocrine system	• Type I diabetes • Type II diabetes
Circulatory system	• Hypertension • Stroke • Heart attack • Heart failure
Nervous system	• Multiple sclerosis • Depression • Alzheimer's disease

Source: Armin Zittermann, Vitamin D Case: Status and impact on healthcare costs. Presentation delivered at University Medical Center Groningen, Netherlands, as part of the symposium "A Century of Vitamins," April 3–4, 2012.

Inadequate levels of vitamin D also have a significant effect on elderly patients. In 2012, it was estimated that the provision of vitamin D supplementation to people aged over 65 in Europe would lead to net healthcare cost savings of EUR 10.5 billion per year.[6]

Though vitamin D deficiency is best known and researched in elderly and in particular hospitalized or institutionalized populations it should be mentioned that micronutrient deficiencies in this group are not limited to vitamin D. Besides inadequate vitamin D a recent review of large-scale dietary intake surveys undertaken in the USA, UK, the Netherlands and in Germany reported lower than recommended daily intakes for vitamins A, E, C and folate. It is of interest that the vitamin status apparently worsens as individuals become more dependent and handicapped/disabled (**Figure 2**).

"Healthy Ageing"

According to the World Health Organization (WHO), by 2050 the proportion of the global population over the age of 60 years will double from its 2000 figure, rising from c. 11% to 22%.[7] Although this may be interpreted as a success story for public health policies and socioeconomic development, it also challenges societies to address the social, economic and health issues of ageing and age-related conditions.

Healthy ageing is key if older people are to remain independent and play an integral part in society. ("Healthy" refers to physical, mental, and social wellbeing as indicated in the WHO definition of health.) Lifelong health promotion, with a clear emphasis on the fundamental role of nutrition and micronutrients to reduce risks of chronic conditions and disability, may prevent or delay the onset of several non-communicable diseases. One example for such an initiative in the European Union is the European Innovation Partnership on Active and Healthy Ageing, which aims to increase the average healthy lifespan by two "healthy" years by 2020.[8]

In the long-term, inadequate micronutrient intake can lead to chronic micronutrient undernutrition and consequent health problems, including lower resistance to development of chronic disease thus reducing health span and longevity. Micronutrient deficiencies (MNDs) are particularly harmful during pregnancy and early childhood due to their impact on the physical and cognitive development of children. Micronutrient requirements also have to be adjusted later in life – for example, to accommodate the specific micronutrient requirements of the elderly and those living in particular settings such as hospitals and institutions.

Chapter 5.3 | Ensuring Good Nutrition for Vulnerable Population
Groups such as Elderly and Hospitalized Individuals in Affluent Societies

268

Figure 2 | **Correlation between growth of micronutrient inadequacy and
increasing dependence on support.**

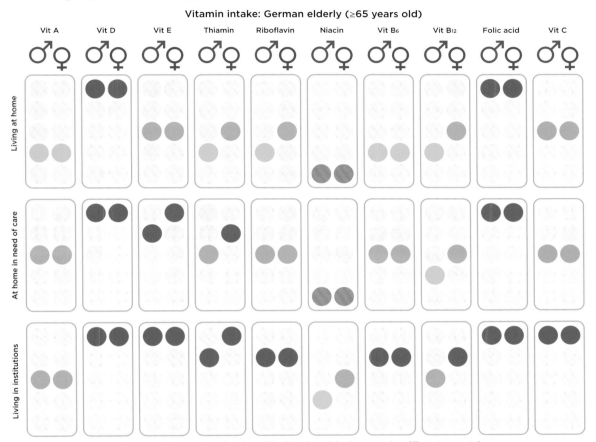

Vitamin intake: German elderly (≥65 years old)

*The nutritional situation is critical in the elderly, even in affluent countries,
and even more so once they become ill or frail*

Source: Verzehrsstudie 2008; Ernährungsbericht 2008 & 2012.

Someone you know is probably malnourished

When you ask advocates why they become champions of a cause, it is usually because of some personal wake-up call. They, or someone close to them, has privately suffered from the condition they are now publicly fighting for. By this rule of thumb, we all should be nutrition champions. That is because every country has a serious public health problem and one in every three people is affected worldwide.

What is malnutrition? It's all around you. It's your friend's baby who just won't grow properly through lack of the right kind of feeding and care; it's your exhausted mother who does not have enough vitamins and minerals coursing through her veins; it's your father's blood pressure that is too high because of too much salt; it's your sibling who has diabetes because of too much sugar; it's your friend who cannot walk up the stairs to your apartment because his joints scream out in pain from carrying too much bodyweight because of an imbalanced diet and too little exercise.

It is too many early graves and it is too much lost potential.

*Source: Lawrence Haddad, Senior Research Fellow in the
International Food Policy Research Institute's Poverty
Health and Nutrition Division, Huffington Post,
September 16, 2015*

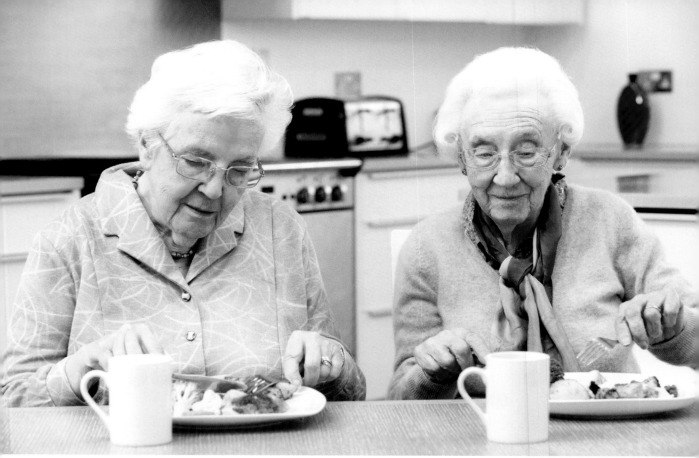

Two elderly women enjoying a meal together. Healthy ageing is key if people are to remain independent and play an integral part in society.

Malnutrition in hospitalized patients

Clinical surveys in hospitalized patients continue to show an unacceptable high frequency of undernutrition from all over Europe. In the words of the Committee of Experts on Nutrition, Food Safety and Consumer Protection, Council of Europe: "There are many adverse consequences of disease-related undernutrition. The patient becomes apathetic and depressed, and this may lead to loss of morale and loss of will to recover. Inability to concentrate means that the patient cannot benefit from instructions about techniques needed for self-care. A general sense of weakness impairs appetite and ability to eat. The respiratory muscles are weakened, making it difficult to cough and expectorate effectively, with increased risk of lung infection. Impaired ventilatory drive may also make it difficult to wean a critically ill patient from a ventilator. Cardiac function is impaired, with reduced cardiac output and risk of heart failure. Gastrointestinal function and structure is injured. Mobility is reduced, delaying recovery and predisposing to thromboembolism and bedsores. The undernourished patient develops impaired resistance to infection, which in turn can worsen nutritional status. Undernutrition, in combination with disease, is thus an insidious factor which prolongs recovery, increases the need for high-dependency nursing care and sometimes intensive care, increases the risk of serious complications of illness and, at its worst, leads to

death either from a preventable complication or from inanition. To all this is added the reduced quality of life of the patients."[9]

The consequences of malnutrition in hospital patients are therefore highly ramified, although not always immediately evident. An inadequate diet in patients whose health may already be compromised by a variety of factors not only increases individual suffering but also greatly increases the costs of attempting to return that individual to a state of relative health and wellbeing. Longer stays in hospital, higher prescription rates and increased demands on medical and nursing staff are just some of the more obvious consequences of inadequate nutrition.

Malnutrition in elderly patients

The elderly are at increased risk of developing both protein-calorie malnutrition and vitamin and mineral deficiencies. The frequency of undernutrition increases with advancing age due to problems such as poor dentition, loss of taste, difficulty swallowing and malabsorption. Drug-nutrient interaction is also a major factor, as many elderly people are on medication, and the actions of numerous active pharmaceutical ingredients can interfere with the body's ability to digest and utilize such nutrients as are ingested.

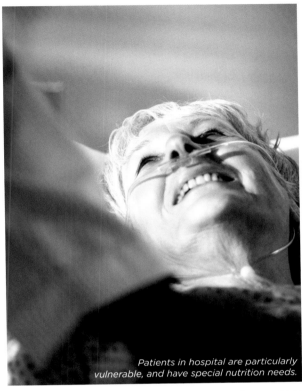

*Patients in hospital are particularly
vulnerable, and have special nutrition needs.*

Table 2 | **Drug-nutrient interaction**

Drug	Reduced nutrient availability
Alcohol (regular consumption > 2 units)	Zinc, vitamins A, B_1, B_2, B_6 folate, vitamin B_{12}
Antacids	Vitamin B_{12}, folate, iron, total kcal
Antibiotics, broad-spectrum	Vitamin K
Digoxin	Zinc, total kcal (via anorexia)
Diuretics	Zinc, magnesium, vitamin B_6, potassium, copper
Laxatives	Calcium, vitamins A, B_2, B_{12}, D, E, K
Lipid-binding resins	Vitamins A, D, E, K
Metformin	Vitamin B_{12}, folate / Vitamin C, folate
Phenytoin / Salicylates	Vitamin D, folate / Vitamin C, folate
SSRIs (Selective serotonin reuptake inhibitors)	Total kcal (via anorexia)
Trimethoprim	Folate

*Source: James T. Birch, Jr., Assistant Clinical Professor – Dept. of Family
Medicine, Division of Geriatric Medicine, Landon Center on Ageing Kansas
University Medical Center, 2007.*

Figure 3 | **Healthy Ageing**

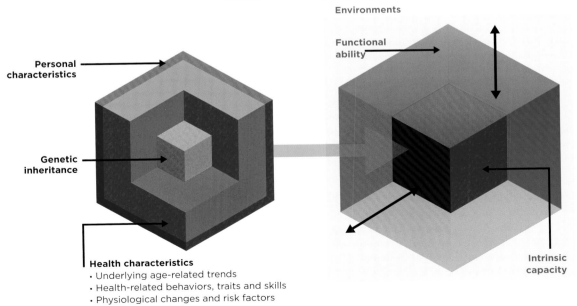

Source: Adaptation of World report on ageing and health: http://apps.who.int/iris/bitstream/10665/186463/1/9789240694811_eng.pdf?ua=1

Chapter 5.3 | Ensuring Good Nutrition for Vulnerable Population
Groups such as Elderly and Hospitalized Individuals in Affluent Societies

271

Figure 4 | **Disease-related malnutrition: Clinical and economic consequences**

In Europe: 33 million people*

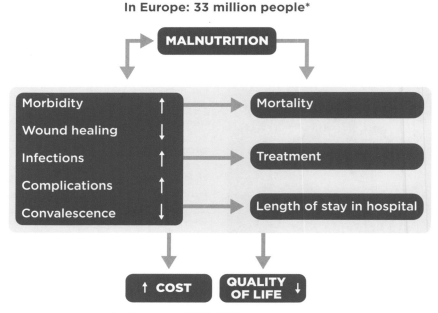

*LjungqvistO, de Man F. NutrHosp2009; 24:368-70.

Source: Health Economics and (Disease-Related) Malnutrition: The Economic value of medical nutrition, Karen Freyer, University of Maastricht, 2013

These (patho)physiological considerations are compounded by a range of practical factors. Elderly people may be less mobile than their younger counterparts, and may experience difficulty walking, driving or carrying shopping. They may be dependent on others for the purchasing and preparation of food, and their purchasing power itself may be limited, forcing them into a narrow range of buying choices. The challenges of shopping for food and preparing it in the home may encourage them to purchase non-perishable, processed foods, which are frequently high in sodium and nitrates and concomitantly low in vitamins.

Even if nutritious food is readily available, the ability of the elderly to consume it may be compromised by a variety of physical limitations. Oral health problems such as poor teeth, ulcers or dry mouth may make it difficult to masticate properly, and may lead to the conscious avoidance of certain nutritious foods. Changes in the senses of taste and smell that may result from illness and age, as well as from the effect of certain drugs and also radiation therapy, may make certain foods unattractive, or may diminish the individual's appetite. Appetite loss may also be caused by a reduction in physical activity resulting

directly from the increased immobility caused by age-related conditions such as arthritis, osteoporosis, sciatica and heart disease. Depression, social isolation and other mental health conditions may also play their part, as may dementia and alcohol or substance abuse. Last but not least, a limited understanding of the importance of good nutrition, and of how to obtain it from the diet, may play a role. For many reasons, a vicious spiral may be initiated, whereby poor diet hampers physical and mental capacity, thus further limiting the individual's capability to access the nutrients that would help that individual to reverse the direction of the spiral.

The anorexia of ageing

Ageing is associated with a wide range of physical changes, including reduction in bone mass, lean mass, and water content, accompanied by an increase in body fat. This may be accompanied by a decline in the function of one or more organs. This loss of physical robustness may lead to a phenomenon known as the "anorexia of ageing," whereby the feedback loops in the elderly person's brain may falsely signal satiety or turn off the stimulation for hunger. The anorexic signals come to predominate over the central feeding drive.

Chapter 5.3 | Ensuring Good Nutrition for Vulnerable Population
Groups such as Elderly and Hospitalized Individuals in Affluent Societies

272

How to prevent malnutrition in hospitals

John E Thomas and David R Morley have observed that: "Nutritional intervention holds the promise of mitigating the growing burden of chronic disease and disability and improving the quality of life of the rapidly growing older population".[10] The Committee of Experts on Nutrition, Food Safety and Consumer Protection list five major factors, common for Europe, that seem to be the major barriers for proper nutritional care in hospitals, and propose remedies for each of them.

Lack of clearly defined responsibilities in planning and managing nutritional care

The responsibilities of staff categories and the hospital management with respect to procuring nutritional care should be clearly assigned. This means that standards of practice for assessing and monitoring nutritional risk/ status of the patient should be developed at a national level, and the responsibility of each task clearly assigned. The responsibility of the hospital with regard to the nutritional care and support of the patient should not be limited to the hospital stay.

Lack of sufficient educational level with regard to nutrition among all staff groups

A general improvement in the educational level of all staff groups is needed. Specifically, a continuing education program on general nutrition and techniques of nutritional support for all staff involved in the nutritional care of patients should be available with focus on the nutritional training of the non-clinical staff members, and the definitions of their area of responsibility.

Lack of influence and knowledge of the patients

The provision of meals should be individualized and flexible, and all patients should have the possibility to order food and extra food – and be informed about this possibility. Also, patients should be involved in planning their meals and have some control over food selection. This should include the possibility of immediate feedback from the patients' likes and dislikes of the served food – and the use of this feedback to develop appropriate, target group specific menus. Patients should be informed of the importance of good nutrition for successful treatment prior to admission and at discharge.

Lack of co-operation between different staff groups

The hospital managers, physicians, nurses, dieticians and food service staff should work together toward the common goal: optimal nutritional patient care – and the hospital management should give priority to co-operation, e.g., by initiating organizational research to optimize co-operation. Also, organized contact between the hospital and the primary healthcare sector should be established.

Lack of involvement from the hospital management

The provision of meals should be regarded as an essential part of the treatment of patients, and not as a hotel service. The hospital management should acknowledge responsibility for food service and the nutritional care of the patients, and give priority to food policy and management of food services. The hospital managers should take account of the costs of complications and prolonged hospital stay due to undernutrition when assessing the cost of food service.

Source: Report and recommendations of the Committee of Experts on Nutrition, Food Safety and Consumer Protection, Council of Europe Publishing, November 2002.

The relationship between NCDs and declining cognition and wellbeing in later life

Physical functioning of older adults has improved from the 1980s onwards, and common diseases such as arthritis have become less disabling. In contrast, prevalence rates of chronic health conditions (e.g., cardio-vascular diseases, cancer) and multimorbidity, both associated with compromised wellbeing, are higher among later-born cohorts. In light of these conflicting findings, indicators of health should be taken into account when examining secular trends in cognition and wellbeing.

Source: Secular Changes in Late-life Cognition and Wellbeing: Towards a Long Bright Future with a Short Brisk Ending? SOEP – The German Socioeconomic Panel study at DIW Berlin 738-2015.

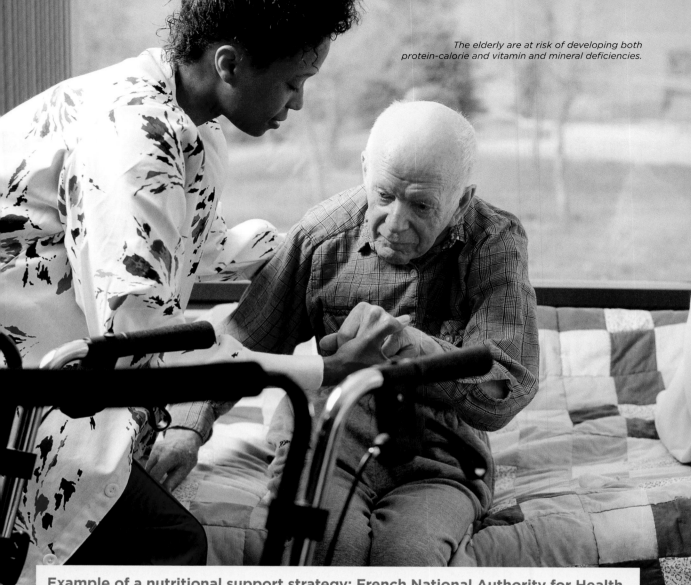

The elderly are at risk of developing both protein-calorie and vitamin and mineral deficiencies.

Example of a nutritional support strategy: French National Authority for Health

Methods of nutritional support

The different methods of nutritional support are:

- Oral nutritional support: this comprises nutritional guidance, assistance during eating, provision of fortified food, and oral nutritional supplements some of which are reimbursed

- Enteral nutritional support

- Parenteral nutritional support, only when the gastrointestinal tract is not functional or the patient is not capable of ingesting food.

The nutritional assessment should include a simple dietary interview of the elderly person or of his/her relatives, to establish whether the person has a varied diet, rich in fruit and vegetables, and if he/she eats protein-containing foods (meats, fish, eggs) regularly. It is also recommended to evaluate the daily fluid intake. In malnourished elderly subjects or when there is a risk of malnutrition, not only should nutritional management be provided, but identified risk factors should be corrected, by proposing for example:

- Technical or human assistance during meals

- Oral and dental care

- A reassessment of the appropriateness of medication and diets

- Management of any underlying diseases.

Nutritional support is all the more effective when it is implemented early.

Source: *Nutritional support strategy for protein-energy malnutrition in the elderly, Clinical Practice Guidelines, Haute Autorité de Santé (French National Authority for Health), France, April 2007, slightly adapted.*

Figure 5 | **A public-health framework for Healthy Ageing: opportunities for public-health action
across the life course**

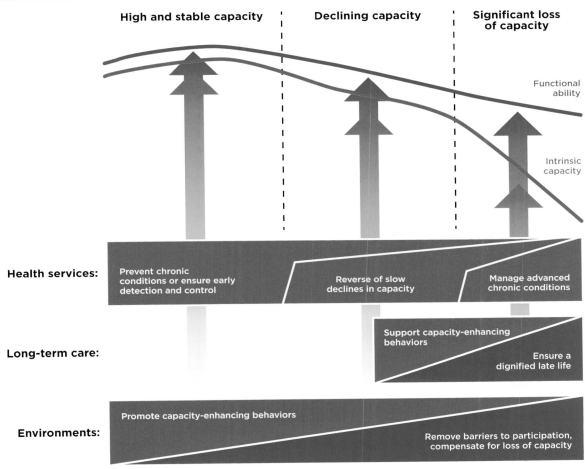

Source: Adapted from WHO World Report on Health Ageing: http://apps.who.int/iris/bitstream/10665/186463/1/9789240694811_eng.pdf?ua=1

My personal view

Peter Weber

Nutrition is very complex, as it comprises a mixture of nutrients acting in concert and dependent on one another. Recent scientific insights have significantly increased scientific and medical understanding of the role and relevance of the various constituents of the diet, and an increasing level of significant scientific agreement exists about the importance of an appropriate level of macro- and micronutrient intake throughout the course of life to support growth, foster health, and prevent the onset of disease. In addition, it is important to realize that micronutrient inadequacies are also a fact in "Western-type" societies and are a growing problem as life expectancy in these societies increases.

Recent changes in life-style and eating patterns, along with increasing dependency on pre-cooked and processed foods, require that more attention should be given to nutrition as a key factor in determining human health.

Nutritional deficiencies are often ignored and underappreciated, despite being a global issue of rising importance with devastating consequences for individuals, communities and national economies.

It is critical to continue developing nutritional solutions and economic models that address the value of nutrition interventions in improving public health as well as the impact of such interventions on healthcare budgets. The evidence is very encouraging, but key stakeholders need to engage to make it happen, and the elderly and their particular circumstances (which include a higher likelihood of taking medications on a regular basis as well as a greater chance of spending time in hospital) should receive much more attention in the future.

The extensive scientific knowledge currently available needs to be translated into cost- effective, practical public health solutions. These may include fortification and/or supplementation, and specific delivery mechanisms should be assessed on a case-by-case. basis The evidence is established, but it needs to be translated into efficient actions, policies and medical practice. Let's make it happen!

Further reading

Péter S, Saris WH, Mathers JC et al. Nutrient Status Assessment in Individuals and Populations for Healthy Aging – Statement from an Expert Workshop. Nutrients 2015;7(12):10491-500. doi: 10.3390/nu7125547.

La Fata G, Weber P, Mohajeri MH. Effects of vitamin E on cognitive performance during ageing and in Alzheimer's disease. Nutrients 2014 ;6(12):5453–72. doi: 10.3390/nu6125453.

References

1   Florence Nightingale, Notes on Nursing: What It Is, and What It Is Not, London, Harrison, London, 1898; republished as Gutenberg EBook #17366, 2005 http://www.gutenberg.org/files/17366/17366-h/17366-h.htm.

2   Nutrients 2014;6:6076-6094; doi:10.3390/nu6126076.

3   Mohajeri MH, Troesch B, Weber P. Inadequate supply of vitamins and DHA in the elderly: Implications for brain aging and Alzheimer-type dementia. Nutrition 2015;31:261–275. DOI: http://dx.doi.org/10.1016/j.nut.2014.06.016.

4   Nutrients 2014;6:6076-6094; doi:10.3390/nu6126076.

5   Stephanie Pappas, Dickensian Diagnosis: Tiny Tim's Symptoms Decoded, Live Science March 5, 2012, http://www.livescience.com/18802-dickenstiny-tim-diagnosis.html. Accessed December 10, 2015.

6   Cashman KD, Dowling KG, Skrabáková Z et al. Vitamin D deficiency in Europe: pandemic? AJCN. First published ahead of print February 10, 2016 as doi: 0.3945/ajcn.115.120873.

7   World Health Organization. Global Age-Friendly Cities. Geneva: World Health Organization, 2007:1–76.

8   Lagiewka, K. European Innovation Partnership on Active and Healthy Ageing: Triggers of setting the headline target of 2 additional healthy life years at birth at EU average by 2020. Arch Public Health 2012;70: doi:10.1186/0778-7367-70-23.

9   Report and recommendations of the Committee of Experts on Nutrition, Food Safety and Consumer Protection, Council of Europe Publishing, November 2002.

10 Morley JE, Thomas DR (eds). Geriatric Nutrition. Baton Rouge: CRC Press 2007.

Nutrition-Specific and Nutrition-Sensitive Interventions

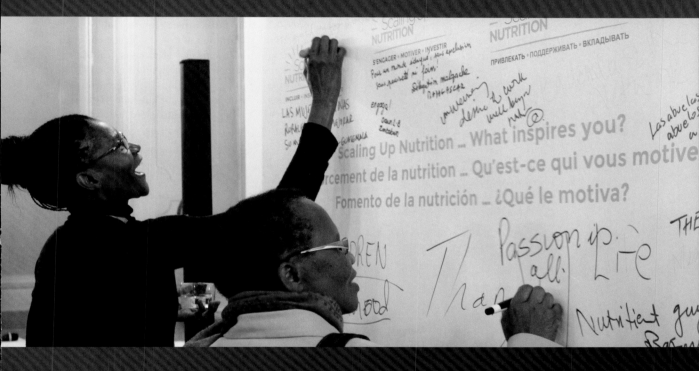

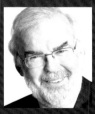

Tom Arnold
SUN Movement Coordinator ad interim and Director General
of the Irish Institute of International and European Affairs

"If you want to eliminate hunger, everybody has to be involved."

Bono (Paul David Hewson), *lead singer of U2 and philanthropist*

Key messages

- The SUN Movement marks its fifth year with 56 countries and the Indian State of Maharashtra committed to scaling up nutrition.

- SUN Countries are proving that to tackle malnutrition, we must recognize that nutrition transcends sectors. It is a multifaceted challenge, which requires a genuine partnership driven by passionate leadership at the highest levels.

- Defeating malnutrition, united with multiple sectors and stakeholders in a truly coherent approach, is no longer an abstract aspiration – it is the new normal.

- The combined power of high-level political commitment paving a path for multisectoral action, a supportive policy environment across sectors essential for improving nutrition, and the scale-up of proven interventions are key ingredients supporting change.

- SUN Countries are proving that building alliances, comprising critical sectors and committed stakeholders, are transforming nutrition. How they share, learn and build a culture of effective partnering is a stepping-stone toward achieving the vision of the SUN Movement.

The 2013 Lancet series on Maternal and Child Nutrition stated that: "Acceleration of progress in nutrition will require effective, large-scale nutrition-sensitive programs that address key underlying determinants of nutrition and enhance the coverage and effectiveness of nutrition-specific interventions."[i] It stated further that "…protection of nutrition, let alone acceleration of progress, will entail more than bringing nutrition-specific interventions to scale. It will require a new and more aggressive focus on coupling effective nutrition-specific interventions (i.e., those that address the immediate determinants of nutrition) with nutrition-sensitive programs that address the underlying causes of undernutrition."

The authors concluded that "Nutrition-sensitive programs can help scale up nutrition-specific interventions and create a stimulating environment in which young children can grow and develop to their full potential."

The concept of nutrition-specific and nutrition-sensitive interventions is now a fundamental element in the discourse of the global nutrition community, helping to distinguish between two types of intervention, each of them essential in the battle to eliminate malnutrition worldwide. This chapter discusses the application of this distinction by the global nutrition community with special reference to the SUN (Scaling Up Nutrition) Movement.

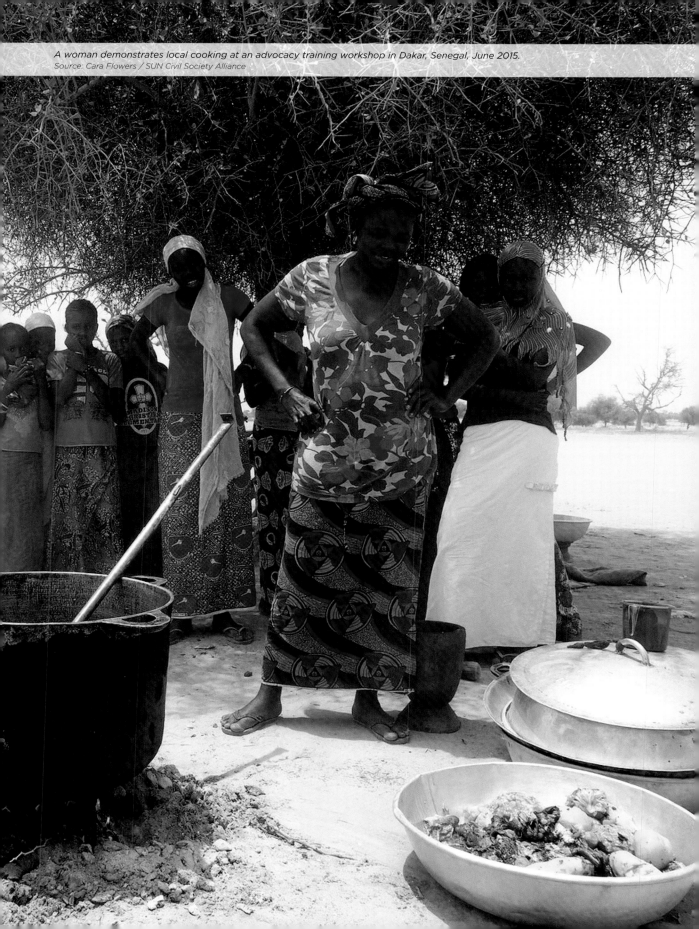

The Lancet and the SUN Movement

The 2013 Lancet series on Maternal and Child Nutrition was a major milestone in the development of a concerted global response to malnutrition. It appeared five years after the 2008 Lancet series on the same topic, which concluded that more than a third of child deaths and 11% of the total disease burden worldwide were due to maternal and child undernutrition. The authors further estimated that stunting, severe wasting, and intrauterine growth restriction together were responsible for 2.2 million deaths and 21% of disability-adjusted life years(DALYs) for children younger than 5 years. "Nutrition is a desperately neglected aspect of maternal, newborn, and child health," the authors wrote. "The reasons for this neglect are understandable but not justifiable." It is to that 2008 publication that the origins of the Scaling Up Nutrition (SUN) Movement may be ultimately traced.

The five-part 2008 Lancet series on nutrition filled a longstanding gap by marshalling systematic evidence of the impact of undernutrition on infant and child mortality and its largely irreversible long-term effects on health and on cognitive and physical development. It also demonstrated the availability of proven interventions that could address these problems and save millions of lives.

The set of interventions proposed by the Lancet focused on the "window of opportunity" from minus 9 to 24 months (i.e., from pregnancy to two years old): this "window" offers the chance to make a high nutritional impact that will reduce death and disease and avoid irreversible harm. The Lancet noted that other studies drawing on a similar set of interventions have demonstrated very high cost-effectiveness, with high returns to cognitive development, individual earnings and economic growth. The authors of the 2008 Lancet series lamented, however, that nutrition was regarded for the most part as an afterthought in development priorities and that it had been seriously underemphasized by both donors and developing countries.

Launch of the SUN

In April, 2010 the governments of Canada and Japan, the United States Agency for International Development (USAID), and the World Bank co-hosted a high-level meeting in Washington, DC on "Scaling up Nutrition" during the Spring Meetings of the World Bank and the International Monetary Fund (IMF). Senior members of delegations from countries with the highest malnutrition burden, high-level representatives from civil society organizations, development partners, bilateral donor governments and the media participated in the meeting, which appealed to governments worldwide to invest more in the attempt to halve the rate of undernourishment (Millennium Development Goal [MDG] 1c).

The primary objective of this meeting was to obtain buy-in from countries and global development partners for an inclusive approach to country ownership and action for scaling up nutrition investments aimed at sustainable development. Opening the meeting, the then President of the World Bank, Robert B Zoellick, said: "Malnourishment not only means children have to suffer, but it also makes them less productive adults. We need to break the vicious cycle of poverty and malnutrition to give people opportunity and to achieve sustained economic growth. The new multipartner Framework for Action represents a united call to action for this 'forgotten MDG.'"

With 2010 marking the five-year countdown to achieving the 2015 Millennium Development Goals (MDGs), and signs that food prices were rising again in developing countries, Dr David Nabarro, Special Representative of UN Secretary General Ban Ki-moon for Food Security and Nutrition at the time, said: "Food and nutrition security is the prerequisite for a decent and productive life and the achievement of all Millennium Development Goals. It is our collective responsibility to ensure food and nutrition security for all through synergy across the full range of sectors. The SUN Framework has the potential to mobilize all of us behind a smart new approach for vastly better development outcomes."

The SUN Road Map

Following on from the Washington meeting, an action planning meeting of key nutrition stakeholders was held in Rome, hosted by the United Nations World Food Programme (WFP). The focus of the discussion was the challenge of moving the SUN framework into action. The meeting acknowledged that it was a matter of urgency to develop concrete recommendations for the wider group of SUN stakeholders on how to scale up nutritional outcomes relevant to the realization of the MDGs.

A Task Team was agreed on to develop the necessary recommendations in the form of a SUN Road Map that would be completed by the September 2010 Summit on the Millennium Development Goals. The function of the Road Map was to answer the question "How to bring the SUN Framework to life and ensure that it leads to real – and sustained – improvements in nutrition in the highest-burden countries?"

The Task Team had five working groups, which focused on the following themes:

1   Stronger national (country-level) capacities and systems for scaling up nutrition actions

2   Effective campaigning and advocacy for the nutrition scale-up

3   Social movements necessary for scaling up nutrition

4   The sustained engagement of development agencies in support for scaled-up nutritional outcomes

5   The successful and appropriate involvement of commercial enterprises in nutrition-sensitive sustainable development.

Speaking on the final day of the meeting, Ms Josette Sheeran, the then Executive Director of the WFP, said: "Today all nutrition roads lead to Rome. Today is a tipping point. This specialty cause of nutrition is becoming a cause for the world. Food security needs to be turned into food and nutrition security. We can make malnutrition history. Globally we have to create a nutrition movement or a nutrition revolution. We have the possibility to do it – it is within our grasp to give the world's children a better future. We know what to do and now we need to do it. We have to put aside our differences and have the 'tribes' come together. We no longer need a scientific breakthrough, we just need to do it – it is a moral imperative!"

Figure 1 | **Evolution of the SUN Movement**

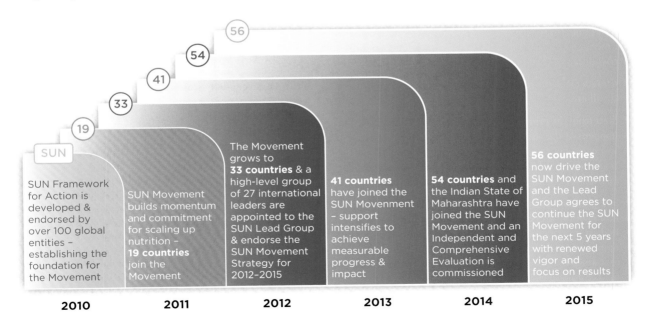

Source: SUN

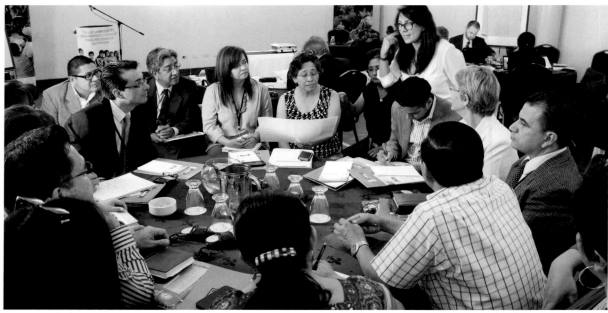

Participants in a regional workshop in Guatemala discuss nutrition allocations in the public budget, April 2015.
Source: SUN Movement Secretariat

The *Scaling Up Nutrition* policy brief

The policy brief on *Scaling Up Nutrition*, which was to give rise to the SUN Movement, had two main purposes. The first was to provide an outline of the emerging framework of key considerations, principles and priorities for action to address undernutrition. The second was to mobilize support for increased investment in a set of nutrition interventions across different sectors.

The main elements of the SUN's framework for action were, and still are:

- **Start from the principle that what ultimately matters is what happens at the country level.** *Individual country nutrition strategies and programs, while drawing on international evidence of good practice, must be country-"owned" and built on the country's specific needs and capacities.*

- **Sharply scale up evidence-based cost-effective interventions to prevent and treat undernutrition, with highest priority to the minus 9 to 24 month window of opportunity where we get the highest returns from investments.** *A conservative global estimate of financing needs for these interventions is $10+ billion per year.*

- **Take a multisectoral approach that includes integrating nutrition in related sectors and using indicators of undernutrition as one of the key measures of overall progress in these sectors.** *The closest actionable links are to*

food security (including agriculture), social protection (including emergency relief) and health (including maternal and child healthcare, immunization and family planning). There are also important links to education, water-supply and sanitation as well as to cross-cutting issues like gender equality, governance (including accountability and corruption), and state fragility.

- **Provide substantially scaled up domestic and external assistance for country-owned nutrition programs and capacity.** *To that end ensure that nutrition is explicitly supported in global as well as national initiatives for food security, social protection and health, and that external assistance follows the agreed principles of aid effectiveness of the Paris Declaration and the Accra Agenda for Action. Support major efforts at the national and global levels for strengthening the evidence base – through better data, monitoring and evaluation, and research – and, importantly, for advocacy.*

Now numbering 56 members worldwide, the SUN Movement recognizes that the causes of malnutrition include both factors that most people would generally associate with nutrition, as well as factors that affect the broader context of life and health. Recognizing this, the SUN Movement looks to implement both specific nutrition interventions and nutrition-sensitive approaches.

SCALING UP NUTRITION

ENGAGE • INSPIRE • INVEST

Philippines

Scaling up
NUTRITION

S'ENGAGER •

SCALING UP NUTRITION IN THE PHILIPPINES:
First 1,000 Days in the context of
Early Childhood Care and Development

SUN Movement delegates from The Philippines with a visitor to their marketplace booth during the SUN Movement Global Gathering, Milan, Italy, October 2015. Source: SUN Movement Secretariat

Nutrition-specific and nutrition-sensitive interventions

The SUN Movement defines these two key concepts as follows:

Specific Nutrition Interventions

- Support for exclusive breastfeeding up to 6 months of age and continued breastfeeding, together with appropriate and nutritious food, up to 2 years of age

- Fortification of foods

- Micronutrient supplementation

- Treatment of severe malnutrition.

Nutrition-Sensitive Approaches

Agriculture: Making nutritious food more accessible to everyone, and supporting small farms as a source of income for women and families

Clean Water and Sanitation: Improving access to reduce infection and disease

Education and Employment: Making sure children have the energy that they need to learn and earn sufficient income as adults

Healthcare: Improving access to services to ensure that women and children stay healthy

Support for Resilience: Establishing a stronger, healthier population and sustained prosperity to better endure emergencies and conflicts

Women's Empowerment: At the core of all efforts, women are empowered to be leaders in Nutrition-Sensitive Approaches.

Nutrition as a development indicator, stunting as a nutrition indicator

Nutrition has always been a key development indicator. Good nutrition allows for healthy growth and development of children, and inadequate nutrition is a major contributing factor to child mortality. Good nutrition is also important for cognitive development, and hence educational success, both of which are important determinants of labor productivity and hence economic growth. Good nutrition also implies balance – neither undernutrition nor overnutrition.

Over the decade or so since the MDGs were set, our understanding of undernutrition and its measurement has advanced further. Underweight (weight for age) is a composite measure, which aggregates two different aspects of undernutrition, namely weight for height (or wasting, a measure of current nutritional status) and height for age (or stunting, a measure of long-run nutritional status).

The underweight goal has served its purpose to focus attention on nutrition. Going forward we can improve on the original MDG target by using stunting as an indicator of nutrition status rather than underweight.

Source: http://www.copenhagenconsensus.com/post-2015-consensus/nutrition, accessed 29 July 2015.

Figure 2 | **The countries driving the SUN Movement**

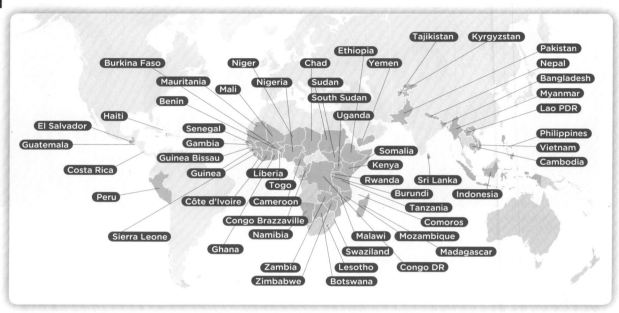

Source: SUN

SUN Country Snapshots: Agriculture and social protection programming for better nutrition

These approaches describe how countries across the SUN Movement are working multisectorally to ensure that nutrition is a key element in agriculture and social protection programs.

Burundi

Burundi is currently integrating nutrition into the nation's sectoral policies and development plans. Backed by high-level political commitment to scale up nutrition, the two main priorities of their multisectoral strategic plan for food security and nutrition (MSPFN) is to improve hygiene practices through a hand-washing initiative as well as to promote dietary diversification through backyard vegetable gardens in schools and households nationwide. Some key challenges impacting multisectoral efforts focusing on agriculture and social protection include the following:

• Harmonizing and aligning points of view, practices and customs between the ministries, non-government organizations and donors.

• The budget for the MSPFN needs to be finalized to pave the way for resource mobilization.

• Certain sectors such as social and environmental protection can still be better represented.

• Promoting behavior change and the adoption of best practices and habits in food and agricultural production is still not easy.

• Understanding the underlying causes of malnutrition and its medium- and long-term effects remains challenging in a context of transition from family subsistence agriculture to intensive agro-pastoral production less dependent on climate conditions

Burundi: Key lessons

The first forum on food security and nutrition, from December 1 to 14, 2011, played a key role in raising awareness and garnering political commitment at a high level regarding the issues of malnutrition and food insecurity. Burundi's involvement in the SUN Movement and the UN Renewed Efforts Against Child Hunger (REACH) initiative have also improved the organization and coordination of national nutrition activities and helped address the multiple causes of malnutrition through a multisectoral and multistakeholder approach. At the local levels, distributing cattle to rural families has significantly increased milk production and consumption, and the promotion of organic fertilizers, kitchen gardens, credit facilities and fertilizer subsidies has helped increase and diversify agricultural production and food consumption in the population. Regarding social protection, identifying the most vulnerable families for the distribution of animals is crucial, and an identification mechanism has been established for future generations.

Lao PDR

In Lao PDR there have been significant efforts to establish a multisectoral committee on nutrition which aims to ensure increasing investment in nutrition as well as to establish all the institutional arrangements needed to improve food and nutrition security. In addition to the committee, the Ministry of Agriculture and Forestry and the Ministry of Health have begun to decentralize the nutrition coordination process. Some key challenges that the government, in partnership with the country's nutrition stakeholders, has been working to overcome include the following:

- Increasing investment from the government and mobilizing resources from external sources for nutrition has worked; however, coordination among stakeholders and donors for the mapping of interventions, resource requirements, implementation coverage and outcomes has been a challenge.

- Limited capacity for implementing nutrition-specific and nutrition-sensitive interventions continues to be a hurdle.

Lao PDR: Key lessons

Lao PDR's experience has proved that recruiting the right coordinators with the right skills and experience at the right institutions can ensure effective coordination. The accelerating levels of commitment and ownership at the local level, with the central level only providing strategic direction, are essential. Decentralizing national-level actions to the village level, including in health and agricultural centers, along with district teams who can provide support and monitoring, is helping. Establishing mechanisms for accountability helps to identify needs. Improving capacity development at all levels is essential for scaling up nutrition, and this all must be viewed as a process of learning by doing.

Nepal

Nepal has developed strategies and plans to address the problem of food insecurity and promote nutrition, attempting to increase the availability of quality food and to increase the income and reduce the workload of women. Social protection schemes are helping to provide sufficient food

and nutritious diets for poor and socially excluded groups.

At present, there are 12 different policies and 21 different acts to guide the agricultural sector in Nepal. Despite this, poor coordination mechanisms among major organizations working to enhance food and nutrition security has led to reduced efficiency and effectiveness. The Multisector Nutrition Plan has been developed to bolster coordination among different relevant sectors. In this context, the agriculture sector in Nepal is attempting to increase the availability of quality foods through homestead food and livestock production; to increase the income of poorer women through credit incentives; to promote increased consumption of micronutrient rich foods; to reduce the workload of women and provide them with healthy and efficient energy; and to develop the capacity of the sector and strengthen linkages with other sectors.

At the same time, the following are some of the social transfer programs in Nepal that target the vulnerable groups, aiming to tackle poverty and improve nutritional status.

- Cash transfer and social protection programs, including safety net programs and in-kind transfers for senior citizens throughout the country, children, people with disabilities and endangered indigenous peoples; scholarships; and food for work and school meal programs

- Free social services, including essential healthcare services

- Poverty reduction and social empowerment programs aimed at various marginalized communities and women, in collaboration with development partners

- Pensions and social insurance, mainly focused on formal sector employees

- Labor market interventions such as labor legislations, vocational and skill development trainings, rural community infrastructure works, and so on.

Nepal: Key lessons

Through Nepal's experience, legal provisions in the acts and regulations make local bodies more responsible for implementing nutrition and social protection programs at the local level. Directives circulated to the local bodies play a vital role in the effective implementation of activities to improve the nutritional status of pregnant women and children. The implementation of interventions and activities jointly, among the relevant sectors and stakeholders, gives multiple outcomes in reducing chronic malnutrition.

Yemen

In Yemen, development partners and the government have been engaged in developing a long-term integrated multi-sectoral action plan for combating undernutrition from 2015 to 2019, with the engagement of all sectors. The agriculture, food security and social protection sectors have agreed on the principle of programmatic and geographic convergence, in that all sectors will work together in approximately half the districts with a high burden of undernutrition.

The SUN Yemen team faced some challenges in the beginning of the process. It took time to build consensus on planning for common results, alignment with the newly emerging political situation and new Government, and capacity constraints in coordination and multisectoral planning. These challenges were addressed with the help of United Nations partners and the SUN Movement Secretariat. As Yemen moves towards implementation, transforming these planning documents into action will be the real challenge, especially implementing the nutrition-sensitive interventions. In the current situation, mobilizing financial resources for this plan will be a huge challenge for the government and the SUN Donor Network.

Yemen: Key lessons

A regression analysis, which was completed by the Maximizing the Quality of Scaling Up Nutrition consortium, was a very important step in the process of preparing the national framework. Understanding the key drivers of malnutrition in Yemen was very helpful in bringing stakeholders toward a collective view of the causes and, most importantly, the response needed. This exercise was particularly useful in helping to understand the role of adolescent girls as caregivers in the home and the consequent potential impact of schooling on nutrition indicators at household level. Through the regression analysis, the costing process and the trajectory analysis, the various sectors and ministries now have a much better grasp of what it means to include nutrition objectives in the planning of interventions which do not necessarily have a nutrition objective.

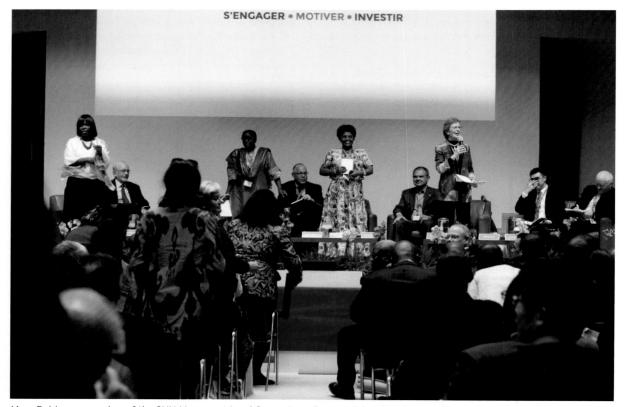

Mary Robinson, member of the SUN Movement Lead Group (standing, on right of podium), calls all women participants of the SUN Movement Global Gathering to rise, Rome, Italy, October 2014. Source: SUN Movement Secretariat

The Future of the SUN Movement 2016–2020

The past five years in the life of the Movement have been a collaborative journey, involving partners from civil society, United Nations (UN) agencies, donors, business and academia. Our conviction and determination to end malnutrition, in all its forms, lights our way toward 2020.

The Independent Comprehensive Evaluation of the Movement that took place in January 2015, the widespread consultation that followed, and the subsequent endorsement of the new SUN Movement Strategy (2016-2020) by the SUN Movement Lead Group in September 2015, have all reinforced the imperative for the SUN Movement to continue with renewed ambition and vigor.

The SUN Movement Strategy (2016–2020) builds on the momentum and progress realized during the first phase of collective action and commitment. Mirroring the ambition of the 2030 Agenda for Sustainable Development, the new strategy calls for greater emphasis on implementation and accountability. The strategic objectives seek to consolidate ground gained since 2012 while setting the bar even higher. They aim to:

1 Expand and sustain the enabling political environment that was instrumental in elevating nutrition to the level of importance it has achieved today

2 Prioritize and institutionalize effective actions that contribute to good nutrition by building and enhancing sound policy and legal foundations;

3 Implement actions aligned with national common results frameworks

4 Effectively use, and also significantly increase, financial resources for nutrition.

The Road Map of the SUN Movement Strategy (2016–2020) will strive to achieve these objectives by:

• Fostering improvements in the management of the policy and budget cycle in SUN Countries

• Strengthening advocacy, social mobilization and communication efforts

• Conducting supporting actions across sectors, among stakeholders, and between levels of government through improved functional capacities

• Strengthening the equity drivers of nutrition, including the roles of women and girls.

A SUN Movement Executive Committee has been formed to provide strategic guidance and help monitor progress toward achieving the Movement's ambitions by 2020. The establishment of an Executive Committee was a key recommendation in the Comprehensive Independent Evaluation aimed at strengthening governance and accountability within SUN. The Committee is chaired by Shawn Baker, Director of Nutrition from the Bill & Melinda Gates Foundation, with Abdoulaye Ka, National Coordinator of the National Committee for the Fight Against Malnutrition, Prime Minister's Office, Senegal as vice-chairman. A new SUN Movement Lead Group, chaired by Anthony Lake, Executive Director of UNICEF, is being formed to ensure nutrition is in the global, regional and country spotlight – and this more than ever before.

Ambassador Gerda Verburg of the Netherlands has been appointed by the UN Secretary General Ban-Ki Moon as the new Sun Movement Coordinator, and will lead the Movement for the next five years. Ms. Verburg was previously the Permanent Representative of the Kingdom of the Netherlands to the Rome-based UN Organizations (FAO, WFP and IFAD), Chair of the Global Agenda Council for Food and Nutrition Security of the World Economic Forum (WEF), and Chair of the UN Committee on World Food Security (CFS).

I am proud to have served as Interim Coordinator of the SUN Movement since September 2014. The SUN Movement stands for nutritional transformation. Millions of girls, women, boys and men are disadvantaged because they are needlessly malnourished. All within the Movement are capable of ending this injustice. The Movement is ready to surge forward with renewed ambition and vigor. It is time to make it happen.

My journey with the SUN

Tom Arnold

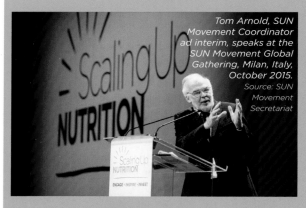

Tom Arnold, SUN Movement Coordinator ad interim, speaks at the SUN Movement Global Gathering, Milan, Italy, October 2015.
Source: SUN Movement Secretariat

The Scaling Up Nutrition (SUN) Movement contributes to the spirit of strengthened global solidarity, focused on the needs of the poorest and most vulnerable, and with the participation of countries, stakeholders and people. The SUN Movement exists as a manifestation of the belief that only by working together – across the diversity of sectoral approaches, stakeholder interests and institutional mandates – will it be possible to achieve the progressive realization of the right to adequate food, and nutrition justice for all.

I have been involved with the SUN Movement ever since it was launched by US Secretary of State Hillary Clinton and Irish Foreign Minister Micheál Martin in 2010, when I was still Chief Executive of Concern Worldwide. SUN has done a great deal to highlight the political importance of nutrition. Many of the world's political leaders are now beginning to appreciate the significance of nutrition for the current and long-term welfare of their people, as well as for their prospects of economic growth. SUN is creating opportunities for this thinking to be shared, focusing on topics such as attracting the necessary resources and building the required capacity.

A determination to end malnutrition

As at the end of 2015, the Movement is led by 56 countries and the Indian State of Maharashtra. Together, along with multiple stakeholders from civil society, United Nations agencies, donors, business and academia, we are all united by our determination to end malnutrition in all its forms. It is within our power to confront and overcome this challenge.

Following the Independent Comprehensive Evaluation (ICE) of the SUN Movement which concluded in January 2015, the SUN Movement Lead Group was unanimous that the Movement should remain inclusive, multi-stakeholder and multisectoral: a "big tent" open to all countries committed to achieving nutrition justice for all.

Guided by the evaluation and subsequent SUN Movement Lead Group decisions, together we are looking forward to the next five years of the SUN Movement. We will ensure that the Movement's unique advocacy for better nutrition is louder and more visible than ever before. We will continue to enrich the Movement's unique ability to catalyze action, ensure and improve our transparency, and strengthen our emphasis on gender and women's empowerment, climate change, and fighting inequity.

The SUN Movement Strategy and Road Map 2016–2020

The development of a the new SUN Movement Strategy and Road Map 2016–2020 will be central to achieving results, but its adoption is just the beginning of a difficult journey ahead. The Strategy will only be meaningful to the extent it is used by SUN Countries and the multiple stakeholders supporting it to become a reality.

It will be vital to build upon current successes with greater ambition for results and impact on stunting in all countries committed to scaling up nutrition. This ambition is the unique quality that has made the Movement a success. The ambition will ensure it remains country-led, inclusive, multistakeholder and multisectoral.

I often think back to the SUN Global Gathering in Rome in November 2014, which brought together some 300 people for a three-day period in the run-up to the second International Conference on Nutrition (ICN2). I thought the exchanges between participants were very significant, because people were standing up and showing what they had achieved in their own countries, and others were asking them detailed questions about how they had managed to do these things. It's not about new ideas as such: it's about doing a few things well, and doing them collectively – ensuring, for instance, that appropriate sanitation is in place, providing the conditions that are conducive to good nutrition. In the longer term, I think it's crucial that women's voices should be heard and that they should help to formulate nutrition policy and shape nutrition programs going forward.

The tremendous energy and enthusiasm that drive the SUN Movement bodes well for the future. Nutrition is in the spotlight – more now than ever before. The political will is growing, and the evidence is stronger than at any time in the past.

Further reading

Changing Food Systems for Better Nutrition

Can food systems be changed for better nutrition? And if they can, how can these changes be achieved?

More information available at: http://www.unscn.org/files/ Publications/SCN_News/SCNNEWS40_final_standard_ res.pdf

The Nutrition Sensitivity of Agriculture and Food Policies

Eight country case studies (Brazil, Malawi, Mozambique, Nepal, Senegal, Sierra Leone, South Africa, and Thailand) as well as a synthesis report were completed which describe and analyze national policies in the area of food and agriculture.

The individual Country Case Studies can be found at: http://www.unscn.org/en/publications/country_case_ studies/ the_nutrition_sensitivity2.php

CAADP Agriculture Nutrition Capacity Development Initiative

The New Partnership for Africa's Development (NEPAD) and the African Union Commission (AUC) have launched an initiative to strengthen capacity for addressing nutrition through the formulation and implementation of National Agriculture and Food Security Investment Plans in collaboration with Regional Economic Communities and with the support of FAO and USAID.

More information available at: http://www.fao.org/food/ fns/workshops/caadp-nutrition/en/http://www.nepad.org/ fr/foodsecurity/news/3153/integratingnutrition-national-agriculture-and-food-security-investment-plans

Agriculture and Nutrition: A Common Future

A Framework for Joint Action by the Technical Centre for Agricultural and Rural (CTA), The European Union, FAO and the World Bank Group.

More information available at: http://cta.int/images/ publications/Agriculture-Nutrition-ICN2%20%281%29. pdf

What Risks Do Agricultural Interventions Entail For Nutrition?

Agricultural development status impacts individual nutrition through food, health, and care practices. This working paper identifies six categories of risks.

More information at: http://www.spring-nutrition.org/ publications/resource-review/updates/what-risks-do-agricultural-interventionsentail-Nutrition

Simulating Potential of Nutrition-Sensitive Investments by the Center for Globalization and Sustainable Development, The Earth Institute, Columbia University

The purpose of this study is to help decision-makers in SUN countries to prioritize key nutrition-sensitive investments across different sectors.

More information at: http://scalingupnutrition.org/ wp-content/uploads/2014/07/SUN-Report-CU_Jan-21-2014.pdf

How Agriculture Can Improve Child Nutrition

This report by Save the Children examines and explores how nutrition can be prioritized within agricultural policies, strategies and investment plans.

More information at: http://www.savethechildren.org.uk/ resources/online-library/nutrition-sensitivity

References

i   *Ruel MT, Alderman H and the Maternal and Child Nutrition Study Group, Nutrition-sensitive interventions and programmes: how can they help to accelerate progress in improving maternal and child nutrition? Lancet 2013; 382: 536–51 Published Online June 6, 2013 http://dx.doi.org/10.1016/ S0140-6736(13)60843-0.*

The Role of Good Governance in Delivering Good Nutrition

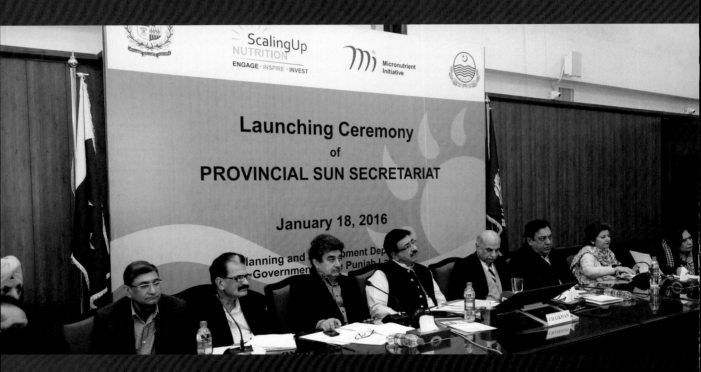

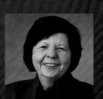

Eileen Kennedy
Tufts University, Friedman
School of Nutrition Science and
Policy, Boston MA, USA

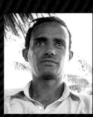

Habtamu Fekadu
Save the Children,
Addis Ababa, Ethiopia

"The time is always right to do right."

Nelson Rolihlahla Mandela (1918–2013), *South African anti-apartheid revolutionary, politician, and philanthropist; President of South Africa 1994–99.*

Key messages

- It is generally agreed that good governance is essential for effective policy and program development and implementation.

- There is no such thing as a formulaic approach to governance that can be applied universally; there are, however, a number of factors that contribute to effective governance, including leadership, advocacy, a legal framework, stakeholder involvement, and enduring commitment.

- Capacity development at all levels – including the individual, institutional and political – is essential.

- Evidence and research are important for policy and program development, but advocacy is key.

- Leadership at all levels is a prerequisite for sustaining the momentum of effective nutrition policies and programs.

Nutrition: A fundamental right of all humanity

There has been a growing recognition of the key role of nutrition in human health and national development. The following quote highlights the importance of nutrition in the Post-2015 Sustainable Development Goals: "Nutrition is, not least, a fundamental right of all humanity. Without good nutrition, the mind and body cannot function well. When that happens, the foundations of economic, social and cultural life are undermined."[1]

With this realization, combined with the confirmation of efficacious and affordable interventions, governments around the world, and their development partners, are currently seeking effective and sustainable ways to implement solutions at scale. The process of designing and implementing nutrition policies and programs within a country has many dimensions, including the technical, logistical, political, economic and social. In addition, increased attention is now being focused on governance, capacity development, and the creation of enabling environments. Each of these terms will be defined in the following sections.

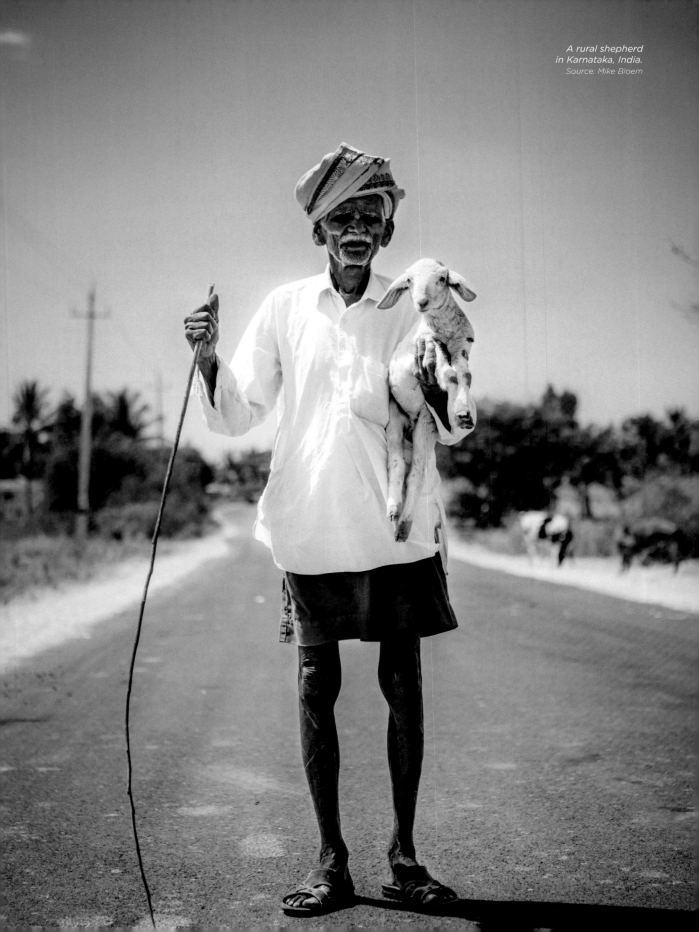

The relevance of governance to nutrition today

The concept of good governance is not new. As far back as 1992, a World Bank Report – Governance and Development – defined the term as "The manner in which power is exercised in the management of a country's economic and social resources for development."[2] Similarly in 1999, the World Bank defined governance as "the traditions and institutions by which an authority in a country is exercised."[3]

Good governance has recently received increased attention as a critical success factor both in the scientific and the implementation literature. This serious attention to a more systematic measurement of governance has been fueled, in part, by a critique of the international "nutrition architecture" as "broken, fragmented and dysfunctional."[4] This observation has prompted lively discussion about international and national models of effective governance.

International governance

The emergence of large-scale initiatives such as the Scaling Up Nutrition Movement (SUN), Renewed Efforts against Child Hunger and Under Nutrition (REACH), and the Committee on World Food Security (CFS) illustrate different models of governance.

SUN was launched at a United Nations annual meeting in 2010. The SUN Movement brings together authorities of countries burdened by undernutrition, a broad range of stakeholders from multiple sectors in-country, and a global coalition of partners. The establishment of SUN also provides a framework for assessing nutrition governance. The elements of nutrition governance include: an inter-sectoral mechanism for nutrition; having a national nutrition plan/strategy; adoption of the nutrition plan/strategy; nutrition in the national nutrition plan; the existence of a national nutrition policy; the adoption of a national nutrition policy; the allocation of budget for the plan; regular nutrition monitoring/surveillance; a line for nutrition in the health budget; a line for nutrition in the agriculture budget; and a line for nutrition in the social development budget.

REACH is a country-led approach to scale up proven and effective interventions, addressing child undernutrition through partnerships and coordinated action on the part of UN agencies, civil society, donors and the private sector, under the leadership of national governments. It has operated in 12 countries. REACH is currently being phased

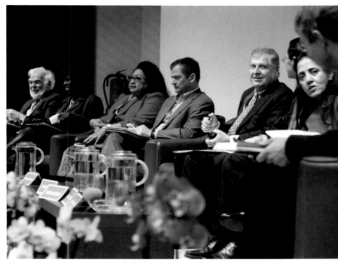

Panel of speakers at the SUN Movement Global Gathering, Rome, Italy, October 2014. Source: SUN Movement Secretariat

out, but the country-level focus for a coordinated approach to nutrition will remain.

The CFS is the UN Governing Body that reviews and follows up on food security and nutrition policies. It uses a multistakeholder platform including UN agencies, bilateral organizations, civil society, and the private sector. The CFS endorses policy recommendations and guidelines on a wide range of food security and nutrition topics. Policy recommendations are based on scientific and evidence-based reports produced by the High Level Panel of Experts on Food Security and Nutrition.

Good governance, capacity development, and an enabling environment: definitions

The renewed emphasis on nutrition, nationally and globally, has focused attention on a linked trio of factors: governance, capacity development, and an enabling environment.

There is almost universal agreement that appropriate governance is essential for effective program and policy implementation. Yet the concept of "good governance" remains elusive. The public policy literature is replete with illustrations of governance; yet the term itself remains open to different interpretations by different audiences. Curiously, it is often easier to identify poor governance than good governance.

Good governance is not unique to nutrition; however, with the renewed emphasis on nutrition through initiatives such as SUN, the nutrition focus in the SDGs and the proliferation of country-level national nutrition plans, governance related specifically to nutrition is front and center.

Capacity development is critical for the effective implementation of policies and programs. When the term "capacity" was first linked to nutrition, some focused narrowly on academic capacity, as measured by the granting of degrees. Capacity is now viewed in a much more holistic perspective and includes individual, institutional, political, advocacy, leadership, communication and delivery capacity. A recent high-level workshop concluded that inherent in effective capacity development is the imperative to simultaneously and consistently address the three interrelated levels of capacity: individual, institutional and systemic.[5]

Similarly, more attention is now being given to the importance of an "enabling environment" for nutrition. In many ways, this term is as nebulous as that of governance. One definition describes it as "A set of interrelated conditions – such as legal, organizational, fiscal, informational, political and cultural – that impact on the capacity of development actors such as civil society to engage in development processes in a sustained and effective manner."[6] Alternatively, at the national level, the word "enabling" means to "make able; give power, means, competence, or ability to; authorize."[7] The examples in this chapter point to the fact that enabling environments can be created. They contain three essential elements.[8] These are:

- Knowledge and evidence;
- Capacity and resources; and
- Politics and governance.

Figure 1 | **The key factors for effective nutritional policy-making and program development. The nine crescents represent ministries relevant for multisectoral coordination. These will vary from country to country.**

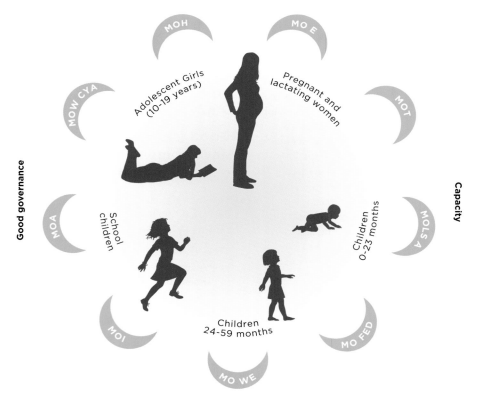

Source: NNP launch presentation, June 2013, Federal Ministry of Health, UNECA Addis Ababa.

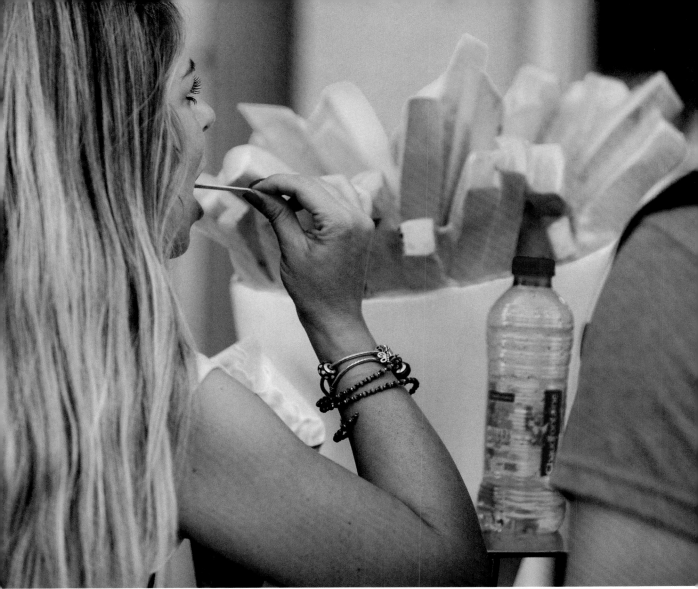

Good policy-making is the basis for improved nutrition, everywhere in the world.
Source: Mike Bloem

From theory to action

Concepts such as good governance and an enabling environment are intrinsically vague. Policy officials essentially want an answer to the questions: "What works, in what context, and at what cost?" No formulaic approach as yet exists that can delineate the specific steps that can provide a menu for success, or the necessary ordering of these steps. What we can do, however, is to learn from a series of examples in this chapter, which may lay out some broader principles.

A first step in the policy cycle for nutrition (broadly defined) is to get issues onto the policy agenda at the international or national level. The presentations at the 2014 Micronutrient Forum Global Conference pointed out that: "having proven solutions to address malnutrition and, more specifically, to eradicate micronutrient deficiencies, does not automatically result in the adoption of these interventions." Much of the literature on public policy emphasizes that, in the final analysis, identifying nutrition as a priority is a political process. Indeed, global forums have highlighted that fact that "Political will and evidence-informed policy are essential for the sustainability of nutrition initiatives at both the national and international levels." Here again, one representative of a bilateral organization commented that "political will is commonly used as a catch-all concept, the meaning of which is so vague that is does little to enrich our understanding of the political and policy processes... We must begin by giving 'political will' a quite specific and narrow meaning."[9] With these observations in mind, this chapter will try to "deconstruct" elements of political will and enabling environments into some core components. How does nutrition get on the policy agenda?

Evidence linked to policy and programs

Former Deputy Executive Director of the World Food Programme Namga Ngonge once said: "The world is replete with good ideas that have never made it off the shelf."[10] So how, if at all, does evidence get translated into action? Some researchers have been rather unimpressed by science's ability to influence the nutrition agenda. For example, as Alfred Sommer once remarked: "The central premise of this symposium, that data can drive public policy, is both laudatory and even vaguely plausible. The historical record, however, is not encouraging."[11] Can evidence influence policy in a sustainable manner? To provide an answer to this question, we use two examples: one is international, the other country-specific.

Hidden hunger

Assumptions following the World Food Conference in 1974 colored the nutrition agenda for decades. There was a basic understanding that agricultural production was needed to increase incomes of smallholders and that this, in turn, would improve energy intake. There was the implicit assumption that most malnutrition was caused by inadequate energy intake at household level. During the 1970s and 1980s, there was a definite food bias towards malnutrition. Indeed, the "green revolution" produced dramatic results in some parts of the world. Agricultural output grew and caloric intakes increased in certain areas, while nuances of the complexity of nutrition also began to emerge. For example, the gains achieved with the green revolution technologies did not necessarily translate into improvements in nutritional status, particularly in preschool-aged children. With this as a backdrop, the early studies on micronutrient malnutrition took on special significance.

Administration of vitamin A. The tip of the red capsule containing a dose of vitamin A is cut with scissors and the contents of the capsule squeezed out into the child's mouth. Source: Mike Bloem

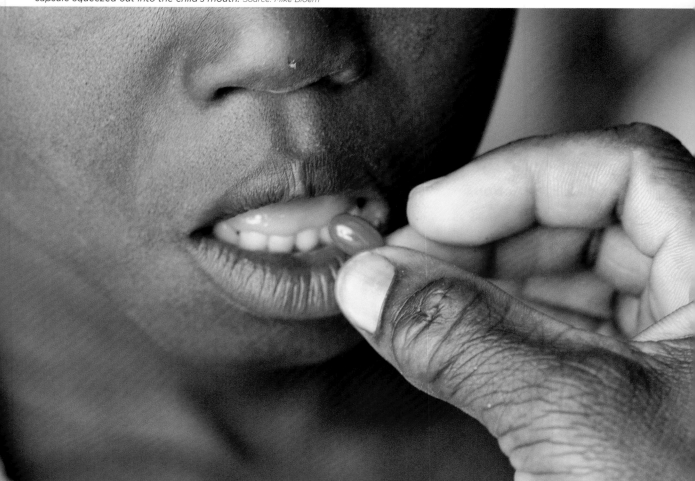

It has been known for years that vitamin A deficiency, if left untreated, can cause blindness. A group of researchers from Johns Hopkins University conducted research in Indonesia in preschool-aged children and found that vitamin A supplementation significantly decreased child mortality. There was incredulity among some in the research community that this postulation of a link between vitamin A and mortality was correct. At a meeting of the Sub Committee on Nutrition in the 1980s in Nairobi at which the findings from the study in Indonesia were discussed, one SCN member noted: "If [the results] were true, we would have known this already."

The novel findings from the Indonesia study set in motion a series of activities. Additional vitamin A supplementation trials were conducted. A meta-analysis of studies was conducted and concluded that there was a 23% reduction in mortality in preschool-aged children who were given vitamin A supplementation. A high-level conference, chaired by UNICEF and WHO, was held in early 1990 in Montreal. A spotlight was shone on micronutrient malnutrition – called "Hidden Hunger." Dramatic increases in funding emerged from donors in developed countries.

Over time, the evidence of a positive impact of vitamin A programs has been widely documented. While there are still disagreements over short-term vs. longer-term strategies for vitamin A treatment and deficiency prevention, vitamin A supplementation is one of the efficacious and effective interventions identified in the 2013 Lancet Series.

The example of vitamin A may appear to be a clear story of research linked to action. That would be an incomplete assessment. The evidence was important, but advocacy in support of these results was key. The researchers involved in the initial work made a concerted effort to reach the policy community. In the USA, hearings were held in Congress, an earmark for micronutrient interventions was passed – and the rest is history. Some might think the vitamin A story is a clear example of leadership in championing nutrition issues.

Hunger in America

The topics of food insecurity and hunger in the USA have had a stormy history. In the late 1960s, attention was focused on the problem of hunger in the USA. Activities such as the Ten State Nutrition Survey, documentaries such as "Hunger in America," and visits by politicians to poverty-stricken areas of the country pointed to the fact that hunger was a problem. However, a Presidential Task Force on Food Assistance could not agree whether, and to what extent, hunger existed in the USA.[12] All the members of the committee agreed that hunger was unacceptable. In addition, there was general agreement that clinical measures of hunger – mainly anthropometrics – did not provide sensitive indicators of the condition: *"In many people hunger means not just symptoms that can be diagnosed by a physician, it bespeaks the existence of a social, not a medical problem: a situation in which someone cannot obtain an adequate amount of food, even if the shortage is not prolonged enough to cause health problems."*

The clear message that there needed to be a definition of hunger delinked from clinical signs prompted attention from the research community. Two events turned out to be critical in the debate about hunger in America. First, legislation was passed under the National Nutrition Monitoring and Related Research Act of 1990, which required the government to recommend a standardized method for defining hunger and food insecurity. Second, the American Institute of Nutrition published a major report[13] clarifying the meaning of hunger from the scientific literature. For the first time, all people defined food insecurity in the US as *access at all times to enough food for an active and healthy life.*

A 1994 Conference on food security measurement built on the AIN report and additional research.[14] The conference brought together a wide constituency including policy officials, researchers and advocates. The conference led to the launch of the US Food Security Module, which has subsequently become a routine part of food security monitoring in the USA. The Food Security Module measures hunger and food insecurity from the perspective of those affected. It was launched by the then US Vice President, Al Gore, and gave the event enormous visibility. The reaction to the Food Security Module was both positive and negative. Opponents – in part, because of the perceived link to the White House – criticized this monitoring approach as a means of inflating the number of hunger- and food-insecure households in the USA. The Food Security Module survived and is used as one method for monitoring food security in the USA. Here again, the leadership linked to evidence was one ingredient that contributed to success.

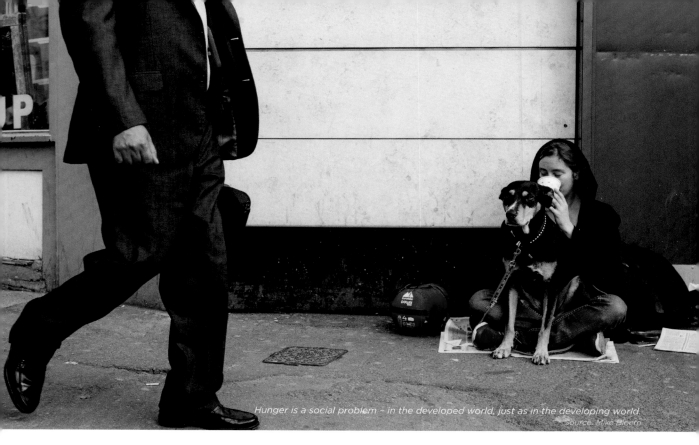

Hunger is a social problem – in the developed world, just as in the developing world.
Source: Mike Bloem

Capacity and resources

Similar to good governance, capacity development is generally agreed as being important in program and policy implementation, but here again, the definition is interpreted in a variety of ways. A guiding principle in the launch of the SUN Movement was that what ultimately matters is what happens at the country level. The phrase that is used within SUN is that policies and programs need to be "country-owned."

The example of Malawi and its commitment to eliminating and preventing acute malnutrition illustrates the power of harnessing sustainable resources and investing in capacity development. Severe acute malnutrition is defined as -3 z-scores below the median weight-for-height. If left untreated, the case fatality rate is extraordinarily high. The Government of Malawi, acting together with two international non-governmental organizations – Valid International and Concern International – embarked on a strategy to promote the community-based management of acute malnutrition (CMAM) in children under the age of five. Using frontline workers, a system of identifying and triaging children with severe acute malnutrition was implemented. The premise of CMAM is that uncomplicated forms of severe acute malnutrition can be successfully treated in the community.

Community-based management of acute malnutrition has been shown to be a very effective way to deal with severe malnutrition in Malawi. Frontline health workers are trained to screen and monitor preschool-aged children; this allows malnourished children to be identified and treated early. The treatment modality is based on a combination of ready-to-use therapeutic foods provided in the form of take-home rations complemented by outpatient care. Community mobilization has been key to the success of treating severe acute malnutrition in Malawi. In addition, a focal point for nutrition in the Office of the Prime Minister in Malawi provides a platform to ensure that community-based management of acute malnutrition continues to be a priority for Malawi. Here again, leadership at the highest level has been an important success factor.

Politics and governance

While the Lancet Series of 2008 and 2013 provided the scientific basis for the SUN Movement, for the concepts they conveyed to become "real," it was imperative to translate the science into action.

As noted earlier in this chapter, SUN identified characteristics that were associated with good governance. These included:

• The existence of a National Nutrition Plan/Program;

• An intersectoral mechanism for nutrition; and

• The existence of a National Nutrition Monitoring System.

Ethiopia was one of the initial countries to join the SUN Movement, and as such was termed an "early-riser" country. It exemplifies the SUN principles outlined above. For Ethiopia, this included a National Nutrition Strategy and National Nutrition Plans of 2008 and 2013. These two National Nutrition Plans were not, however, the first endeavor to launch strategies for improving nutrition in Ethiopia. Decades earlier, the Government of Ethiopia had participated in the Joint Nutrition Support Programme funded by UNICEF and WHO. The Joint Nutrition Support Programme was not viewed by the Government of Ethiopia as a long-term success, yet it shares some elements with the country's more recent activities within the framework of the SUN Movement. A recent study attempted to ascertain what has contributed to the Government of Ethiopia's enthusiasm for the SUN Movement and the palpable energy supporting the implementation of the National Nutrition Plan.[15]

The SUN Movement has always stressed that nutrition programs must be "country-owned." Various steps were taken by the Government of Ethiopia to ensure a sense of inclusion in preparation for implementation of the second National Nutrition Plan. One seminal event that created awareness of the importance of investing in nutrition was a 2010 Workshop on accelerating the reduction of stunting. This was followed by the formation of a technical working group which included all sectors involved in nutrition; as noted in a recent study, this working group turned out to be influential in guiding the 2013 National Nutrition Plan.[16] Finally, a 2013 meeting which included all ministers in the Government of Ethiopia provided a high-visibility forum for showing the importance of nutrition. In addition to having a National Nutrition Strategy and two National Nutrition Plans, the Government of Ethiopia established a National Nutrition Coordinating Body chaired by government and donors and including representatives of civil society. In the early years of operation, this body was criticized for being a board on paper only, and for failing to provide the necessary level of coordination across varied sectors. The National Nutrition Coordinating Body has since been revitalized so as to better bring together the major players to implement a multisector nutrition program.

Going forward, there are clearly challenges in maintaining the momentum of the National Nutrition Plan. First, senior government officials as well as other key stakeholders identified leadership – at all levels and across all stakeholders – as critical.[16] Without this leadership, it is unlikely that the enthusiasm for the plan will continue. There is, however, reason for optimism that nutrition will continue to receive support. The National Nutrition Coordinating Board, acting together with higher-level

government officials and parliamentarians, renewed the commitment to end hunger and undernutrition in Ethiopia by 2030. The ambitious declaration that resulted is called the "Seqota" declaration. It is a clear indication of a policy commitment to keep the momentum for nutrition vibrant in Ethiopia. In addition, the Government of Ethiopia recently launched its second five-year Growth and Transformation Plan, which includes stunting as an indicator, and emphasizes the importance of multisector approaches to improving nutrition.

What will success of the National Nutrition Plan look like? Curiously, answers from each of the stakeholder groups involved stress the importance of taking the timeframe into account when formulating such a judgment. Early success can be measured by awareness of the National Nutrition Plan. As noted by respondents, it may take time for the elements of the plan to filter down from the national to sub-national level. As the present book is being written, the next five-year National Nutrition Plan is under revision, with a view to aligning it with the goals of the Growth and Transformation Plan; this is a further indication that the Government of Ethiopia is utilizing a holistic approach to improving nutrition. Ultimately, improvement in the health and nutrition of Ethiopians will be the true litmus test of success.

Figure 2 | **The Seqota Declaration articulates the Government of Ethiopia's renewed commitment to end undernutrition and hunger by 2030**

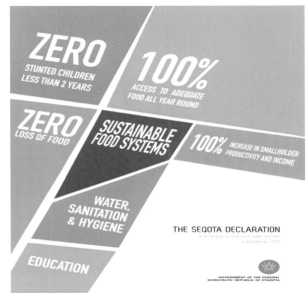

Source: Federal Ministry of Health of Ethiopia

Summary

There are proven, effective nutrition interventions for
improving the nutritional status of at-risk populations.
There is also a growing understanding of the need to attend
to certain aspects of governance in order to ensure the
successful implementation of policies and programs.
Research in the area of good governance is still in its early
stages. The recognition of the vital importance of good
governance has sparked serious attention to research in this
area. This is an exciting time for nutrition, and more
attention to governance and the enabling environment is a
giant leap forward.

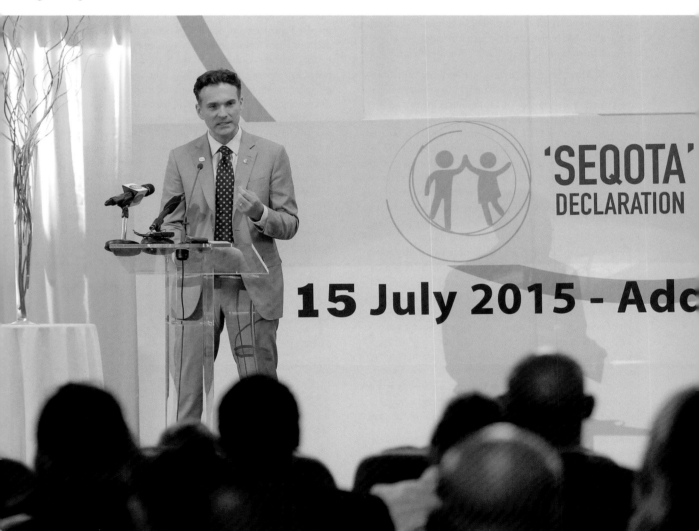

Joel Spicer, CEO and President of the Micronutrient Initiative (MI), addresses delegates in Addis Ababa, Ethiopia, at the event that launched the Seqota Declaration, July 15, 2015.
Source: Micronutrient Initiative (MI)

My personal view

Eileen Kennedy

Having been involved in nutrition as a policy official, program implementer and researcher, I have seen at first hand the critical need for good governance. Its constituent elements may take many forms. Without leadership combined with advocacy, however, there will be missed opportunities for making a positive difference in nutrition.

Further reading

Hauck, K Smith P. The Politics of Priority Setting in Health: A Political Economy Perspective. 2015 www.cgdev.org. Accessed January 12, 2016.

Global Nutrition Report. 2015. www.global nutrition report.org. Accessed January 12, 2016.

References

1 Webb, Patrick, Nutrition and the Post-2015 Sustainable Development Goals. Boston, MA: United Nations System, 2014. http://unscn.org/en/publications/nutrition-and-post-2015-agenda.

2 World Bank, Governance and Development. Washington, DC: World Bank Publications, 1992. http://documents.worldbank.org/curated/en/1992/04/440582/governance-development.

3 Kaufmann D, Kraay A, Zoido-Lobaton P. Governance Matters: Policy Research Working paper. http://info.worldbank.org/governance/wgi/pdf/govmatters1.pdf. Accessed December 16, 2015.

4 Morris S, Cogill B, Uauy R. Effective International Action Against Undernutrition: Why has it proven so difficult and what can be done to accelerate progress? Lancet 2008;371:608–621.

5 Fanzo J, Graziose MM, Kraemer K et al. Education and Training a Workforce for Nutrition for a Post-2015 World. Advances in Nutrition Journal 2015;6:639–647.

6 Open Forum for CSO Development Effectiveness. "Issue Paper 8: Enabling Environment." http://www.ccic.ca/_files/en/what_we_do/osc_open_forum_wkshop_2009-10_paper_8_e.pdf. Accessed December 16, 2015.

7 Micronutrient Forum. Bridging Discovery and Delivery: Micronutrient Forum Global Conference, Addis Ababa, Ethiopia, 2-6 June 2014. http://micronutrientforum.org/wp-content/uploads/2014/04/Micronutrient-Forum-Global-Conference-Ethiopia-2014-Proceedings.pdf. Accessed December 16, 2015.

8 Open Forum for CSO Development Effectiveness. "Issue Paper 8: Enabling Environment." http://www.ccic.ca/_files/en/what_we_do/osc_open_forum_wkshop_2009-10_paper_8_e.pdf. Accessed December 16, 2015.

9 Micronutrient Forum. Bridging Discovery and Delivery: Micronutrient Forum Global Conference, Addis Ababa, Ethiopia, 2-6 June 2014. http://micronutrientforum.org/wp-content/uploads/2014/04/Micronutrient-Forum-Global-Conference-Ethiopia-2014-Proceedings.pdf. Accessed December 16, 2015.

10 Ngonge N, personal communication.

11 Sommer, Alfred. How Public Health Policy is Created: Scientific Processes and Political Reality. Am J Epidemiol 2001;154:S4–S6.

12 Sommer, A, Tarwotjo I, Djunaedi E et al. Impact of Vitamin A Supplementation on Childhood Mortality: A Randomized Controlled Community Trial. The Lancet (1986): 1169–1173.

13 Anon.

14 Beaton GH, Martorell R, Aronson KJ et al. Effectiveness of Vitamin A Supplementation in the Control of Young Child Morbidity and Mortality in Developing Countries – Nutrition Policy Discussion Paper No. 13. United Nations (1993): 1–166.

15 Pear R. US Panel Says Hunger Cannot be Documented. New York Times, February 9, 1984. http://www.nytimes.com/1984/01/09/us/us-panel-says-hunger-cannot-be-documented.html?pagewanted=all&_r=0. Accessed December 17, 2015.

16 Anderson, S.A. Core Indicators of Nutritional Status for Difficult to Sample Populations. J Nutr 1990;170:1557–1600.

17 Radimer KL, Olsen CM, Campbell CC. Development of Indicators to Assess Hunger. J Nutr 1990;120:1544–1548.

18 Kennedy Eileen et al (Dec 2015). Multisector Nutrition Program Governance and Implementation in Ethiopia: Opportunities and Challenges. Food and Nutrition Bulletin (in press).

What Gets Measured Gets Done: How nutrition monitoring, impact evaluation, and surveillance can support program improvement and policy development

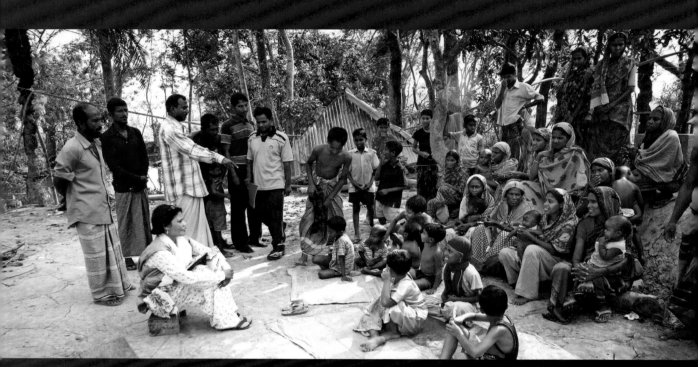

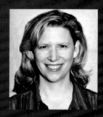

Maria Elena D Jefferds

Behavioral Scientist with the International Micronutrient Malnutrition Prevention and Control (IMMPaCt) Team in the Division of Nutrition, Physical Activity and Obesity, Centers for Disease Control and Prevention, Atlanta, GA, USA

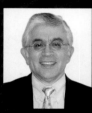

Rafael Flores-Ayala

Team Lead of the International Micronutrient Malnutrition Prevention and Control Program, Centers for Disease Control and Prevention, Atlanta, GA; member of the Global Nutrition Report's Independent Expert Group; Co-Chair of the Micronutrient Forum; Adjunct Associate Professor at the Rollins School of Public Health, Emory University, Atlanta, GA, USA

"If you can't describe what you are doing as a process, you don't know what you are doing."

William Edwards Deming *(1900–1993), American engineer, statistician, professor, author, lecturer, and management consultant.*

Key messages

- Most countries are currently not on track to meet the global nutrition targets agreed by the World Health Assembly (WHA) in 2013.

- The release of the World Health Assembly 2025 global nutrition targets and the Global Nutrition Report can represent strategic opportunities for improving nutrition worldwide.

- Various monitoring, evaluation and surveillance frameworks exist to guide the development, implementation and evaluation of nutrition programs and systems.

- Countries and nutrition programs benefit from nutrition monitoring and surveillance systems that are used for decision-making, program improvement, accountability and policy development.

- Supporting capacity development is a key opportunity for action.

Key concepts

Monitoring, Evaluation and Surveillance

- "Monitoring is the ongoing collection, analysis, and interpretation of data on the program (inputs, activities, outputs, and outcomes). The primary purpose of monitoring data is to enable program managers to assess the performance of programs for program improvement."[1]

- "Program evaluation is the assessment, as systematic and objective as possible, of a planned, ongoing, or completed program that covers its need, design, implementation, impact, efficiency and sustainability, so as to incorporate lessons learned into the decision-making process about the program and inform and guide public policy."[1]

- "Public health surveillance is the ongoing, systematic collection, analysis, interpretation, and dissemination of data regarding a health-related event for use in public health action to reduce morbidity and mortality and to improve health."[2]

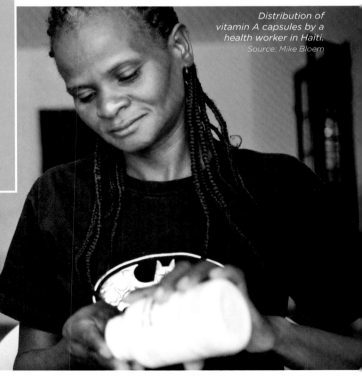

Distribution of vitamin A capsules by a health worker in Haiti.
Source: Mike Bloem

The importance of monitoring, evaluation and surveillance

The world is rallying around the global nutrition targets agreed by the World Health Assembly (WHA) in 2012,[3] but currently most countries are not on track to meet them or do not have sufficient data to ascertain whether they are meeting nutrition targets. There is modest global progress on stunting and exclusive breastfeeding but little progress on low birth weight, wasting, overweight and anemia. Among the 193 countries, 94 do not have data to monitor the WHA targets, and coverage data for nutrition-specific interventions are very scarce. There are not enough high-quality, country-driven and country-owned nutrition data, and this weakens nutrition accountability.[4]

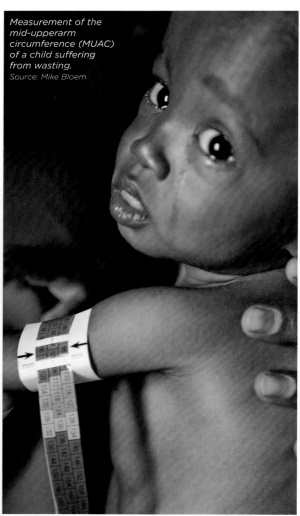

Measurement of the mid-upperarm circumference (MUAC) of a child suffering from wasting.
Source: Mike Bloem

Monitoring is a key component of program management, as both monitoring and managing use data to examine and oversee program inputs, activities and outputs. Within a country, monitoring of a public nutrition program is essential to understand the effectiveness of program operations, identify and address problems, and improve program performance. As a result, it is virtually impossible to have effective programs without internal monitoring systems that are managed by program staff. While not always required, evaluation of a specific program can be useful for documenting whether the program is achieving the expected outcomes and impacting on the population in an efficient and sustainable way.

Nutrition surveillance systems within countries provide timely information about the nutritional status or nutrition programs in the country in order to make policy and programmatic decisions to improve the nutrition situation of a population. Global surveillance that documents the number and types of programs in countries, as well as other key indicators such as coverage, are important to support global coordination, understand and develop global guidelines and technical resources, and mobilize resources.

Often it is the case that 'what gets measured gets done'. It is not feasible or appropriate to continuously collect data on all possible indicators. As a result, the indicators included in monitoring, impact evaluation or surveillance systems may be given priority. They thus have greater chance of being accomplished, compared to other inputs, activities, outputs or outcomes that are not similarly prioritized. This can make the selection of, for example, nutrition program indicators or global targets that must be periodically reported, into catalyzing events that energize programs and countries to especially focus on these areas and document their performance. The release of the World Health Assembly 2025 global nutrition targets[3] and the Global Nutrition Report,[4] for example, can represent strategic opportunities for improving nutrition worldwide. With a global interest in improving country-owned and country-driven data and accountability, this chapter describes existing frameworks and tools, as well as key areas on which to focus and strategic opportunities to improve nutrition monitoring, evaluation and surveillance.

Frameworks and tools useful for monitoring, evaluation and surveillance

Fortunately, various monitoring, evaluation and surveillance frameworks exist to guide the development, implementation and evaluation of nutrition programs and systems. In addition, there are many specific tools that serve as technical resources, such as manuals,[1, 5, 6] compilations of existing systems,[7] global program surveillance databases,[8, 9] and indicators such as those found in the WHO/CDC eCatalogue of indicators for micronutrient intervention programmes,[10] World Health Assembly 2025 global targets,[3] or the Global Nutrition Report,[4] for example.

The CDC Framework for Program Evaluation in Public Health[11] is one framework useful for designing monitoring, evaluation or surveillance systems, and includes six steps:

1 Engage stakeholders

2 Describe the project

3 Focus the design

4 Gather credible evidence

5 Justify conclusions

6 Ensure use and share lessons learned (**Figure 1**).

The Framework also defines the standards of utility, feasibility, propriety, accuracy and accountability that should inform the development and implementation of a monitoring, evaluation, or surveillance system.[11] Other characteristics important for many systems to be useful and feasible include: timeliness, simplicity, flexibility, acceptability, representativeness, stability and sustainability.[2]

Figure 1 | **Framework for program evaluation in public health**[11]

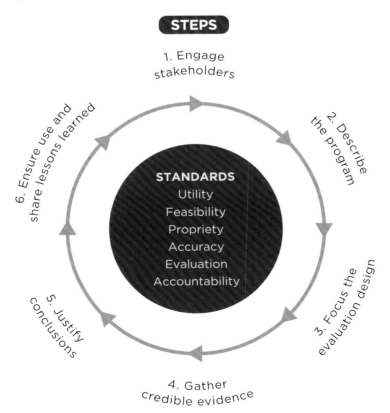

Chapter 5.6 | What Gets Measured Gets Done: How nutrition monitoring, impact evaluation, and surveillance can support program improvement and policy development

305

Figure 2 | **WHO / CDC logic model for micronutrient interventions in public health**[13]

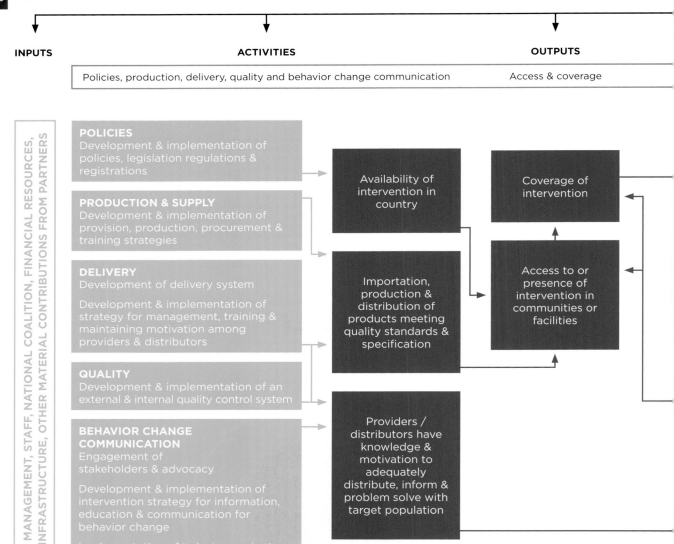

© World Health Organization 2011

Logic models are useful tools that visually organize information and describe the "program logic" by portraying the expected processes and effects of multiple, coordinated actions.[12] While often limited to a single page, they can also be more than one page; simple or complex; linear, unidirectional, circular or developed in any way that best describes the program logic for the audience and purpose of developing the logic model. Logic models are key tools for designing monitoring, evaluation or surveillance systems as they help diverse stakeholders understand how a nutrition program is supposed to work and contribute to achieving public health goals. They can

Chapter 5.6 | What Gets Measured Gets Done: How nutrition monitoring, impact evaluation, and surveillance can support program improvement and policy development

306

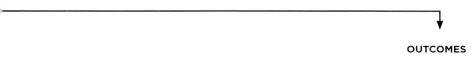

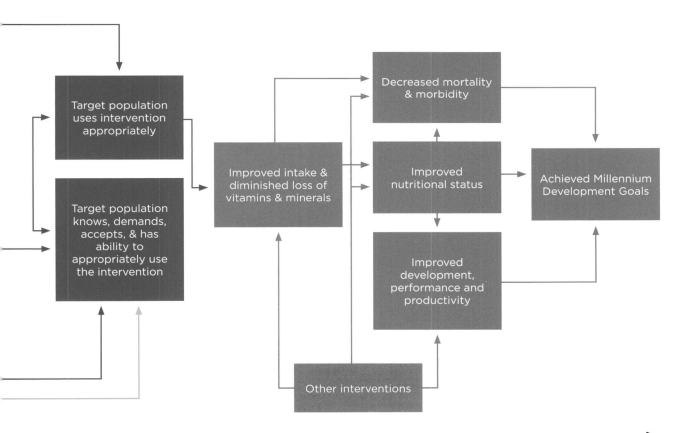

WHO/NMH/NHD/MNM/11.5

serve as a framework for program design and implementation, and for developing monitoring, evaluation and surveillance tools and indicators. The Logic model for micronutrient interventions in public health[13] was developed as a generic logic model tool that already identifies for the user priority areas, expected processes, and concepts that apply to most public health micronutrient interventions (**Figure 2**). Adaptable versions of the logic model are available in the six official languages of WHO on their website. The logic model can be adapted to any public health program context to support program planning, implementation, monitoring, impact evaluation and surveillance.

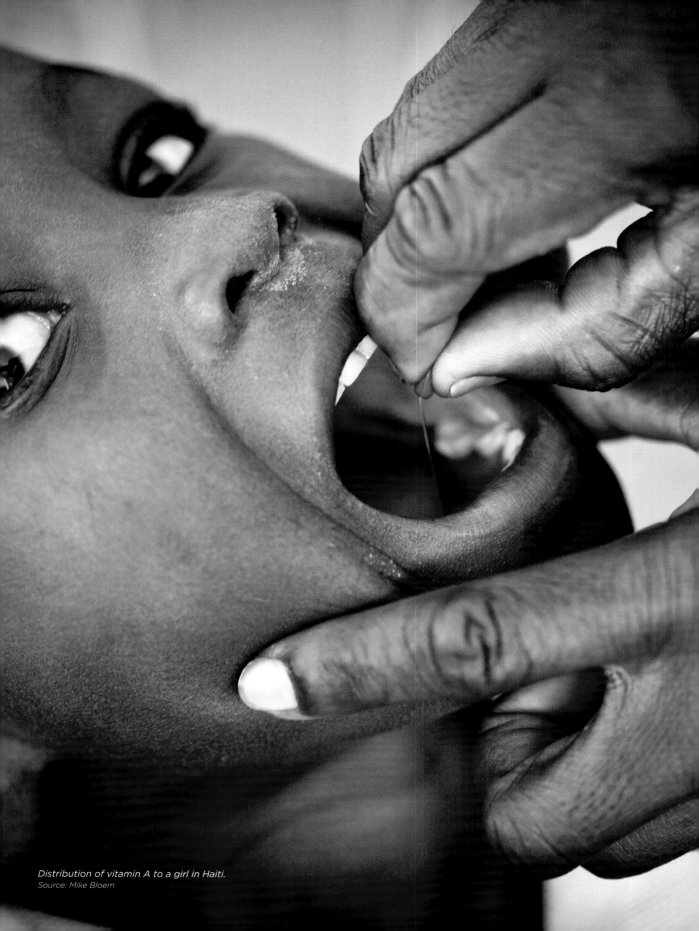

Distribution of vitamin A to a girl in Haiti.
Source: Mike Bloem

Key areas to focus monitoring, evaluation and surveillance

Countries and nutrition programs benefit from having timely, high-quality information collected routinely through nutrition monitoring and surveillance systems that are used for decision-making, program improvement, accountability and policy development. Effective internal monitoring systems that program staff either collect or are able to access provide information necessary to manage the program and resolve issues for program improvement. Programs might also have external monitoring systems that are collected and managed independently of program staff. Further, when specific questions about program performance occur, it might be necessary to collect additional focused, specialized information to better understand the question, issue, or problem, and identify appropriate solutions and changes. Within countries, nutrition surveillance data are important for policy and program decisions. They can be used to track progress in reducing malnutrition, assist in nutrition planning and advocacy, promote accountability for government and agency actions, respond promptly to rapid changes in nutritional status, and inform and influence nutrition programming decisions. Data may be collected through the management information systems of government ministries with this mandate, or by systems developed by other stakeholders in-country. Ideally all relevant stakeholders and users of the data are involved in these systems, so they meet the data needs and are valued with sustained support and commitment over time.

Evaluating nutrition programs can be complex and expensive, and this procedure is usually not necessary for most public nutrition programs to consider, particularly when global policies and guidelines exist, or if there are not enough resources and expertise to design and implement the evaluation, which is the norm for most nutrition programs. Keeping these issues in mind, evaluations provide useful information to develop public health policy with a view to improving nutrition. Three types of evaluation useful for developing public policy include impact evaluation, cost-effectiveness, and sustainability evaluation.

Under real-world programmatic conditions, an impact evaluation measures the effects of the program on specific outcomes and expected program objectives in the population (e.g., reduce the prevalence of stunting or iron deficiency among young children). Cost-effectiveness examines the efficiency of a program by comparing program costs and effects (impacts) with the costs and effects of alternative interventions. Sustainability evaluation assesses whether positive public health outcomes are maintained over time, and in addition to measuring the public health impacts, may consider funding stability; political support; partnerships; organizational capacity; program improvement; surveillance, monitoring and evaluation; communication; and strategic planning.[14]

While this information is critical for developing policies and guidelines at a global level, it is not necessary or appropriate for most nutrition programs in countries to undergo these types of evaluation. Deciding whether to conduct an evaluation is always context-specific and depends on many factors.

At a global level, surveillance of nutrition programs, supporting global databases, and filling data gaps are increasingly emphasized as key components necessary to meet the worldwide commitment to the global nutrition targets of the World Health Assembly.[3] The Global Nutrition Report highlighted the critical need to fill global data gaps by including it as one of the 10 recommendations in the report, in particular emphasizing the need for more data on micronutrient status, intervention coverage and other process and outcome data from interventions.[4] The Global Monitoring Framework for Maternal, Infant and Young Child Nutrition has a core set of indicators to be reported by all countries; there is also an extended set of indicators from which countries can draw to design national nutrition surveillance systems fitting their specific epidemiological patterns and program decisions.[3]

Identify the data gaps that hinder effective action – and fill them

Countries, donors, and agencies should work with the technical nutrition community to identify and prioritize the data gaps that are holding back action and then invest in the capacity to fill the gaps. *All countries, including high-income countries*, should reach out to UN agencies to facilitate the conversion of their own data into international databases convened by the UN agencies.

Source: 2015 Global Nutrition Report: Actions & Accountability to Advance Sustainable Development, p. xxviii, http://ebrary.ifpri.org/ utils/getfile/collection/p15738coll2/id/129443/filename/129654.pdf.

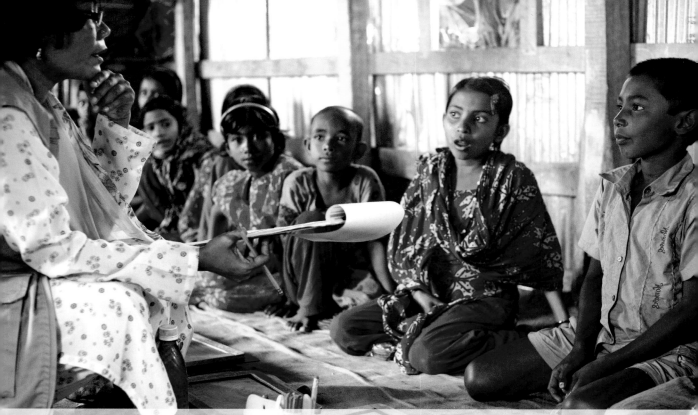

Schoolchildren at BRAC School at East (Purba) Mostofapur, Nilgonj Union, Bangladesh receiving fortified biscuits from WFP and being interviewed by WFP staff. *Source: Mike Bloem*

Strategic opportunities to improve monitoring, evaluation and surveillance

Supporting capacity development is a key opportunity for action, as nutrition capacity is interdependent at the individual, organizational, and system levels, and all these levels are necessary to carry out effective nutrition programs, monitoring, evaluation, and surveillance systems (**Figure 3**[15]).

Figure 3 | **Capacity pyramid**

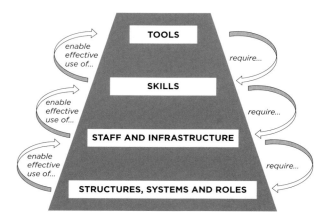

Source: Potter C and Brough R. Systemic capacity building: a hierarchy of needs. Health Planning and Policy 2004; 19(5) page 340. Used by permission of Oxford University Press.

Short-term capacity building goals include the development and dissemination of tools (e.g.,[1, 5, 10]), as well as technical assistance, training, and supportive supervision to strengthen staff skills.

In addition to technical tools and frameworks for monitoring, evaluation and surveillance, there are existing models in countries for capacity transfer to other countries or settings of feasible and useful data collection systems that are used to improve nutrition programs and policies (e.g., Case Study), as well as agencies that specialize in nutrition monitoring, evaluation and surveillance. Tools, frameworks and other global technical resource documents are useful and necessary, but are not sufficient by themselves to develop, implement and maintain systems for monitoring, evaluation or surveillance in the absence of capacities at individual, organizational, and systems levels, making this a priority area of focus.

Furthermore, supporting innovation in new methods for monitoring, evaluation and surveillance – including integration and harmonization with innovative technology, spatial analyses, and sampling approaches – can potentially help address the existing bottlenecks and capacity issues that occur with many programs and countries.

Case Study

Sugar fortification with vitamin A in Guatemala – Commercial and household monitoring and surveillance

By Carolina Martinez and Mónica Guamuch, Nutrition Institute for Central America and Panama (INCAP)

In Guatemala, sugar is fortified with vitamin A, and results from monitoring and surveillance systems show that the program complies with legal regulations for fortification. The monitoring system includes internal monitoring, which is carried out by the producers in packaging plants; commercial monitoring, carried out by the Food Regulation and Control Department from the Ministry of Health; and external social monitoring, carried out by the League of Consumers Association (LIDECON, its acronym in Spanish). Household monitoring data are also collected through surveillance systems in the country.

For commercial monitoring, the Ministry of Health and LIDECON collect sugar samples in retail stores in order to assess compliance of their vitamin A content with regulations. LIDECON also provides education to consumers about the importance of food fortification. Sugar samples collected by the government are analyzed by the Guatemalan National Laboratory, and the samples collected by LIDECON are analyzed by the Nutrition Institute for Central America and Panama's laboratory (INCAP, its acronym in Spanish). During 2015, over 90%[1] of the retail samples collected by government complied with the regulations.[2] In 2013, LIDECON reported that 87% of the retail samples collected met the national requirements.[3]

Household-level fortification monitoring data have been collected in several ways, including through school-based sentinel surveillance and household surveillance. From the mid-1990s until 2012, school-based sentinel surveillance was supported by the Ministry of Education, UNICEF and INCAP. Official rural public schools were randomly selected around the country, and students were asked to bring in sugar samples from their homes. The sugar samples were used to assess household coverage of fortified sugar, including the vitamin A content and whether the samples contained an adequate level of vitamin A to have a positive nutritional impact on population health. In 1995, coverage was less than 60% with an average 6.6 mg retinol/ kg sugar, but coverage improved over time. In

2011, the average vitamin A content of sugar nationwide was 9.4 mg / kg, with 86% of samples above the minimum level expected of 3.5 mg / kg.[4] In 2013, an evaluation[5] was conducted in the western highlands region because of the proximity to Mexico, where sugar fortification is not mandatory and there is a high risk of unfortified sugar crossing into Guatemala. Samples were collected in randomly selected schools, and 70% of the samples met the criteria of acceptable fortification; 91% in the metropolitan area and 73% in the northeast area showed vitamin A levels at or above the expected minimum household levels.[6] In 2012, as part of a prototype for a nutrition surveillance system, sugar samples were collected from a representative sample of households in five departments of the western area of the country. They showed that 93% of the samples had vitamin A levels above 3.5 mg / kg with an average of 9.6 / kg.[7]

References

1   Datos del Departamento de Regulación y Control de Alimentos del MSPAS.

2   Acuerdo Gubernativo 021-2000. REGLAMENTO PARA LA FORTIFICACIÓN DEL AZÚCAR CON VITAMINA A.

3   Informe final. Proyecto colaborativo Nutrisalud, LIDECON, INCAP. Monitoreo social externo y vigilancia de alimentos fortificados en hogares en Quiché, San Marcos, Huehuetenango, Totonicapán y Quetzaltenango. 2013.

4   LIDECON, INCAP, CONAFOR. Situación de los programas de fortificación de alimentos. 2012.

5   Informe final. Proyecto colaborativo Nutrisalud, LIDECON, INCAP. Monitoreo social externo y vigilancia de alimentos fortificados en hogares en Quiché, San Marcos, Huehuetenango, Totonicapán y Quetzaltenango. 2013.

6   C. Martinez, D. Mazariegos. Contenido de yodo en sal y vitamina A en azúcar en muestras del programa de Escuelas Centinela Regiones Metropolitana y Suroriente. 2013 Estudio colaborativo, INCAP, UVG, LIDECON.

7   Sistema de Vigilancia de la Malnutrición en Guatemala (SIVIM), Congreso Latinoamericano de Nutrición. (presentación). Habana, Cuba; 2012. Disponible en: http://www.incap.int/index.php/es/publicaciones/doc_view/287-presentacion-sivim-slan-final.

"Nutrition needs a data revolution" This call to action in the Global Nutrition Report[4] highlights the need at global level for funders to increase resources available for collecting data, to invest in capacity building, to support the comparability of data collected, and to update and maintain national and global nutrition databases for accountability. They emphasize that data on intervention coverage and other key process and outcome indicators must be prioritized.[4] Related to this, harmonization across institutions to support new global databases of nutrition indicators and the global infrastructure for nutrition will strengthen evidence-based decision-making for global policy, development of technical resources, mobilization of resources, and global coordination for improved accountability. This makes supporting "a data revolution" another priority area of focus to improve nutrition.

Our personal view

Maria Elena D Jefferds & Rafael Flores-Ayala

The World Health Assembly nutrition targets,[3] Global Nutrition Report,[4] and similar initiatives highlight the unique opportunity and global focus at this point in time to improve nutrition worldwide. Countries, global donors, partners, and other stakeholders recognize that high-quality and timely monitoring, evaluation and nutrition surveillance data are critical to improve the nutrition situation of populations.

We have tools, frameworks and models of useful systems, as well as agencies with expertise in monitoring, evaluation and surveillance, to help fill these data gaps. Focusing on capacity building, innovation, and investing to support a "nutrition data revolution" are strategic opportunities at this point in time to improve nutrition and health worldwide.

Further reading

Website of the WHO the Vitamin and Mineral Nutrition Information System (VMNIS): www.who.int/vmnis.

Global Nutrition Report (GNR) website: http://globalnutritionreport.org/.

Potter C, Brough R. Systemic capacity building: a hierarchy of needs. Health Planning and Policy 2004;19(5):336–345.

Home Fortification Technical Advisory Group. A Manual for Developing and Implementing Monitoring Systems for Home Fortification Interventions. Geneva: Home Fortification Technical Advisory Group, 2013.

Website of the International Initiative for Impact Evaluation: http://www.3ieimpact.org/en/.

Disclaimer: The findings and conclusions in this report are those of the authors and do not necessarily represent the official position of the Centers for Disease Control and Prevention.

References

1   Home Fortification Technical Advisory Group. A Manual for Developing and Implementing Monitoring Systems for Home Fortification Interventions. Geneva: Home Fortification Technical Advisory Group, 2013.

2   Centers for Disease Control and Prevention. Updated Guidelines for Evaluating Public Health Surveillance Systems: Recommendations from the Guidelines Working Group. MMWR; 2001. Report No.: 50, p2.

3   World Health Assembly. Comprehensive implementation plan on maternal, infant and young child nutrition. Geneva, 65thWorld Health Assembly, 2012.

4   Global Nutrition Report. 2014. Available at http://globalnutritionreport.org/. Accessed August 25, 2015.

5   Global Alliance for Vitamin A (GAVA). Data-Driven Monitoring of Vitamin A Supplementation Programmes: A Guide for District (Area-based) Managers. Ottawa: Micronutrient Initiative, 2015.

6   World Health Organization. Nutritional surveillance. Geneva: World Health Organization, 1994.

7   Friedman, Gregg. Review of National Nutrition Surveillance Systems. Washington, DC: FHI 360/FANTA, 2014.

8   UNICEF. Nutridash 2013: Global report of the pilot year. UNICEF, New York, NY, 2014.

9   Food Fortification Initiative (FFI). Global Progress on legislation to mandate fortification of at least one industrially milled cereal grain. Available at http://www.ffinetwork.org/global_progress/. Accessed August 25, 2015.

10 WHO/CDC. eCatalogue of indicators for micronutrient intervention programmes. Available at: https://extranet.who.int/indcat/. Accessed August 25, 2015.

11 Centers for Disease Control and Prevention. Framework for Program Evaluation in Public Health. Centers for Disease Control and Prevention; 1999.

12 W. K. Kellogg Foundation. Logic Model Development Guide, pp. 1–62. Battle Creek, MI: W. K. Kellogg Foundation, 2004.

13 WHO/CDC. WHO/CDC logic model for micronutrient interventions in public health. Available at www.who.int/entity/vmnis/toolkit/logic_model/en/. Accessed August 25, 2015.

14 Center for Public Health System Science, Washington University. Program Sustainability Framework and Domain Descriptions v2. St. Louis, MO: George Warren Brown School of Social Work, 2013.

15 Potter C. and Brough R. Systemic capacity building: a hierarchy of needs. Health Planning and Policy 2004;19(5):336–345.

The Critical Role of Food Safety in Ensuring Food Security

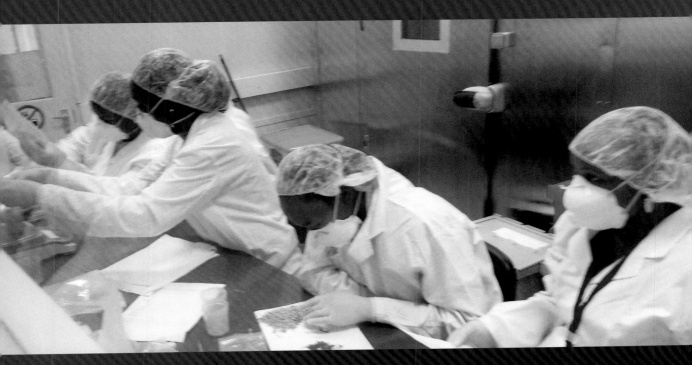

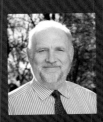

Dave Crean
Vice President of Corporate
Research and Development,
Mars, Incorporated

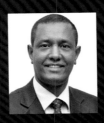

Amare Ayalew
Program Manager of the
Partnership for Aflatoxin Control
in Africa (PACA), the African
Union Commission

Acknowledgments:

Thanks to all those involved in the production of this document especially
Rebecca Bieniaszewska and Oakland Innovation, without whom it would not

"Partnership with the private sector to improve food safety globally is critical. FAO recognizes this and engages with the food industry at national and international levels to both leverage and disseminate knowledge that will promote effective food safety practices along the food chain. Food safety is complex, and addressing food safety issues requires a multisectorial approach."

Ren Wang, *Assistant Director-General of FAO's Agriculture and Consumer Protection Department.*

Key messages

- Today's global food supply chains make the food safety landscape more complex and challenging than ever before. Food safety management has not kept pace with this development.

- Unsafe food cannot sustain human health and has tragic social and economic consequences.

- New food safety threats are emerging. Aflatoxin is a particularly good example: the health and economic effects of aflatoxin cause devastation, especially for the world's poorest.

- Improving levels of food safety globally requires the development of new technologies, sustainable commitments, and human and institutional capacity, especially among farmers.

- Collaboration among all stakeholders is necessary to leverage the right food safety knowledge, risk management methods and interventions across the global food supply chain.

Food safety: the context

Ensuring safe and nutritious food for all is arguably one of the key public health challenges of our time. The safety of the food we consume directly influences our health, but its significance within the broader food supply system can scarcely be overstated. The economic implications (and impacts) of food safety are clear, and have been extensively documented.[1, 2]

While the discipline of food safety has long been discussed and researched, its link to food security has yet to be fully appreciated. The UN Food and Agriculture Organization (FAO) defines food security in the following terms: "Food security exists when all people, at all times, have physical, social and economic access to sufficient, safe and nutritious food which meets their dietary needs and food preferences for an active and healthy life."[3]

This is a deeply insightful definition, and should not be simplified. Food security has often been conceived merely in terms of having sufficient food. Nutrition and safety – critical components of that definition – are often afterthoughts, and in some instances are simply forgotten. The decoupling of food safety and food security is sometimes so overt that terminology such as "nutrition security" has emerged, perhaps in an attempt to compensate for the lack of focus on anything more than the sufficiency aspect of food security. Yet all the elements of food security, including safety, must be addressed simultaneously in order to achieve the goal implicit in the FAO definition.

Food safety: the global impact

The latest data from the World Health Organization (WHO) suggests that each year, foodborne illnesses cause almost one in 10 people on the planet to fall ill (**Figure 1**). Some 420,000 deaths a year are believed to result from foodborne illnesses, a significant proportion of these in children less than five years old.[4] Contaminated food causes some 230,000 diarrheal deaths a year; this is the best estimate of the global impact of foodborne illness that we have yet seen, and represents a heroic effort on the part of the WHO, having required 10 years to compile. This figure may nevertheless still be an underestimate.

The US Centers for Disease Control and Prevention (CDC) report from 2011, which focused on the United States, and attempted to compensate for the under-reporting inherent in the data, estimated that one in six people in the US is a victim of foodborne illness, with 3,000 related deaths each year.[5] If we were to simply extrapolate the CDC data to the globe, that would suggest that approximately a billion people suffer from some variety of foodborne illness each year. Obtaining a clear view of the global impacts of unsafe food is a very complex undertaking. What is clear, however, is that even the latest data are likely to be an underestimate.

The food safety landscape: then and now

Understanding our progress in the management of foodborne disease depends on having the prerequisite baseline surveillance data. Few countries routinely collect such data, and such data as are available depend on affected individuals coming forward for treatment and being correctly diagnosed. Even the most advanced medical systems struggle to obtain consistent and comparative data, especially data that permit the identification of trends over past decades. Nevertheless, some devastating outbreaks have been well documented.

The headlines 20 years ago

One of the deadliest Salmonella outbreaks in American history occurred in 1985 in Chicago, USA, as a direct result of tainted milk produced at Hillfarm Dairy (operated by that city's Jewel Companies Inc.). At least 16,000 cases of *Salmonella enterica serovar Typhimurium* were documented, but the outbreak is estimated to have affected between 150,000 and 250,000 people in total; it caused nine deaths.[6]

In 1985, an outbreak of Listeriosis in Los Angeles County led to the deaths of pregnant women and babies. Contaminated Mexican-style fresh cheeses resulted in the deaths of 28 people, including 10 newborns and 18 adults. There were also 20 miscarriages.[7]

Figure 1 | **WHO Estimates of the global burden of foodborne diseases. 2015**

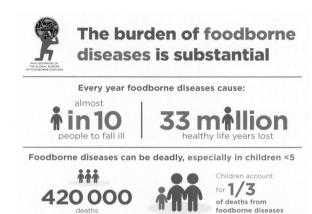

Source: WHO Estimates of the Global Burden of Foodborne Diseases. 2015.

In 1988 in the UK, the presence of *Salmonella enterica serovar Enteritidis pt4c* in eggs hit the headlines. This type of Salmonella was a new issue, and due to a change in its pathogenicity, it actually managed to penetrate hens' ovaries, allowing Salmonella to get inside the egg for the first time.[8]

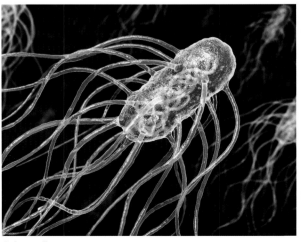

Salmonella.
Source: SDAVID MACK/Science Photo Library/Getty Images

A number of high-profile food safety outbreaks occurred in the 1990s linked to a range of foods, including smoked mussels (1992; New Zealand); "rillettes" or potted pork (1993, France); pasteurized chocolate milk (1994, USA); raw milk soft cheese (1995, France); frankfurters (1998–99, USA); and butter (1998-9, Finland) to name a but few.[9]

In 1993 an outbreak of E. coli O157, a new serotype in the USA, caused 700 people to fall sick. Four children died. Hamburgers from the fast-food chain Jack in the Box were thought to be the cause.[10]

A previously unknown variant of Creutzfeldt-Jakob (new version Creutzfeldt-Jakob, nvCJD) rocked the world in 1996.[11] NvCJD was attributed to the consumption of meat contaminated with scrapie, a prion disease of sheep. With it came the discovery that the disease had jumped species and was causing Bovine Spongiform Encephalopathy (BSE), or "mad cow disease," as it became commonly known. BSE wreaked havoc on agricultural exports, and led to the rapid implementation of new traceability systems and the practice of removing high-risk materials from the food and feed supply chain. Improvements across the industry often result from a devastating failure or event. This is clearly an inefficient, and somewhat tragic, approach to progress.

The recent past

An incident in 2004, originally believed to be due to mycotoxin contamination and affecting an estimated 6,000 dogs in Asia, was later found to be the result of melamine adulteration. It took years to understand exactly what had happened and why, but these incidents highlighted the risk of the tangible impact of an "unknown," a new hazard, forcing a revision of food safety globally.[12]

In 2007 the chemical melamine was detected in pet food in North America, causing kidney failure in thousands of dogs and cats. The tragic impact of melamine poisoning on humans was revealed in the Chinese milk scandal of 2008, in which milk, infant formula and other food materials were commercially adulterated with melamine. An estimated 300,000 individuals developed kidney stones and suffered kidney damage. Six infants died, and an estimated 54,000 babies were hospitalized.[13]

In 2014 the use of gutter oil in food was linked to pastries sold in Hong Kong in stores including Maxim's Cakes, 7-Eleven and Starbucks. Gutter oil is oil extracted from a variety of waste streams such as food waste, offal from slaughterhouses and the by-products of leather processing plants.[14]

The months immediately prior to the drafting of this chapter were marred by significant food safety issues. Blue Bell Creamery, a US purveyor of ice cream for over 100 years, experienced Listeria contamination in 2015, resulting in 10 reported cases, with three deaths. Despite suspending manufacturing in two facilities for several months, Blue Bell Creamery continued to experience issues in other facilities and was reportedly unable to identify the sources of the contamination.[15]

Again in 2015, Chipotle Mexican Grill – a US fast food business which positioned its offering as natural, transparent and simple recipes – experienced multiple food safety issues, including outbreaks of illness due to Shiga toxin-producing Escherichia coli 026 and Norovirus. The crisis led to the closure of over 40 restaurants in the American Northwest for an extended period.[16] Hundreds of people fell ill in California and the Southwest, and an outbreak at a college campus in Boston prompted regulators and the Justice Department to subpoena the company in order to understand its food safety protocols. Following the crisis, Chipotle stated that they intend to become a leader in food safety, closing all their restaurants for a day in order to conduct extended food safety training.

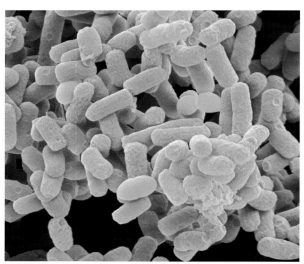

Colored scanning electron micrograph (SEM) of Escherichia coli bacteria (pink). A few cocci bacteria (yellow) are also present. Magnification: x40,000 when printed at 10 centimeters wide.
Source: Science Photo Library – Steve Gschmeissner / Getty Images

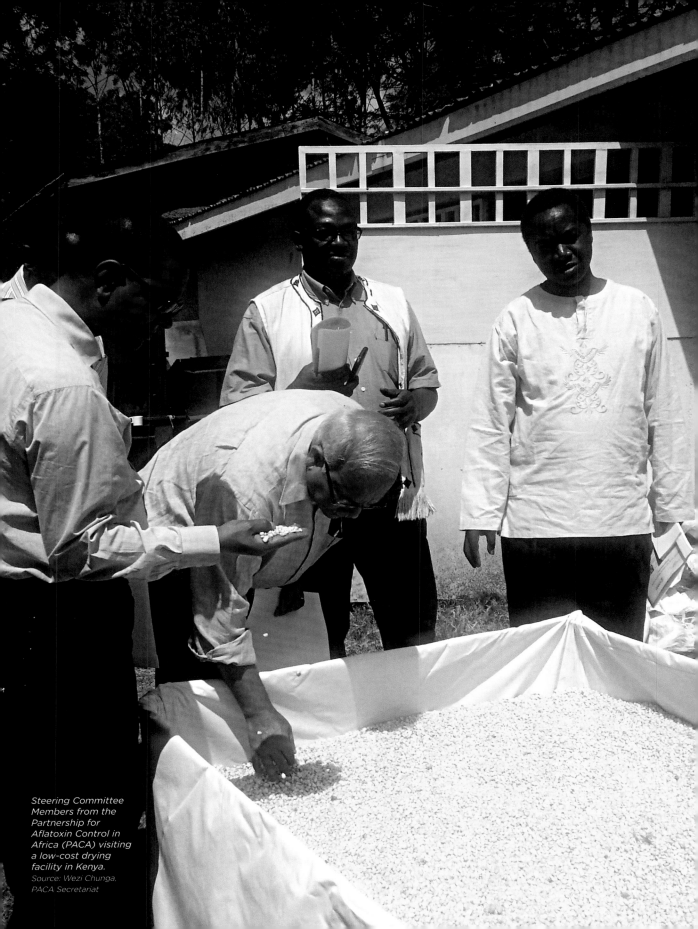

Steering Committee Members from the Partnership for Aflatoxin Control in Africa (PACA) visiting a low-cost drying facility in Kenya.
Source: Wezi Chunga.
PACA Secretariat

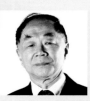

Dr Junshi Chen

Chief Adviser, China National Center for Food Safety Risk Assessment (CFSA)

Food safety in China

Over the past 30 years, China – as a developing country with a large population and considerable geographical heterogeneity – has experienced rapid progress, eliminating food shortages and rendering hunger a thing of the past. Like many other developing countries, China today experiences the inevitable conflict between traditional, small-scale farms and small food businesses on the one hand and increasingly stringent consumer demands for a safe, high-quality food supply on the other.

Microbial contamination, mycotoxins, heavy metals, pesticide residue, veterinary drug residues and environmental pollutants in foods are the major food safety concerns in China. In addition, food fraud erodes consumer confidence in the food system and challenges the government's ability to control food safety. Food producers, distributors and retailers, as well as the government, all have a responsibility to meet consumer expectations and ensure that food produced and consumed in China is safe. This can only be done by following the risk analysis framework, with the support of all stakeholders.

Aflatoxin contamination offers a good example of food safety challenges in contemporary China. Because small-scale farming still predominates in the country, aflatoxin contamination in corn, milk, nuts and even certain types of tea continues to be a major food safety issue. Moreover, the effects of climate change have made it more difficult to control aflatoxin contamination in agricultural products. The introduction of improved crop production and handling practices and the deployment of appropriate technologies are the prerequisites for bringing aflatoxin contamination in China under control.

Globalization of the food supply: a new level of risk?

For the general public, the impression is one of an increasing number of food safety scares, and new threats on top of old. Not only do food safety threats remain today; the list of hazards that food safety practitioners must manage has continued to grow, and has become more complex. New organisms are adapting, causing illness in the food supply chain, and prompting consumers to question the ability of industry and regulators to cope with these issues. Commercial adulteration, evolving consumer attitudes and increasing pressure from a 24-hour social media environment are all compounding the challenges faced by food manufacturers.

The world increasingly depends on a global supply chain to source key raw materials. Global supply chains are not in themselves new: spices have travelled across the world from Asia for centuries; sugar has been a key export from South America; and cocoa has been distributed worldwide from West Africa. What *has* changed is the volume and pace at which ingredients are traded in response to a growing global demand that now must satisfy consumers in all corners of the world.

The Transnationality Index (TNI), which measures the extent to which companies operate outside their home country borders, shows that food manufacturing became more trans-nationalized over the period 1990–1999. One food and beverage company featured in the top 10 non-financial companies ranked by TNI for the final year of that decade.[17,18] By 2013, the food and beverage companies in the top 10 by TNI had increased from one to three, demonstrating the international scale at which we are operating today and the increased requirements concerning risk management and governance.[19]

The food and beverage industry is one of the most global non-financial business sectors in terms of the number of companies that feature, with eight companies in the top 100 most transnational companies ahead of telecommunications, mining and quarrying, utilities and wholesale trade.

Table 1 | **Number of companies in the top 100 per sector as ranked by TNI in 2013**[19]

Sector	No. of companies in top 100 in 2013
Petroleum	12
Motor vehicles	11
Electrical and electronic equipment	9
Pharmaceuticals	9
Food and beverage	8
Telecommunications	5
Mining and quarrying	5
Utilities (electricity, gas and water)	5
Wholesale trade	5

Source: Based on data from the United Nations Conference on Trade and Development World Investment Report 2014

Figure 2 | **The well-traveled salad**[20]

In a recent analysis of a simple American salad plate, researchers traced the ingredients' origins and generated a surprising picture:

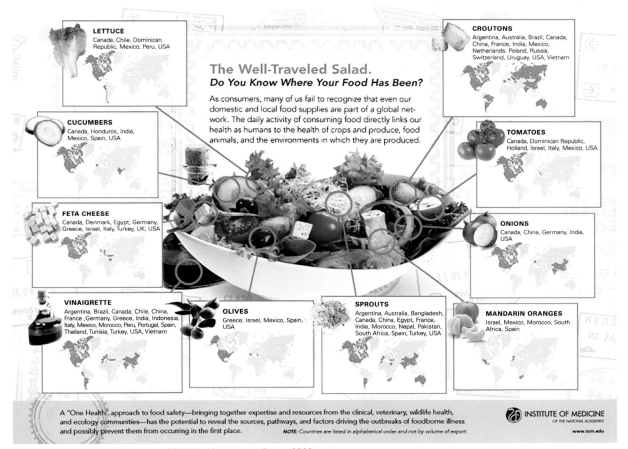

Source: IOM (Institute of Medicine), UNCTAD World Investment Report 2002.
Reprinted with permission from the National Academies Press, Copyright 2002, National Academy of Sciences

Today, many ingredients travel hundreds or even thousands of miles before being consumed. Great concern has been caused by supply from China,[21] although, interestingly, global demand for Chinese raw materials is increasing faster than China's supply to the world.[22]

Food safety incidents are caused by supply from countries with different standards, but while this adds to the complexity of the global food supply, it is not the core issue. Both developed and developing countries experience food safety outbreaks that are domestic in origin, as the CDC data has shown.[5,14,15] The key challenge is that not all food safety management is created equal, and today's global supply chains are being managed to varying levels of food safety capability, often lacking the infrastructure and validation methods necessary to keep pace with the volume

of trade. The food supply chains, globally, are insufficiently robust. The lack of harmonization of food safety management not only makes it difficult for food companies to control risks; it also hinders the development and application of cohesive and standardized global food safety standards and governance – in which business should be a partner. All of this translates into tangible economic costs, which cannot be afforded by most business models, health systems or economies.

Additional burdens on today's already overstretched global food supply systems are food loss and food waste. Not all food produced for human consumption is eaten. FAO estimates that around one third of the food produced in the world every year – approximately 1.3 billion tons – is lost or wasted, with quantitative food losses and waste per year estimated at around 30% for cereals and 40–50% for root crops.[23, 24] These figures do not include the unsafe food that is being consumed: we are probably significantly overestimating the global food supply because the unsafe food is not extracted from the data. And much bigger challenges lie ahead.

According to the FAO: "Over the next four decades, the world's population is forecast to increase by 2 billion people and to exceed 9 billion people by 2050. Recent FAO estimates indicate that to meet the projected demand, global agricultural production will have to increase by 60 percent from its 2005–2007 levels."[25]

To meet this demand, we will have to optimize food supply systems in an unprecedented way. In 2011 Scientific American stated that: "The world must solve three food issues simultaneously. End hunger, double food production by 2050, and do both while drastically reducing agriculture's impact on the environment."[26] Sustainable food production expert Jason Clay states that: "We have to produce as much food in the next 40 years as we have in the last 8,000… And if we want to do it without expanding further into the environment, we're going to have to produce twice as much food on the same amount of land."[27]

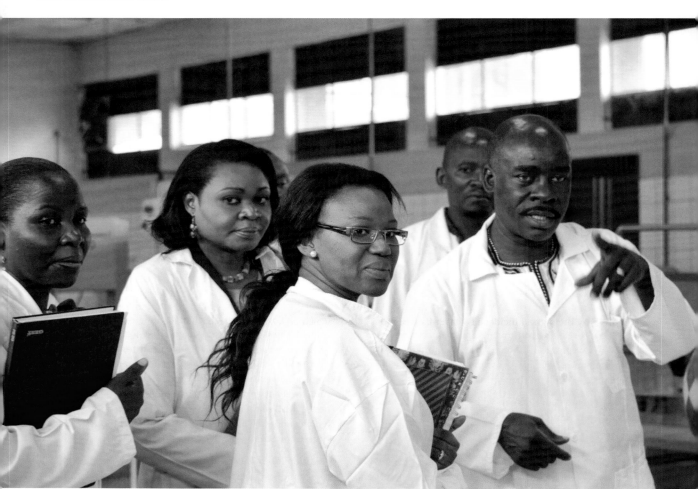

A visit to a PACA-partner lab in Uganda by teams from the African Union (AU) and the New Partnership for Africa's Development (NEPAD), an African Union strategic framework for pan-African socioeconomic development. Food safety is a complex problem, and there is still a long way to go in effectively addressing it on a global scale.
Source: Wezi Chunga, PACA Secretariat

Counting the cost of unsafe food: a focus on aflatoxin

The impact and challenges of aflatoxin perhaps exemplify better than anything else the interplay of food security and food safety.

Aflatoxins are invisible poisons that contaminate many staple food and cash crops (including maize, tree nuts, cassava, millet, peanuts, wheat and a range of spices) and animal feeds. They are produced by the related fungal species *Aspergillus flavus* and *Aspergillus parasiticus*. Aflatoxin contamination can occur throughout value chains, making it difficult to target interventions. Pre-harvest occurrence of aflatoxin increases when crops are subjected to stress factors such as drought and attacks from pests. Post-harvest contamination spikes with poor drying, storage and handling. Aflatoxin is virtually indestructible, since normal food processing practices do not affect aflatoxin levels to any appreciable extent. The aflatoxin problem is so complex that it straddles three sectors: public health, agriculture, and trade.

Health and nutrition impact of aflatoxins

Aflatoxins cause liver cancer in humans.[28] Aflatoxin B₁ is the most potent naturally occurring liver carcinogen so far known. There is an up to 30 times greater risk of acquiring liver cancer from chronic infection with Hepatitis B virus and dietary exposure to aflatoxin as compared to exposure to either of the two factors alone.[29] The number of liver cancer cases continues to increase year by year, with 748,000 new cases and 695,900 deaths from the tumor occurring in 2008, making it third in the world and first in Africa in terms of annual cancer mortality rates. Aflatoxin may play a causative role in 5–28.2% of all global liver cancer cases.[30] Both aflatoxin exposure and chronic Hepatitis B infection predominate in rural Africa, which explains why the highest incidence of liver cancer (40%) occurs in Africa.

In addition, mounting evidence indicates that ingestion of aflatoxin-contaminated food is associated with stunting in children, as well as maternal anemia and mortality. A recent report concluded that the consistency of human epidemiological studies and the mechanistic data in animal models suggest that mycotoxin (the general name for toxins from fungi) exposure contributes to stunting.[28] Aflatoxin exposure is also linked to immune system suppression and increased susceptibility to infectious diseases such as malaria and HIV-AIDS.

Exposure to high levels of aflatoxins is fatal. This is tragically evidenced in outbreaks of acute aflatoxin poisoning, such as the outbreak in Kenya in 2004 that killed 125 people due to consumption of maize contaminated with aflatoxins.[31]

Aflatoxins also affect the volume and value of agricultural output, and can directly impact food and nutrition security. For instance, about 10% of the 2010 Kenyan maize harvest was withdrawn from the food supply in a responsible move taken by the Kenyan government to protect public health.

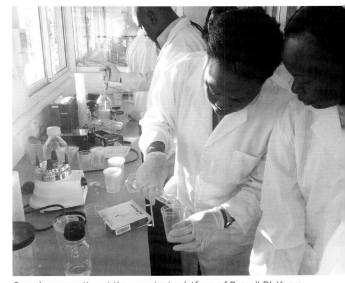

Sample preparation at the mycotoxin platform of Beca-ILRI, Kenya.
Source: Wezi Chunga, PACA Secretariat

Economic impact of aflatoxins

Due to the serious health effects of aflatoxins, legislation around the world limits their presence in food and feed, which adversely affects market access for many developing countries. Related to this, the geographical scope for sourcing a reliable supply of safe, quality raw materials such as groundnut has shrunk in the past four decades because of aflatoxin contamination. Africa could earn up to US$1 billion per year from groundnut exports by regaining the 77% share of the global groundnut export market it enjoyed in the 1960s instead of the current share of 4%, which is valued at just US$64 million. Despite the general decline in the demand for groundnuts for crushing to oil, the demand for edible groundnuts has been steadily increasing globally. The groundnut industry in Africa has been thrown into disarray – partly due to the difficulty of meeting aflatoxin standards and the consequent loss of attractive export markets, and partly due to unfavorable public policies.

The lack of consistency in aflatoxin standards among countries hampers export. Countries are likely to trade with each other if they have similar sanitary and phytosanitary standards (SPS). Moreover, developing countries with weak SPS capacities find it difficult to meet the diverse standards of importing countries. Investment by developing countries in strengthening SPS capacities, and in particular, food safety capacities, needs to be commensurate with the cost of weak capacities in these areas. The costs are: exclusion from export markets with associated lost opportunity for economic development and unacceptably high dietary exposure of local consumers to mycotoxins. Preliminary studies commissioned by the Partnership for Aflatoxin Control in Africa (PACA) reported Disability Adjusted Life Years (DALYs) ranging from 93,639 in the Gambia to 546,000 in Tanzania, with US$94 million to be saved in the Gambia alone if efforts were to be made to reduce aflatoxin exposure.

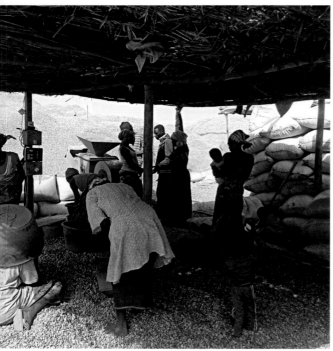

Women shelling groundnuts in Senegal, a PACA partner country. The women and their children are fully exposed to the dust emanating from the groundnut shells, which is laden with fungal spores containing aflatoxins. A bowl and a bag are being used as protective head-coverings.
Source: Winta Sintayehu, PACA Secretariat

Why is aflatoxin a threat to smallholder farmers of Africa?

Aflatoxins are a worldwide problem because of the global movement of affected produce. However, the challenge is more serious in Africa, and the burden on smallholder farmers far more pressing, for a number of reasons (**Figure 4**). First, prevalence of the toxin is higher in Africa and South East Asia. Second, subsistence farmers cannot afford to diversify their diet and are often heavily dependent on high-aflatoxin-risk staple crops such as maize and groundnuts. They consume 70% of what they produce, selling the better-quality produce to generate income. Third, weak policy and organizational support, coupled with limited awareness of the importance of aflatoxin control to public health, aggravate the problem – more so in the case of smallholder farmers.

Figure 3 | **Factors contributing to the serious aflatoxin problem in Africa**

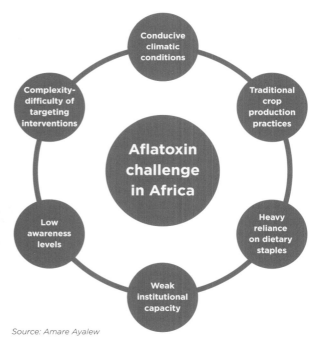

Source: Amare Ayalew

Aflatoxin mitigation

Systemic thinking is called for in order to manage the complex problem of aflatoxin contamination. Possible solutions require multidisciplinary and multistakeholder actions. Effective aflatoxin control relies on: integrating measures aimed at reducing aflatoxin contamination (pre- and post-harvest technology solutions which are suitable for adoption by small-scale farmers and which have the highest potential for impact); minimizing the risk of human or animal exposure in the event that contamination does occur (regulatory solutions); and creating a policy and institutional environment which enables technology solutions and regulation to be effective in abating the aflatoxin problem. Moreover, developing countries should proactively invest in making their agricultural sectors more competitive. Increased productivity and responding to market requirements enables farmers to afford aflatoxin control technologies while improving their food and nutrition security and their market income.

The Partnership for Aflatoxin Control in Africa (PACA) and governments of six pilot countries on the continent (Gambia, Malawi, Nigeria, Senegal, Tanzania and Uganda) generated empirical evidence on the nature and impact of aflatoxin contamination, and developed comprehensive yet feasible Aflatoxin Control National Plans. These plans take the multisectoral approach and aim at empowering consumers and protecting them from the devastating effects of aflatoxins both within Africa and beyond, resulting in economic gains, increased smallholder incomes, enhanced agribusiness, and reduced poverty. The Partnership for Aflatoxin Control in Africa has launched a unique one-stop portal known as Africa Aflatoxin Information Management System to provide comprehensive information ranging from aflatoxin levels in key crops in different countries to testing methods and data on trade volumes, losses and rejections, and aflatoxin-related health impacts. This unique resource will support policy and interventions toward more effective aflatoxin control in agriculture and food systems in Africa. Testing and scaling of pre-harvest (biocontrol) and post-harvest (storage and drying) technologies are being conducted by PACA partners in Africa. Like most food safety burdens, aflatoxin contamination is preventable and manageable.

The critical role of food safety in ensuring global food security

The food safety landscape is more challenging than it was 20 years ago. At the same time, there has been arguably very little progress over the past 20 to 30 years in terms of our ability to ensure safe food. Today, the environments within which food suppliers, producers and manufacturers operate continue to evolve at an ever-increasing rate, with new hazards and pathogens regularly emerging, exacerbated by the globalization of the food supply chain. The added pressures of climate change and population growth compound the problem.

While great strides have been made in data collection – of which the WHO Estimates of Foodborne Diseases report is an excellent example – the lens through which food safety is viewed needs to change. The health and economic impacts of unsafe food continue to cause devastation, especially for those who are already most vulnerable. Aflatoxins are a notable example, with disastrous consequences both medically and economically. However, although the devastating impacts are widely acknowledged, the crops affected are not currently counted as part of food waste estimates, leading to a potentially skewed view. We know that some 30–50% of all food produced is either lost or wasted, as described in chapter 3.4 of this book. At the same time FAO estimates that 4.5 billion people are exposed to aflatoxins annually, many of them having consumed "food" considered unfit for onward distribution. The way we look at unsafe food, and at food waste, must change.

It is clear that we cannot achieve food security unless we tackle food safety on a global scale. The question is, are we doing enough to mitigate threats to the food supply in light of the challenges we face? The answer is no. If we are to tackle these global threats head-on, our approach to food safety management must adapt to the changing environment. We must become better connected, collaborate, and openly share food safety knowledge and expertise. Only through collaboration among all stakeholders will we ensure that the right food safety knowledge, risk management methods and interventions are successfully applied across the global food supply chain.

J B Cordaro

Global Food Security, Nutrition and Safety Consultant, Mars, Incorporated, McLean, VA, USA

How Business Partnerships Can Help Achieve Food Security

The value of business partnerships

Growing awareness of the significant human, economic and social impacts of global food safety problems has led decision-makers to think in new ways in order to increase the likelihood of food security. At the center of this thinking is the recognition that:

1 no single entity can raise the bar to ensure safe food at all times for all people;

2 the private sector possesses tools, capabilities and expertise that can effectively be deployed to foster food safety;

3 food safety is a pre-competitive matter; and

4 multisector, multidisciplinary partnerships and collaborations are required to manage food safety challenges.

The private sector is participating in food safety collaborations, working in close partnership with governments and other stakeholders. These uncommon partnerships have become necessary as public resources for addressing food safety have dwindled.

Events of recent years have demonstrated the need for, and the value of, expanded and inclusive private-sector participation in this area. Three contemporary entities are especially notable for their trailblazing commitment to engage the private sector in pursuit of higher food safety standards. They are: (1) the Global Alliance for Improved Nutrition (GAIN), established in 2002; (2) the UN Committee on World Food Security (CFS), established by the World Food Conference in 1974 and reformed in 2009 to ensure that the voices of many stakeholders, including the private sector, should be heard in policy formulation; and (3) the African Union Commission's Partnership for Aflatoxin Control in Africa (AUC PACA), established in 2012 to eliminate the harmful impacts of aflatoxins.

GAIN, the UN CFS and PACA emphasize the strategic role that the private sector plays in fulfilling their missions.

• With GAIN, the private sector includes local and multinational food companies, especially those producing fortified foods for micronutrient-deficient populations. These companies support country food fortification programs by sharing their technical expertise, including their expertise on food safety and quality.

• With the UN CFS, the Committee's Private Sector Mechanism (PSM) provides the platform for interested businesses to help shape the outcomes of the food security, nutrition and safety discussions and to help formulate recommendations for consideration by member states.

• With PACA, the private sector, international organizations, foundations and other stakeholders seek to deploy resources to manage aflatoxins from farm to fork.

In addition to the leading role exercised by the UN CFS, other parts of the UN System, such as FAO, have increased calls for collaboration with the private sector during the past decade. Under the leadership of UN Secretary General Ban Ki-moon, major events in 2014 and 2015 defined frameworks for global food security, nutrition and safety agendas. These frameworks have specific targets and activities to fulfil the hypothesis that hunger and malnutrition can be ended by 2030. In each of the Secretary General's interrelated, global milestone events, essential roles for the private sector were emphasized:

1 the International Conference on Nutrition (ICN2), with strong participation from business, approved the Rome Declaration – a political statement of the problems and Framework for Action and a technical guide for policy implementation that underscores the essential role of the private sector;

2 the Third Financing for Development Meeting (FfD3) detailed innovative ways to assemble financial, policy, governance and leadership resources for implementation, and called for extensive roles for business and partnerships in mobilizing human and financial resources, expertise, technology and knowledge;

3 the Sustainable Development Goals (SDGs) build on the Millennium Development Goals (MDGs) to transform economic, human and social development by means of 17 goals and 169 targets across food systems, through directives to multistakeholder partnerships;

4 the Climate Change Conference (COP21) forged agreements among countries and obtained commitments from the private sector to stabilize global warming, including actions to address the negative impacts of global warming on agriculture and food production and to partner in finding solutions;

5 the FAO Strategy for Partnerships with the Private Sector recognizes that the fight against hunger – to meet the Zero Hunger Challenge – can only be won if the private sector utilizes its knowledge, data and scientific innovation capabilities to increase sustainable food production, eliminate waste and provide the most vulnerable people with access to food; and

6 the profile of Partnerships, as one of the 5Ps of Agenda 2030, places multistakeholder Partnerships alongside People, Planet, Prosperity and Peace.

The September 2015 UN Private Sector Forum, led by Secretary-General Ban Ki-moon and with a commentary from Bono, illustrated the shift in thinking that has taken place. Bono said: "I'm late to realizing that it's you guys, it's the private sector, it's commerce that's going to take the majority of people out of extreme poverty." He added: "As an activist, I almost found that hard to say."

Linkages among food security, nutrition and safety

Sustainable and resilient global food security systems must be developed to provide consumers regular access to diverse diets with adequate amounts of nutritious foods that are safe and affordable. Each of these components is essential, and no single one is sufficient to overcome food insecurity; however, safety drives the ultimate availability and nutritional values such that without safe food, nutrition insecurity will persist for consumers, especially in Africa. The vision of ending hunger and malnutrition by 2030 will remain unfulfilled unless the challenges of unsafe food are brought under control and solutions are implemented to manage their harmful impacts.

For too long, food safety was viewed as an afterthought to production and nutrition, but now linkages among safety, availability and nutrition are widely recognized, and are generating increasing attention. At the same time, the many safety challenges in food systems – from production to consumption – have been claiming more and more attention, as the present book's chapter on Food Safety by Crean and Ayalew demonstrates.

An example of collaboration: Mars, Incorporated and the Partnership for Aflatoxin Control in Africa (PACA)

Business can responsibly deploy, and strategically leverage, its storehouses of tools, capabilities, knowledge, insights, research, technologies, management tools and expertise for safer, better quality foods. For example, Mars, Incorporated has stepped forward to collaborate in multisector and multidisciplinary ways. Mars cooperates with the UN Committee on World Food Security (UN CFS) to increase awareness of food safety challenges by sponsoring food safety side events. In addition, the Mars Global Food Safety Center (GFSC) was established as the world's first center of excellence to address food safety problems on a pre-competitive basis. The GFSC benefits over 60 other Mars partnerships with UN agencies, universities, and international organizations such as the World Food Programme (WFP); the Food and Agriculture Organization (FAO); the GAIN Business Platform for Nutrition Research (BPNR); and a unique focus on aflatoxins with the Partnership for Aflatoxin Control in Africa (PACA).

Mars and PACA agreed to share food safety resources and expertise to control aflatoxins – the most serious food safety problem in African food crops. To date, the partnership has:

1 facilitated the sharing of research, knowledge, and best practices, and will enhance capability for aflatoxin testing and controls;

2 raised awareness among global policy-makers of aflatoxin issues; and

3 identified opportunities to pilot and implement practical efforts to harmonize food safety management in Africa.

On the signing of the PACA-Mars agreement, H.E. Rhoda Peace Tumusiime, Commissioner for Rural Economy and Agriculture of the African Union Commission, stressed: "The cooperation between the African Union Commission and Mars is in line with our efforts to tackle the complex aflatoxin challenge by working together with a wide array of stakeholders. We value the competencies of the private sector, and particularly the experience of Mars in food safety and quality and the creation of preemptive food safety research platforms, all of which are of direct relevance to aflatoxin control…This Memorandum of Understanding should serve as a launching pad for collaborations to improve food quality and safety standards that eventually benefit millions of small-scale farmers in Africa, who depend on crops such as maize and groundnuts for their income and food."

The value of global food systems will not be defined simply by whether more food is produced, but rather by whether critical food safety deficiencies are more effectively managed from farm to fork so as to provide vulnerable populations sustainable, regular access to nutritious, affordable, safe and wholesome food products. Improving the safety of foods helps ensure that food systems sustain food security, and that better nutrition is available to those who need it, now and in the future.

Our personal view

Dave Crean & Amare Ayalew

Economically developed and developing countries may be vastly different, but they broadly share the same food supply system, and perhaps nothing illustrates this better than the challenges of ensuring the safety of the world's food supply. The classic approaches to food safety whereby stakeholders operate in isolation must be changed: they are not sufficient, and will only become worse in the face of increasing population growth, economic pressure and global warming.

We must establish transparent and rigorous systems and enhance the relationships among farmers, processors, distributors and retailers in all countries. Food safety data today are viewed as a decision-making tool by businesses, but we are missing their true value: they are a public health asset. How can regulators organize and equip themselves to create a system that allows for use of that data, and how can business mobilize to provide that data? Rigorous data and surveillance can become the platform to drive interventions, the interventions that will fix and protect the food supply.

Food safety challenges cannot be addressed by a single entity or discipline. Thus multidisciplinary and multisector partnerships and collaborations are required on a continuous, permanent basis. Without safe food, the world will not achieve global food security and improved nutrition. After all, if it's not safe, it's not food.

References

1   McLinden T, Sargeant JM, Thomas MK et al. Component costs of foodborne illness: A scoping review, BMC Public Health 2014;14;509.

2   Minor T, Lasher A, Klontz K et al. The Per Case and Total Annual Costs of Foodborne Illness in the United States, Risk Analysis 2015;35;1125–39.

3   FAO World Food Summit, 1996.

4   WHO Estimates of the Global Burden of Foodborne Diseases, 2015.

5   US Centers for Disease Control and Prevention (CDC), Estimates of Foodborne Illness in the United States, 2011.

6   Ryan C, Nickels MK, Hargrett-Bean NT et al. Massive Outbreak of Antimicrobial-Resistant Salmonellosis Traced to Pasteurized Milk, JAMA 1987;258;3269–3274

7   Linnan MJ, Mascola L, Lou XD, et al. Epidemic listeriosis associated with Mexican-style cheese. N Engl J Med. 1988;319(13);823–8.

8   Coyle EF, Ribeiro CD, Howard, AJ et al. Escherichia enteritidis phage type 4 infection: association with hens' eggs, The Lancet. 1988;332;1295–1297.

9   Lawley R, Curtis L, Davis J. The Food Safety Hazard Guidebook, 2nd Edition, RSC 2012.

10 Golan E, Roberts T, Salay E, Caswell J, Ollinger M, Moore, D. Food Safety Innovation in the United States: Evidence from the Meat Industry. Agricultural Economic Report No. (AER-831), 2004.

11 Will RG, Ironside JW, Zeidler M, et al. A new variant of Creutzfeldt-Jakob disease in the UK. Lancet. 1996;347;921–925.

12 Brown CA, Jeong KS, Poppenga RH et al. Outbreaks of Renal Failure Associated with Melamine and Cyanuric Acid in Dogs and Cats in 2004 and 2007, J. Veterinary Diagnostic Investigation 2007;19;525–531.

13 Gossner CM, Schlundt J, Embarek PB, et al. The Melamine Incident: Implications for International Food and Feed Safety. Environmental Health Perspectives 2009;117;1803-1808

14 Wee HM, Budiman SD, Su, LC, et al. Responsible supply chain management – an analysis of Taiwanese gutter oil scandal using the theory of constraint. Int J Logist-Res App 2015,1–15.

15 Multistate Outbreak of Listeriosis Linked to Blue Bell Creameries Products (Final Update), Centers for Disease Control and Prevention, June 10, 2015.

16 Multistate Outbreaks of Shiga toxin-producing Escherichia coli O26 Infections Linked to Chipotle Mexican Grill Restaurants (Final Update), Centers for Disease Control and Prevention, February 1, 2016.

17 UNCTAD World Investment Report 2001.

18 UNCTAD World Investment Report 2002.

19 UNCTAD World Investment Report 2014.

20 The Well-Traveled Salad Infographic from Institute of Medicine. Improving Food Safety Through a One Health Approach: Workshop Summary. Washington, DC: The National Academies Press, 2012.

21 Where Does Our Food Come From? Texas A&M Today, January 30, 2014.

22 Wang X, Evans EA, Ballen FH; Overview of US Agricultural Trade with China, FE902, Food and Resource Economics Department, UF/IFAS Extension 2012.

23 Gustavsson J, Cederberg C, Sonesson U et al. Global food losses and food waste, Extent Causes and Prevention. Study conducted for the International Congress SAVE FOOD! at Interpack 2011 Düsseldorf, Germany, Food and Agriculture Organization of the United Nations, Rome, 2011.

24 www.fao.org/save-food; Accessed March 10, 2016.

25 Part 3 Feeding the world, FAO Statistical Yearbook 2013.

26 Foley JA. Can we feed the world and sustain the planet? Scientific American, 2011;305;60–65.

27 Jason Clay: More Food Less Impact, Momentum Magazine, Winter 2012.

28 Some Traditional Herbal Medicines, Some Mycotoxins, Naphthalene and Styrene. IARC Monographs on the Evaluation of Carcinogenic Risks to Humans, IARC Press, Lyon, France 2002;82.

29 Groopman JD, Kensler TW, Wild CP. Protective interventions to prevent aflatoxin-induced carcinogenesis in developing countries. Annu Rev Public Health 2008;29;187–203.

30 Liu Y, Wu F. Global burden of aflatoxin-induced hepatocellular carcinoma: a risk assessment. Environ Health Perspect 2010;118;818–824.

31 Probst C, Njapau H, Cotty PJ. Outbreak of an acute Aflatoxicosis in Kenya in 2004: Identification of the causal agent. Appl Environ Microbiology 2007;73;2762–2764.

Further reading

Buckley N, Albright MK, Daschle TA et al. Public and Private Sector Interventions for Global Food Security, A Report of the Aspen Food Security Strategy Group , March 2016

Pitt JI, Wild CP, Baan RA et al. Improving public health through mycotoxin control. Lyon, France: International Agency for Research on Cancer, IARC Scientific Publications Series, 2012;158

WHO Estimates of the Global Burden of Foodborne Diseases, 2015

Putting the Sustainable Development Goals into Practice

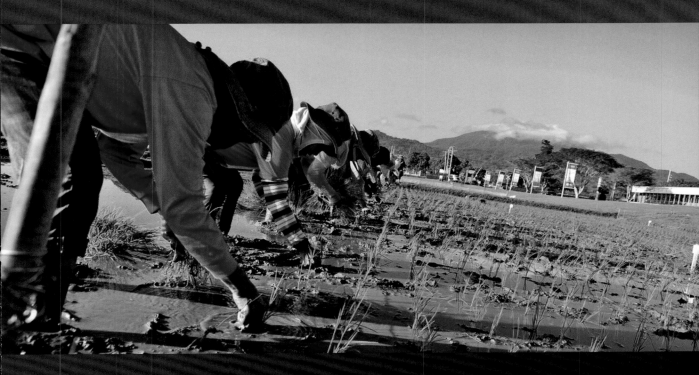

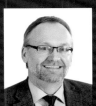

Achim Dobermann
Director & Chief Executive, Rothamsted Research,
Harpenden, Hertfordshire, United Kingdom

"When tillage begins, the other arts follow. The farmers, therefore, are the founders of human civilization."

Daniel Webster (1782–1852), *American senator and statesman.*

Key messages

- The new Sustainable Development Goals (SDGs) and their Targets provide a framework for **all** countries to develop roadmaps for sustainable development in all its dimensions.

- Agriculture contributes to many of the new SDGs and Targets, and therefore needs to receive particular attention.

- SDG 2 on sustainable agriculture is among the most challenging goals to achieve. Transformative changes will be required regarding how food is produced, processed and consumed in order to meet multiple needs.

- Agro-food systems in developed, as well as developing, countries need to be managed with greater precision. Many solutions exist, but new ways of working are necessary in order to achieve faster and greater impact.

- Long-term investment in public R&D is required to ensure that ground-breaking innovations continue to be developed and are widely accessible to all farmers, processors and other businesses.

1. The Sustainable Development Goals: Challenges and opportunities

The advent of agriculture was, in many ways, the advent of civilization as we know it. It was also the beginning of the human manipulation of natural systems on a large scale. It is from this transformation, occurring over thousands of years, that many of our modern challenges originate. What is needed to address these challenges is a dramatic change in the way mankind produces, processes, and consumes food and other agricultural products, but within a significantly shorter time frame than ever before. A new sustainable development agenda is called for that will spur rapid progress in developing as well as developed countries, with an even emphasis on social, economic, and environmental issues. We look for an agenda that is transformative and will encourage new ways of thinking and models of development, rather than business as usual. It must be ambitious, and it must inspire people of all ages and at all levels to act.

The 17 Sustainable Development Goals (SDGs) that were endorsed at a historic summit of world leaders in September 2015 provide the overall new framework for all countries to develop roadmaps towards sustainable development in **all** its dimensions.[1] They push the envelope by bringing together a great diversity of interconnected development issues. The SDGs are the most inclusive agenda the UN has delivered to date, with millions of people submitting input from around the globe and the Targets and Indicators applying in their entirety to all countries.

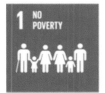 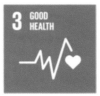 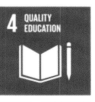
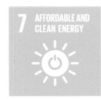 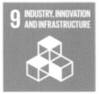
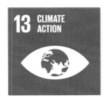   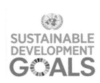

The new SDG 2 (Zero Hunger) on achieving food and nutrition security through sustainable agriculture is the most complex of all of the SDGs. Sustainable agriculture means at least six very different things:

- Agriculture that offers a viable income and livelihood for farmers and business along the whole value chain in any country.

- Agriculture that provides nutritious foods for the entire world population, including the right mix of grains, legumes, vegetables, fruits, nuts, livestock and fish products to ensure adequate supply of energy, protein (with essential amino acids), micronutrients, omega-3 fatty acids, etc.

- Agriculture that will be resilient to future climate change.

- Agriculture that comprehensively reduces greenhouse gas emissions from energy use, deforestation, methane and nitrous oxide.

- Agriculture that reduces other environmental depredations (loss of biodiversity, invasive species, freshwater depletion, soil degradation, destruction of habitat, chemical pollutants from pesticides and herbicides, etc.)

- Agriculture that sustains local cultures, cuisines, etc.

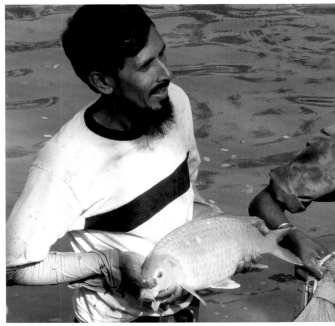

Aquaculture is an integral component of farming systems in Bangladesh, generating extra income and contributing to better nutrition. Source: Achim Dobermann

Agriculture is the central contributor to food security, food quality and dietary diversity, and also to many improvements in nutrition. Investments made in agriculture, along with other sectors in rural societies, can be a key growth engine. Such investments are therefore also central to sustainable development, particularly in low-income settings. Although not always the case, economic growth within poor communities can have beneficial direct and indirect impacts on food and nutrition security through various pathways. Some observers therefore argue that agricultural growth is a precondition for broader growth. Recent evidence has also shown more clearly that household agricultural production has direct and important linkages with dietary patterns and nutrition, and that these are difficult to achieve and sustain through many alternative interventions.

In the coming decades, we need to see a truly transformative change, a Sustainable Agricultural Intensification (SAI). In essence, SAI means producing more food and other agricultural products on the same amount of land, while also using natural resources efficiently and preventing their degradation. As the world population grows, we will need to produce a greater volume of food, as well as more nutritious food, and we will also need to explore new opportunities for how agriculture can help grow the bio-economy as a whole. We also need to limit the expansion of agriculture into forests, wetlands, and grasslands, and to halt the loss of farmland to urbanization. We cannot continue current practices of over-using inputs such as water and pesticides, and must reverse soil degradation and make agriculture more resilient to climate shocks. We need to ensure that future generations of farmers will be able to carry out their fundamental role of feeding humanity, while also supporting their own families and communities. For this, all farmers need to be enabled to be part of a virtuous circle of highly productive agriculture (**Figure 1**).

Figure 1 | **Enhancing food system productivity and value is the entry point for enabling farmers to take their place within a virtuous circle of sustainable agricultural production and livelihood**

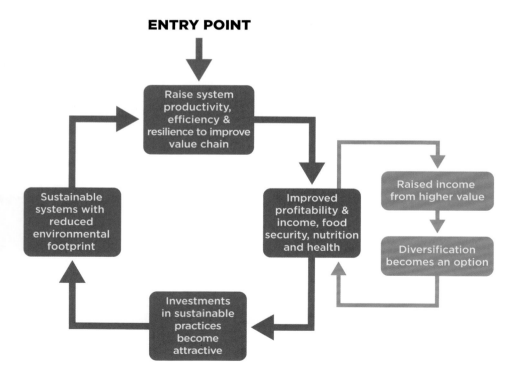

Source: Dobermann A, Nelson R, Beever D et al. 2013. Solutions for sustainableagriculture and food systems. Technical report for the post-2015 development agenda.Sustainable Development Solutions Network (SDSN), New York. http://unsdsn.org/resources/

2. Solutions available for action

Achieving such a transformation of agriculture and food systems on a global, regional and national scale is a massive challenge because of the huge diversity of agriculture. It will require a menu of solutions, as well as good choices that are tailored to the specific environmental and socioeconomic conditions. Farming systems are complex and highly heterogeneous at all scales, from regional and national to village or farm. So too are farming objectives, solutions and tradeoffs. Strategies for Sustainable Agricultural Intensification must provide viable options for farms that can produce substantial surpluses as well as for small farms that support the livelihood of millions of rural people. The specific policies and technology solutions for implementing SAI depend on the socioeconomic and biophysical contexts under which farmers operate, with resource endowment and market access being two main drivers across different scales in any country (**Figure 2**).

The real new challenge is to move to better business models by choice. At the core of devising solutions for this lies a thorough understanding of the socioeconomic and biophysical factors that drive the needs of farmers, agribusinesses, small entrepreneurs, consumers, and many other actors. Solutions need to be flexible in terms of offering a suite of technologies and support systems provided by different sectors in a complementary mode, with a particular emphasis on business-driven models.

All farmers need help in obtaining good access to inputs, markets, information and other supporting services. Strategies that provide the necessary support base, as well as timely market information, will lower the barriers for participating in domestic and export markets.

Governments, civil society, the private sector and international agencies must work together with local extension services and farmers to support the tailoring of SAI solutions to the needs of farmers by:

- Understanding the context in which an effort or an intervention will be implemented, and also understanding its links to the best available scientific and local knowledge

- Identifying the right economic, social and ecological principles of relevance to farmers' needs

- Empowering local communities to improve the performance of the farming system or value chain based on scientific principles as well as local preferences

- Expanding the scope of the effort or intervention and creating the necessary value chains, services, support systems and self-sustained business models

- Monitoring and documenting the performance, as well as lessons learned, in order to enrich the local, national and global knowledge base and thus support further implementation.

Figure 2 | **Resource endowment and access to markets are key determinants for tailoring different solutions to the local context in order to overcome current constraints and establish better business models for agriculture.**

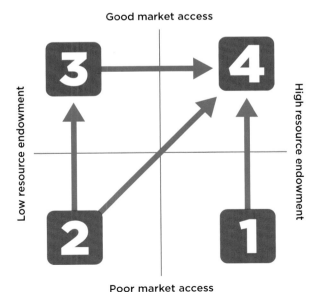

Good market access

Low resource endowment

High resource endowment

Poor market access

Source: Dobermann A, Nelson R, Beever D et al. 2013. Solutions forsustainable agriculture and food systems. Technical report for thepost-2015 development agenda. Sustainable Development Solutions Network(SDSN), New York. http://unsdsn.org/resources/

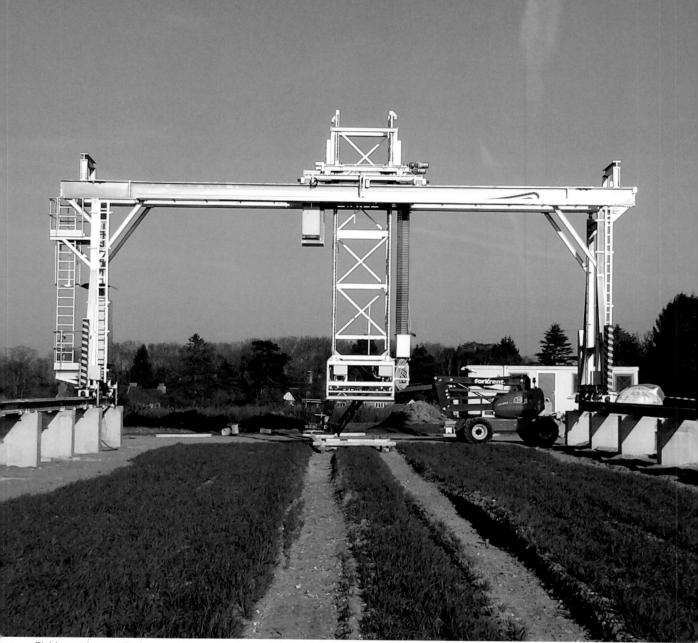

Field scanalyzer at Rothamsted Research – the world's first fully automated field facility for measuring crop growth and health.
Source: Achim Dobermann

3. Solutions for early action

Practical solutions for transforming world agriculture need to address innovation, markets, people, and political leadership, and they also need to enable concrete action for change. Sharp focus must remain on solutions for reducing poverty and improving the livelihoods of rural households and communities, including more resilient crop and livestock systems that can stand extreme heat, drought, floods and other climatic extremes. Small farmers, service providers, processors, marketers and other local entrepreneurs must be central to any investment and policy strategy that enables the development and widespread adoption of new solutions.[3,4]

An important way to solve problems is through practical initiatives involving new technologies, business models, institutional mechanisms and/or policies that are promising, can take place in any country, and can also generate learning elsewhere. They need to address various components of Sustainable Agriculture Intensification and its enabling systems, but many are connected and must be integral parts of a systematic approach to SAI, from creating sustained change, to food production and consumption (Box 1).

Box 1 | Ten key actions for improving nutrient use efficiency in food systems.

Improving the full-chain Nutrient Use Efficiency (NUE) of nitrogen and phosphorus, defined as the ratio of nutrients in final products to new nutrient inputs, is a central element in meeting the challenge to produce more food and energy with less pollution and better use of available nutrient resources.

Nutrient flow is a cycle from resources through stages of use (blue arrows) and recycling (green arrows). The system is driven by the 'motors' of human consumption (red), which are thus also a key part of the solutions needed for achieving future nutrient targets.

The poorest need to be allowed to increase their food and other nutrient consumption, while the richest must realize that it is not in their own interest to over-consume. There are significant differences in the cycles of nitrogen, phosphorus or other nutrients and in the current status of nutrient use among and within countries that need to be taken into account for determining specific targets and

interventions. Hence, the targets for nutrient use and NUE will vary among countries, and so will the pathways for achieving them by addressing any of the specific components of the full-chain NUE relative to their current state.

Possible actions include (numbers in the graph): 1 Improve NUE in crop production; 2 Improve NUE in animal production; 3 Increase the fertilizer equivalence value of animal manure; 4 Low-emission combustion and energy-efficient systems; 5 Develop NOx capture and utilization technology; 6 Improve efficiency in fertilizer and food supply and reduce food waste; 7 Recycle N and P from waste water systems; 8 Energy and transport saving; 9 Lower personal consumption of animal protein and 10 Spatial and temporal optimization of nutrient flows.

Of the 10 solutions proposed, the first three are directly related to agricultural systems management. Specific targets and indicators can be defined for each of these steps.

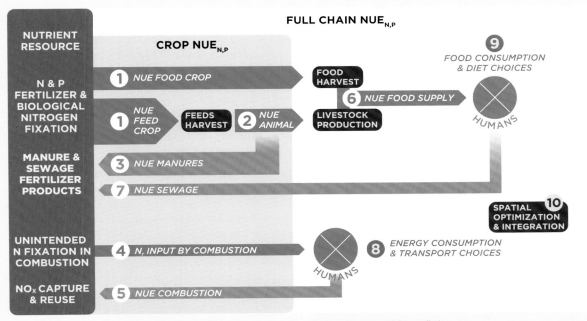

Source: Sutton, M.A. et al. Our nutrient world: the challenge to produce more food and energy with less pollution. (Center for Ecology and Hydrology, Global Partnership on Nutrient Management, INI, Edinburgh, 2012).

Below we provide a few illustrative examples of solutions for early action, i.e., interventions that could be of high priority for many countries in the coming five to 15 years. The examples shown would all make major contributions to SDG 2, but also to various other SDGs. They are a basket of options for countries to consider and adapt to their specific needs. Many more exist and should be pursued.

3(a) New, more productive crop varieties

Crop yield growth rates in many farms remain too low, and farmers often experience periods of food or income insecurity due to yield losses caused by abiotic and biotic stresses. Every farmer should have access to affordable, quality seed from a wide range of well-adapted crop varieties or hybrids via government, private-sector and community seed systems. Enhanced breeding methods such as marker-assisted precision breeding or genetic engineering through genome editing can be deployed to speed up the rate of genetic gain, shorten the time it takes to develop new varieties, and breed new varieties more precisely for specific environments and market segments, thus better meeting farmers' needs.[5,6]

3(b) More nutritious food crops

A few staple food crops dominate the food supply of two billion people suffering from hidden hunger caused by deficiencies in iron, zinc, vitamin A and other micronutrients. Achieving better nutritional balance involves a wide range of measures, diversification of

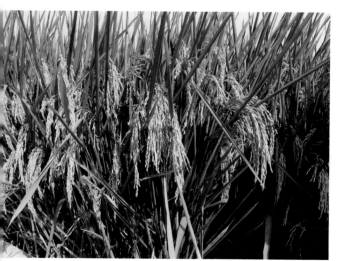

New super rice cultivars have been bred in China to accelerate yield growth.
Source: Achim Dobermann

agricultural systems (crops, livestock and fish products), external mineral and vitamin supply, optimal feeding and caring practices, the breeding of more nutritious crops, agronomic biofortification, and other measures.[7] The promotion of home gardens or livestock and fish are limited in their ability to reach all of the poor; many poor people do not even have the land or other resources to grow their own more nutritious food. While the health benefits of a balanced diet are clear, biofortification is another effective strategy for overcoming specific nutritional deficiencies within rural populations in developing countries. Advances in crop genetics will also enable the growing of crops with health benefits for consumers in higher-income segments. This will help address problems such as the spread of type 2 diabetes, overweight and obesity through interventions such as the development of grains high in resistant starch or soluble fiber.

3(c) New models for agricultural extension

Many unexploited gaps in income, productivity and resource efficiency can be closed by accelerating the transfer of new knowledge and technologies, enhancing farmers' access to markets and information, facilitating better interaction among farmers and knowledge providers, and assisting farmers and small businesses in developing their own technical, organizational and management skills and practices. This is the essence of good agricultural extension, and it has been the driving force for productivity enhancements in the most successful countries.[8]

3(d) Nutrient management and stewardship – from science to local solutions

Improving nutrient management is a central element in meeting the challenge to increase food production, increase farm incomes, improve soil quality, reduce nutrient losses to the environment, and protect natural ecosystems. Both governments and businesses play an important role in this process. Science-based principles for the integrated, site-specific use of fertilizers, organic materials and other nutrient sources have been developed through research. The site-specific nutrient management of crops such as rice, wheat and maize has demonstrated significant benefits in terms of yield, farm profit, increased nitrogen use efficiency, and better nutrient balances.[9] Countries, businesses and international donors should invest in initiatives that seek to systematically improve nutrient management for increased crop production, sustainability and associated benefits.

3(e) Micro-irrigation for smallholder farmers

Many smallholder farms in Sub-Saharan Africa, Asia, and other regions are trapped in poverty, and experience periods of food insecurity due to low cropping intensity and productivity caused by water stress. Irrigation is a key entry point for doubling or tripling crop yields and enabling diversification of cropping systems. Large-scale irrigation systems are capital-intensive and are restricted to lowland areas with suitable conditions. Solar-powered drip or other micro-irrigation technologies, on the other hand, can be customized to meet the needs of small farmers operating in diverse environments with limited capital. Micro-irrigation systems precisely deliver water, nutrients and other inputs directly to the root zone, resulting in high yields and high efficiency of these inputs. Equipped with additional filters, these systems can also supply clean drinking water. Smart-metered, local solar and wind power utility models can provide the electricity needed for irrigation pumps, as well as local households, schools, and small village enterprises, including processing or storing of food.

3(f) New livestock vaccines

Medical and veterinary vaccines inventions are among the most cost-effective disease control interventions ever deployed. They have enabled the global eradication of two lethal diseases: smallpox in humans (1979) and rinderpest in cattle and wild ungulates (2011). Vaccines against livestock diseases have the power to reduce livestock mortality, sustainably increase productivity, increase food and nutritional security,

enhance the livelihoods of the poor, and help developing economies to grow. Extensive quarantine, diagnosis and slaughter of livestock are not sustainable disease control options in developing countries. Diseases of tropical origin are now threatening developed countries. Despite the importance of vaccines, many of the diseases that affect livestock in developing countries are neglected. In countries with a highly industrialized livestock production system, the management of animal health through a variety of interventions is required, thus reducing the dependence on antibiotics and the concomitant build-up of antimicrobial resistance.

3(g) Sustainable grazing – livestock systems

The increasing consumption of animal protein is generally considered at odds with the Earth's ability to feed its people. The 1 billion tonnes of wheat, barley, oats, rye, maize (corn), sorghum and millet poured annually into livestock troughs could feed some 3.5 billion humans. But such reasoning discounts the health benefits of eating modest amounts of animal-source foods and the fact that foraging animals can consume foods that humans cannot eat. A key solution lies in more productive, more sustainable livestock-grazing systems, which can be achieved through (i) improving pastures and feeding animals less human food, (ii) raising regionally appropriate animals, (iii) keeping animals healthy, (iv) adopting smart supplements, (v) eating quality not quantity, (vi) tailoring practices to local culture, (vii) tracking costs and benefits, and (vii) studying and exchanging best practice.[10]

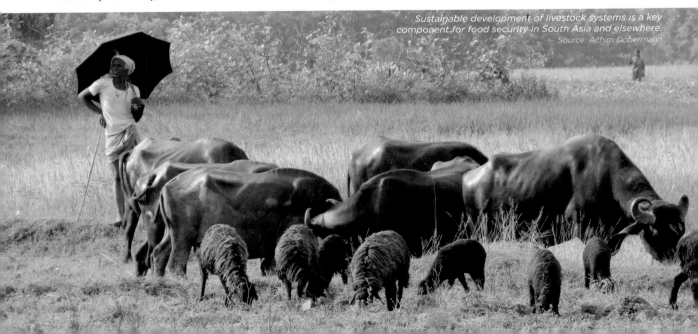

Sustainable development of livestock systems is a key component for food security in South Asia and elsewhere.
Source: Achim Dobermann

Case Study

"Clean Cow" technology

Cows digest their food in four-part stomachs, including a "rumen," which is a site that allows for fermentation – a process that gives off a lot of carbon dioxide and methane gas, since microorganisms assist the process of digestion. Approximately 132 to 264 gallons of ruminal gas are belched daily by every cow on the planet, according to the Penn State College of Agricultural Sciences. Overall, the livestock supply chain emits 44% of the globe's human-induced methane, according to the UN's Food and Agriculture Organization – and a large slice of that comes from methane burps emanating from cattle.

One fundamental way of fixing the problem involves trying to change the chemistry of what's happening in cows' rumens. For some time now, the Dutch Life Sciences and Material Sciences company DSM has been pursuing such a solution, which it appropriately calls its "Clean Cow" project. The company has created a powder that can be added to cow feed that, it says, can produce "a reduction of over 30% in methane emissions with no negative impact on animal welfare, performance, or the amount of feed the animals consume."

DSM worked with a top dairy sciences researcher who focuses on methane emissions, Alexander Hristov of Penn State University, in order to study the clean cow. Hristov and colleagues, including several researchers from DSM, designed and carried out a trial in which 48 cows, receiving varying amounts of the inhibitor in their feed, were observed over 12 weeks. Their methane emissions were measured when they put their heads into feeding chambers which also had atmospheric measurement sensors, and also through nostril tubes attached to canisters on the backs of the cows.

The result was that the inhibitor "decreased methane emissions from high-producing dairy cows by 30%," the research found. The substance "blocks one of the steps of the enzymatic process that produces methane from carbon dioxide and hydrogen," explains Hristov. And he notes that in that process, energy is actually being lost in the form of methane. So with less methane generated, Hristov says, the cow has more energy that can instead be converted to growth and milk production.

Adapted from: Mooney C. Meet the "clean cow" technology that could help fight climate change. Washington Post, July 31, 2015.

3(h) Climate-smart agriculture

Climate-smart agriculture is not a single, specific agricultural technology or practice that can be universally applied. It is an approach that requires site-specific assessments in order to identify suitable agricultural technologies and practices that aim to increase productivity in an environmentally and socially sustainable way, strengthen farmers' resilience to climate change, and reduce agriculture's contribution to climate change by reducing GHG emissions and sequestering more carbon.[11] Typical climate-smart agriculture investment areas include:

- implementation of sustainable land management practices;
- climate risk management; and
- transformation of whole production systems.

3(i) Smart crop protection

As cropping systems intensify, the potential for losses due to insects, diseases and weeds will grow if it is not actively managed. Moreover, levels of resistance to currently available chemicals for insect, disease or weed control have been increasing dramatically in recent years, making it more and more difficult to achieve cost-effective control. This problem may be further exacerbated by climate change and increased climate variability, which could favor the rapid buildup of pest and disease populations. Pest risk will be compounded by increased movement of humans, food and natural products among countries. Over the past four decades, integrated pest management has emerged as a widely accepted approach to manage pests using host plant resistance combined with cultural, biological and chemical control methods. New solutions for next-generation crop protection require the integration of real-time surveillance and forecasting systems with agronomic, genetic and chemical control measures, including new, safer and more durable modes of action. Science is advancing fast in this direction.

The Long-Term Continuous Cropping Experiment (LTCCE) recently marked its 150th rice cropping season. It measures trends in yield and soil properties over its lifetime as indicators of the sustainability of continuous rice cropping on flooded soil. Source: Achim Dobermann

3(j) Innovative smallholder technologies to increase crop value, reduce post-harvest losses, and improve food safety

Because farmers are often unable to dry, store and process their produce, losses are high and there is widespread contamination of foodstuffs with microbes and mycotoxins. For example, most vegetables and high-value food crops are at peak quality at harvest but start to deteriorate soon afterwards. Moisture depletion and physical damage during harvest, packing, storage and transportation causes losses of 20–80%.[12] The loss of produce volume and the losses in nutritional content and quality mean that consumers pay more for products which are less beneficial to their nutritional security. Reducing post-harvest losses of these products will increase the incomes of the producers and the availability of micronutrients for all.

3(k) New business models for smallholder farming and marketing

Where structural transformation processes in urban and rural areas proceed fast, traditional smallholder farming will increasingly be supplemented by, or replaced with, the outsourcing of farming operations, the formation of small and medium-size farmer cooperatives or agribusiness enterprises, and contract farming.[12] Value chains for major agricultural commodities will become more tightly integrated because processors and consumers will demand more information and control over how food is being produced, with supermarket chains playing a particularly important role. For farmers, this

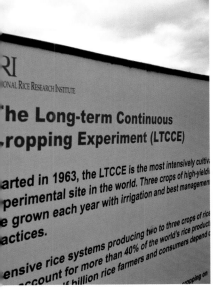

is a chance to connect with rapidly growing domestic and export markets and thus become more direct beneficiaries of competitive food systems. The food industry in particular has increased investments in the direct sourcing of agricultural produce from small farmers worldwide. This trend is expected to continue due to increasing industry and consumer demands for tracing food and meeting certified, as well as non-certified, production standards.

The growth of malls in Nigeria

Delta Mall opened in Warri, Nigeria, last spring, bringing to about a dozen the number of Western-style shopping malls catering to 180 million people in Nigeria, Africa's most populous nation. The emergence of malls – and mall culture – in Nigeria reflects broad trends on the continent, including a growing middle class with spending power and the rapid expansion of cities like Warri that are little known outside the region.

The malls, like the new cars that have replaced the beat-up *tokunbos* (roughly, "used cars") on Nigerian roads, provide visible confirmation that, despite the country's many problems, life has become materially better for many in recent years. Besides shops, the malls have brought leisure activities, like going to the movies and dining at food courts.

Nigeria's population, which is growing and urbanizing at one of the fastest rates in the world, is expected to increase from 180 million to 400 million by 2050, according to projections by the United Nations. That would place Nigeria behind only India and China.

The size of Nigeria's middle class, as well as Africa's, varies according to the definitions used. But many experts agree that Nigeria's size and population growth will drive the expansion of Africa's middle class. Standard Bank, a South African bank with branches across the continent, estimated that Nigeria's middle class grew by 600% from 2000 to 2014. While 4.1 million Nigerian households are now considered middle class, or 11% of the total population, an additional 7.6 million households would make it into that category by 2030, according to the bank's projections.

Informal shops, individually run, are still thriving. Street hawkers sell food, clothes and home appliances on sidewalks, or wherever they can find a captive audience, like Nigeria's epic traffic jams, known as go-slows. The hawkers often compete directly with the malls, selling their wares to people driving into parking lots next to retailers like Game, a discount superstore owned by Walmart.

Adapted from: Onishi N. *Nigeria Goes to the Mall. The New York Times, January 5, 2016.*

3(l) Digital agriculture

Digital technologies will be a key enabler to grapple with the complexity of Sustainable Agriculture Intensification and taking it to scale. Mobile phones, interactive radio, video and internet can enable farmers to access location-specific and timely recommendations that are actionable, but also to contribute to gathering large-scale datasets on the performance of different agricultural options (varieties, planting dates, biological information, etc.) Crowdsourcing can help fill data gaps and thus improve the tailoring of recommendations. Mobile technologies in particular are a vehicle not only to integrate improved varieties, agronomy and policies to support food systems, but also to integrate other key services such as credit, insurance, education and health. Digitally-enabled technologies can drive transparency that in turn supports accountability and ultimately leads to good governance – an essential ingredient for development.

3(m) Promoting integrated landscape management

To successfully address the challenges of food insecurity, persistent poverty, climate change, ecosystem degradation and biodiversity loss, it is critical to move beyond zero-sum strategies that solve one problem but exacerbate others. "Integrated landscape management" aims to realize synergies and reduce trade-offs among these multiple objectives. Farmers and land managers around the world are reaching out across traditional sectoral boundaries to forge partnerships with conservation organizations, local governments, businesses and others to solve problems that are interconnected. More than 107 such initiatives have been documented in Latin America, over 85 in Africa, and an Asian inventory is under way.[13] However, current institutions provide only weak support for these efforts.

3(n) Monitoring the world's agricultural systems

The development of effective monitoring networks is essential to track, anticipate and manage changes in the biophysical, economic, and social aspects of different farming systems around the world.[14] A global agricultural monitoring system should be established as a well-designed and well-directed network of partners engaged in collecting high-quality data required by a wide range of stakeholders. It would provide up-to-date information on the status of agriculture and progress toward meeting the agreed future SDG Targets, including environmental targets affected by agriculture. Simultaneously measuring indicators across SDGs in an integrated monitoring system will allow scientists, land managers and other decision-makers to find solutions to the most pressing problems facing global food security.

4. Investing in long-term change

Foresight is needed to avoid running into another food crisis 20 or 30 years from now. In addition to investing in early solutions or technologies that are likely to become available in the next five to ten years, strategic investments are needed to sustain, and even accelerate, the rate of progress over time. Besides significant private-sector investments, this requires large, stable investments in public-sector research to ensure that ground-breaking innovations continue to be developed and are widely accessible to all farmers and businesses. Open innovation and open access will be needed to achieve broader and faster impact.

There is a need to (i) move from supply-driven to demand-driven agricultural innovation systems that focus on the right priorities, including active participation by key stakeholders, and (ii) simplify the increasing complexity, fragmentation and lack of coordination of agricultural R&D funding that persists in many countries. New, visionary R&D funding models are needed that:

- are founded in strategic long-term thinking;
- have a clear outcome-focus and reward quality science and proven impact;
- enable public-private collaboration in R&D and extension to cover all areas sufficiently and make faster progress;
- encourage open access to information, data and other intellectual property;
- create a viable market for R&D outputs and innovation services;
- enhance cross-border learning, cooperation and technology spillover;
- stimulate more private investments in R&D and direct it to areas of public interest, including attracting new investors such as venture capital and social impact investors;
- systematically improve public R&D infrastructure; and
- build human capital.

Countries should also consider the following general targets:

- Low-income countries and agriculture-based or transition economies, particularly ones with significant food security concerns, should aim to spend at least 10% of their national budgets on accelerating agricultural growth.
- Annual government spending on agricultural research and extension should be at least 1–2% of agricultural

GDP, and should increase by at least 5% per year in low- and medium-income countries.

- All high-income countries should aim to meet the 0.7% of Gross National Income (GNI) target for ODA (Official Development Assistance), and spend at least 10% of their ODA funding on agriculture.

5. Planning and implementing action

Implementation of the new SDGs through targets, indicators, planning and investments should be scalable from local to global levels, and must also be measureable at all levels and scales. The pathways towards more sustainable agriculture and food systems will vary by country as well as within countries, but could follow some common principles.

Planning for success requires a roadmap to realize strategic goals. Action planning needs to be goal-oriented and systematic. National and local governments should apply structured assessment and business planning methodologies to analyze how various solutions could help meet one or more specific targets, and to assess the cost of different options. Researchers must play an important role in guiding that process. A structured assessment typically includes five steps:

1 Background analysis: data collection, past trends and future projections, possible scenarios

2 Analysis of data for problem relevance; definition of key problems/opportunities

3 Assessment of different technology / policy solutions;

4 Estimation of outcomes and effects at scale

5 Modeling of large-scale impact on development goals/targets.

Political will is needed to implement a more coordinated and business-minded approach to development, including behavior change on the part of all participants. One of the major challenges is the alignment of many actors who play different roles in development to ensure strategies are translated into tangible outputs and outcomes to improve food security and nutrition for the rural and urban poor.

One initiative which has shown some success is the development of "Innovation Platforms" to foster linkages between the many players in a given value chain. These "Innovation Platforms" or "Innovation Hubs" bring together the public and private sectors, research and development, and other actors at different places in the value chain to contribute to local innovation and strengthen

links in the chain. Local and national governments are often overwhelmed by disparate programs operating within their borders, but such platforms can give a solid base from which to drive well-coordinated action. The range of relevant organizations includes:

- national governments and local authorities;

- national agricultural research and extension systems;

- universities;

- civil society organizations, including farmers' associations;

- private companies and industry associations;

- sustainable agriculture platforms, think tanks and round tables;

- UN organizations;

- global and regional political bodies and organizations;

- global, regional and national initiatives;

- large business-led initiatives, platforms and development corridors;

- donors, development banks and funds, private foundations, and social/impact investors; and

- international agricultural research centers.

Implementation of the new SDGs through targets, indicators, planning and investments should be scalable from local to global levels, and must also be measurable at all levels and scales. Source: Achim Dobermann

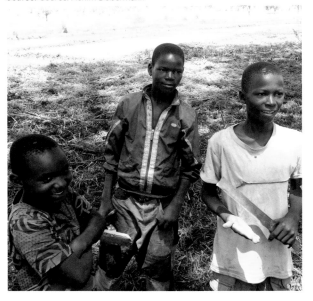

339

My personal view
Achim Dobermann

I have done research on agricultural systems on all continents and in very different political systems. I have visited and worked with well-supported, large commercial growers as well as farmers who have never seen an extension worker in their entire life. I have met many people who are extremely committed to the development of agriculture and nutrition and the protection of the environment. I have never met a farmer who did not care about the quality of the land, the quality and safety of food, or the condition of the environment.

I am convinced that it is possible to feed the growing world population in a sustainable manner, even in a time of climatic changes and extremes. Many of the requisite solutions already exist or could, with wise investments, become available in the next 10–20 years. Early action is good and important, but we also need political will and concrete mechanisms for long-term thinking and action. We need to leave behind national or personal interests as well as unproductive philosophical or ideological debates as to what is right and what is wrong. Instead, let us embrace science and focus on the positive changes that need to be made. We will have to adopt many new ways of working in order to generate new ideas and translate these into real-world impact. Everyone should have that ambition and a role in bringing it about. Only people can make the difference, at all levels.

Further reading

United Nations. *Transforming our world: the 2030 Agenda for Sustainable Development. 2015. https:// sustainabledevelopment.un.org/post2015/ transformingourworld.*

SDSN. *An action agenda for sustainable development. Report for the UN Secretary General. New York: Sustainable Development Solutions Network 2013. http:// unsdsn.org/resources/.*

Dobermann A, Nelson R, Beever D et al. *Solutions for sustainable agriculture and food systems. Technical report for the post-2015 development agenda. New York: Sustainable Development Solutions Network 2013. http:// unsdsn.org/resources/.*

SDSN. *Indicators and a monitoring framework for sustainable development goals: launching a data revolution for the SDGs. New York: Sustainable Development Solutions Network 2015. http://unsdsn.org/resources/ publications/indicators/.*

The Royal Society. *Reaping the benefits: science and sustainable intensification of global agriculture. London: The Royal Society, 2009.*

Bertini C, Glickman D. *Advancing global food security: the power of science, trade, and business. Chicago: The Chicago Council on Global Affairs, 2013.*

References

1   *https://sustainabledevelopment.un.org/post2015/transformingourworld.*

2   *Conway G. One billion hungry: can we feed the world? Ithaca/London: Comstock Publishing Associates, 2012. http://www.cornellpress.cornell.edu/ book/?GCOI=80140100695530*

3   *FAO. The state of food and agriculture. Rome: FAO, 2012. http://www.fao. org/publications/sofa/2012/en.*

4   *Vorley B, Cotula L, Chan M-K. Tipping the balance. Policies to shape agricultural investments and markets in favour of small-scale farmers. Oxford: IIED & Oxfam, 2012. http://www.oxfam.org/sites/www.oxfam. org/files/rr-tipping-balance-agricultural-investments-markets-061212-summ-en.*

5   *Xu Y and Crouch JH Marker-assisted selection in plant breeding: from publications to practice. Crop Sci 2008;48:391-407. https://www.crops.org/ publications/cs/abstracts/48/2/391.*

6   *Jena KK, Mackill DJ Molecular markers and their use in marker-assisted selection in rice. Crop Sci 2008;48:1266–276. https://www.crops.org/ publications/cs/abstracts/48/4/1266.*

7   *Graham RD et al. Nutritious subsistence food systems. Adv Agronomy 2007;92:1–74. http://oar.icrisat.org/4800.*

8   *Labarthe P, Laurent C. Privatization of agricultural extension services in the EU: Towards a lack of adequate knowledge for small-scale farms? Food Policy 2013;38:240–252. http://www.sciencedirect.com/science/article/pii/ S0306919212001054.*

9   *Dobermann A. Et al. Site-specific nutrient management for intensive rice cropping systems in Asia. Field Crops Res 2002;74:37-66. http://www. sciencedirect.com/science/article/pii/S0378429001001976 .*

10 *Eisler MC, Lee MRF, Tarlton JF et al. Steps to sustainable livestock. Nature 2014;507:32–34.*

11 *FAO. Climate-smart agriculture sourcebook. Rome: FAO, 2013. http://www. fao.org/docrep/018/i3325e/i3325e.pdf .*

12 *Reardon T, Timmer CP, Minten B. Supermarket revolution in Asia and emerging development strategies to include small farmers. Proc Natl Acad Sci U S A 2012;109:12332–12337. ttp://www.pnas.org/content/ early/2010/12/01/1003160108.*

13 *Milder JC, Hart, AK, Dobie P et al. Integrated landscape initiatives for African agriculture, development, and conservation: a region-wide assessment. World Development 2014;54:68–80. http://www.sciencedirect. com/science/article/pii/S0305750X13001757.*

14 *Sachs JD et al. Monitoring the world's agriculture. Nature 2010;466:558–560. ftp://ftp.fao.org/agl/agll/docs/wsr.pdf.*

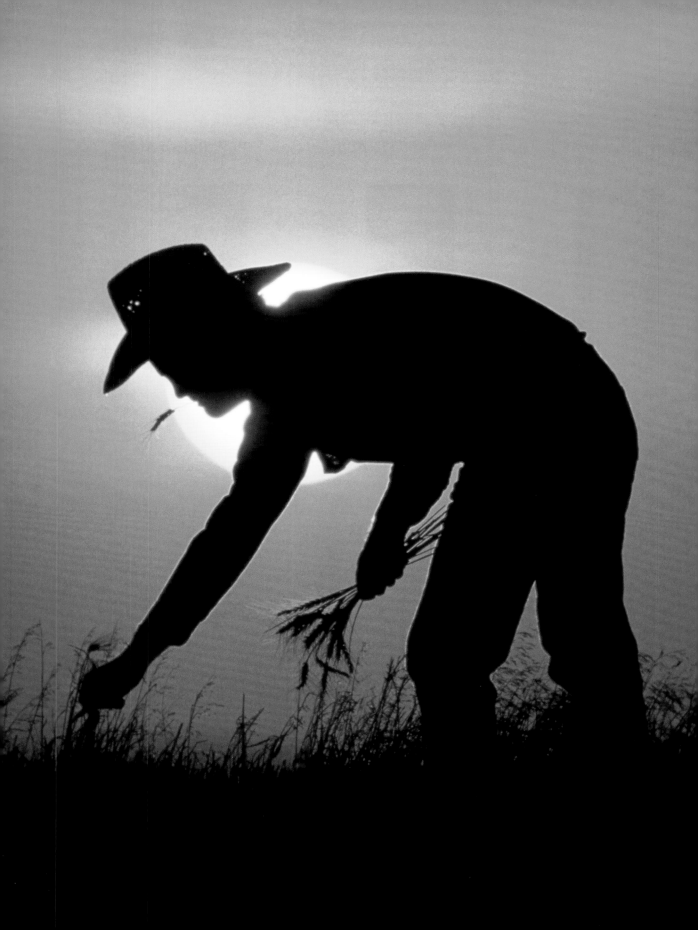

Biographies

Nana Ackatia-Armah

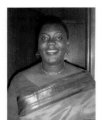

Postdoctoral Fellow, McGill Center for the Convergence of Health and Economics (MCCHE), Desautels Faculty of Management, McGill University, Montreal, Quebec, Canada

Dr Nana Ackatia-Armah is an educational anthropologist, practitioner and evaluation consultant who has worked extensively on topical issues aimed at improving the lives of vulnerable populations – specifically children, young people and women. She has conducted in-depth ethnographic research in which she attempts to understand cultural phenomena from the subject's point of view across multiple disciplines (public health, anthropology, nutrition, sociology, women's studies) and multiple spaces (in schools, on the streets, in post-conflict settings, within communities, and at health centers) in several contexts: Ghana, Sudan, Kenya, India, the United States and Canada. Dr Ackatia-Armah has worked on UN-funded research aimed at evaluating, as well as influencing, national policy on gender equality and equity in national governance. She has also led program design workshops and conducted evaluations for several organizations including World Vision International, Womankind Worldwide, and American Jewish World Services. She is a post-doctoral scholar at McGill University, Montreal, Quebec, Canada.

Nii Antiaye Addy

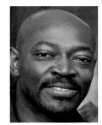

Assistant Professor (Research), Desautels Faculty of Management, McGill Center for the Convergence of Health and Economics, McGill University, Montreal, Quebec, Canada

Dr Nii Antiaye Addy works on partnerships spanning the social economy, the private sector, and the public sector. His areas of expertise include strategy and policy formulation, implementation and evaluation in cross-sector partnerships, with applications in public health, nutrition, and education. His research combines qualitative and quantitative approaches. His recent research and teaching focus on how social innovation emerges from interactions between the beliefs and knowledge of functionally diverse decision-makers in partnerships, and the institutional contexts within which they are embedded. His projects include a study of knowledge-sharing processes in cross-sector food partnerships that are promoting healthy eating behaviors in Quebec. Dr Addy has worked as a consultant and researcher for a number of organizations, including the World Bank, the Hewlett Foundation, Mathematica Policy Research, Inc., and ICF International. He has extensive interdisciplinary experience across multiple contexts, including Ghana, Botswana, South Africa, Madagascar, Guinea, Canada, and the United States.

Prof. Robyn Alders, AO

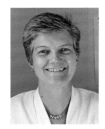

Associate Professor and Principal Research Fellow with the Faculty of Veterinary Science within the University of Sydney, Australia

For over 20 years, Dr Robyn Alders has collaborated closely with smallholder farmers in subsaharan Africa and south-east Asia as a veterinarian, researcher and colleague, working in support of food security and poverty alleviation and focusing especially on the development of sustainable infectious disease control in animals in rural areas. Dr Robyn Alders' current research and development interests include domestic and global food and nutrition security, One Health/Ecohealth, gender equity, and Science Communication. She leads the Charles Perkins Centre/Marie Bashir Institute Healthy Food Systems: Nutrition–Diversity–Safety Research Node. In January 2011, Dr Alders was made an Officer of the Order of Australia for her distinguished service to veterinary science as a researcher and educator, and to the maintenance of food security in developing countries through livestock management and disease control programs.

Tom Arnold

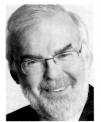

Director General of the Institute of International and European Affairs (IIEA) and Interim Coordinator of the Scaling Up Nutrition (SUN) Movement September 2014 –September 2016

Tom Arnold is a member of the Global Panel on Agriculture and Food Systems for Nutrition and the Agriculture for Impact Montpellier Panel. He was Chairman of the Irish Constitutional Convention (2012–14) and CEO of Concern Worldwide (2001–13). Tom has served on a number of governmental and non-governmental bodies, including the UN Millennium Project's Hunger Task Force, the Irish Hunger Task Force, the Irish Government's Commission on Taxation, and the Consortium Board of the Consultative Group for International Agricultural Research. He is Chairman of the *Irish Times* Trust and a member of the Board of the *Irish Times*. In his earlier career, he was Chief Economist and Assistant Secretary General with the Irish Department of Agriculture and Food and Chairman of the OECD Committee for Agriculture (1993–98). He has a degree in agricultural economics from University College Dublin and Masters degrees from Leuven University and Trinity College, Dublin. He was the recipient of the 2014 Helen Keller International Humanitarian Award.

Amare Ayalew

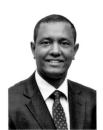

Program Manager of the Partnership for Aflatoxin Control in Africa (PACA), the African Union Commission

Dr Amare Ayalew has led PACA's strategic planning process and the launch of regional and country programs. He has researched the occurrence, epidemiology, and management of aflatoxins and other mycotoxins as well as plant health for over 20 years. Prior to joining PACA, Dr Ayalew had served as Associate Professor of Plant Pathology and Head of the School of Plant Sciences at Haramaya University, Ethiopia. He received a PhD *(summa cum laude)* in plant pathology from the University of Göttingen, Germany, in 2002, and Bachelor's and Master's degrees from Haramaya University in Ethiopia. In 2008, he was a USDA Fellow and Visiting Professor on sanitary and phytosanitary topics at Texas A&M University, USA. Dr Ayalew had five separate research stays at the Bavarian State Research Center in Freising/Munich, Germany between 1993 and 2012.

Brigitte Bagnol

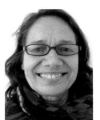

Senior Lecturer, Faculty of Veterinary Science and Charles Perkins Centre, The University of Sydney, Australia; and Research Associate, Department of Anthropology, University of the Witwatersrand, Johannesburg, South Africa

Dr Brigitte Bagnol is a medical anthropologist and gender specialist. She is involved in research in nutrition, One Health and gender. She has extensive international experience in Newcastle disease control and gender issues in Southern Africa. During the global avian influenza response, she worked at the Food and Agriculture Organization of the United Nations, looking specifically at communication issues. Dr Bagnol has brought a gender perspective to a range of sectors, including education, health and agriculture. Her most recent work is a study into early marriage in Mozambique.

343

Shawn Baker

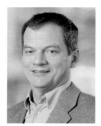

Director of Nutrition,
Bill & Melinda Gates
Foundation, Seattle,
WA, USA

As Director of the Nutrition team,
Shawn Baker leads the efforts of the
Bill & Melinda Gates Foundation to
ensure that women and children
receive the nutrition they need for
healthy growth and development.

Before joining the foundation in 2013,
Shawn served as Vice President and
Regional Director for Africa for Helen
Keller International. In that role, he
oversaw an expansion from 4 to 13
country programs and an 80-fold
increase in program funding. He
shaped flagship programs, including
vitamin A supplementation through
child health days (reaching more than 50
million children twice a year) and food
fortification (reaching more than 130
million people). He led the development
of strategic regional relationships,
particularly with the 15-nation West
African Health Organization.

Shawn received a Master's degree in
public health from the Tulane
University School of Public Health and
Tropical Medicine.

Jenifer Baxter

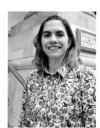

Head of Energy
and Environment,
Institution of
Mechanical
Engineers,
Westminster,
London, UK

Dr Jenifer Baxter is responsible for
providing expert guidance and support
on all mechanical engineering aspects
of energy and the environment. Prior
to joining IMechE, Jenifer was Head
of Enterprise and Innovation at the
University of East London, responsible
for developing collaborative
relationships with businesses,
academics and the wider UEL
community. She has been a Research
Project Manager and Lecturer in
research methods in the Engineering
Department at the University of South
Wales, specializing in advanced
engineering and materials; and before
undertaking her PhD in 2009, she
spent six years working for the Welsh
Government as a Waste Strategy
Advisor. Dr Baxter has a PhD from
Cardiff University in technological
innovation systems examining
hydrogen from waste technologies, an
MSc in Sustainability, Planning and
Environmental Policy, and a BEng in
Environmental Engineering, also
from Cardiff University. She is a
member of both the Institution of
Mechanical Engineers and the Energy
Institute in the UK.

Zulfiqar A Bhutta

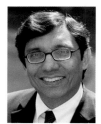

Founding Director,
Centre of Excellence
in Women and Child
Health, The Aga
Khan University,
Karachi, Pakistan;
and Co-Director &
Director of Research,
Center for Global
Child Health, The
Hospital for Sick Children, Toronto, Canada

Dr Zulfiqar Bhutta also holds adjunct
professorships at several leading
Universities globally and is a recipient
of various global awards. He was
educated at the University of Peshawar
(MBBS) and obtained his PhD from the
Karolinska Institute, Sweden. He is a
Fellow of the Royal College of
Physicians (Edinburgh & London), the
Royal College of Pediatrics and Child
Health (London), the American
Academy of Pediatrics, and the Pakistan
Academy of Sciences. Prof. Bhutta's
research interests include newborn and
child survival, maternal and child
undernutrition and micronutrient
deficiencies. He leads large research
groups based in Toronto, South Asia
and East Africa with a special interest in
research synthesis, scaling up evidence-
based interventions in community
settings, and implementation research
in health systems.

Martin W Bloem

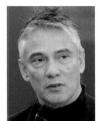

Senior Nutrition Advisor and Global Coordinator HIV/AIDS at the United Nations World Food Programme, Rome, Italy

Dr Martin Bloem holds a medical degree from the University of Utrecht and a doctorate from the University of Maastricht (both in the Netherlands), and has joint faculty appointments at both Johns Hopkins University and Tufts University (both in the USA). With more than two decades of experience in nutrition research and policy, he was the Senior Vice President Chief Medical Officer of Helen Keller International prior to his appointment at the World Food Programme. Dr Bloem has devoted his career to improving the effectiveness of public health and nutrition programs through applied research. He has participated in task forces convened by many organizations, including Columbia University, international non-governmental organizations, the Scaling Up Nutrition Movement, the United Nations Children's Fund (UNICEF), the United States Agency for International Development (USAID), and the World Health Organization (WHO).

Prof. Parul Christian

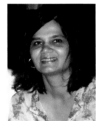

Senior Program Officer, Women's Nutrition, Bill & Melinda Gates Foundation; Professor, Department of International Health, Johns Hopkins Bloomberg School of Public Health, Baltimore, MD, USA

Until 2016 Dr Parul Christian was Professor of International Health and Human Nutrition at the Johns Hopkins University Bloomberg School of Public Health, Baltimore, MD, USA. Dr Christian has advanced the field of maternal and child nutrition and micronutrient deficiency prevention in South Asia and Africa. As an experienced nutritionist, epidemiologist, and community trialist, her research has contributed policy relevant knowledge related to the impact of maternal nutrition and micronutrient supplementation in improving pregnancy-related outcomes, including fetal growth, maternal and infant health and survival, as well as long-term outcomes of child cognition, and cardio-metabolic risk. She has also conducted trials of locally developed complementary food supplements to examine impact of linear growth and stunting in less than 2 year-olds and carried out impact evaluation studies of child nutrition programs in India and Malawi. She has over 150 peer-reviewed publications, 12 invited letters and commentaries, and 8 book chapters to her name.

John B Cordaro

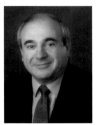

Global Food Security, Nutrition and Safety Consultant, Mars, Incorporated

Since 2007, J.B. Cordaro has served as a consultant to Mars, Incorporated, focusing on assembling networks of influential decision-makers to stimulate collaboration and partnerships to improve food quality, eliminate hunger and enhance food security. J.B. has five decades of experience and has worked in approximately 40 countries in positions with the US Agency for International Development (USAID); as staff representative for Senator Hubert H. Humphrey; as Food Program Manager, US Congress Office of Technology Assessment; as Executive Director, Food Safety Council; and as President-CEO, Council for Responsible Nutrition (CRN). He was a Congressional staff delegate at the 1974 World Food Conference and remains involved in nutrition and food systems initiatives with the UN Committee on World Food Security (UN CFS) and other stakeholders. J.B. holds a BSS from Loyola University, New Orleans, LA, USA and an MS from Cornell University, Ithaca, NY, USA.

345 **Dave Crean**

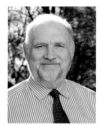

Vice President of Corporate Research and Development, Mars, Incorporated

Dr Dave Crean has over 30 years' experience in food safety, having worked in many countries and most Mars businesses. Dr Crean leads Quality and Food Safety at Mars, developing operational and research strategies to address current and future business challenges. He has spoken extensively about the linkages between food safety, food security and the critical role of multistakeholder collaboration. Dr Crean led the establishment of the Mars Global Food Safety Center in Beijing, China – a collaborative food safety platform designed to capture, generate and share food safety knowledge globally. He is also a lead partner in the IBM-Mars Consortium for Sequencing the Food Supply Chain.

Dave graduated with a BA (Hons) Degree in Applied Biology from Liverpool Polytechnic, UK in 1982.

Julian Cribb

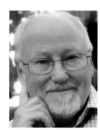

Author, journalist, editor and science communicator

Julian Cribb is Principal of Julian Cribb & Associates, who provide specialist consultancy in the communication of topics related to science, agriculture, food, mining, energy and the environment. His career includes appointments as a newspaper editor, scientific editor for The Australian newspaper, Director of National Awareness for the Commonwealth Scientific and Industrial Research Organisation (CSIRO), member of numerous scientific boards and advisory panels, and President of various Australian professional bodies for agricultural journalism and science communication.

Prof. Jai K Das

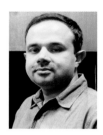

Assistant Professor for the Division of Women and Child Health, Aga Khan University, Karachi, Pakistan

Dr Jai Das has been actively involved in research and conducting evidence-based systematic reviews. He is currently Pakistan's Site Director for the Cochrane Collaboration and Coordinator for the Maternal Child Link on the Global Health Network. His research interests include interventions to address maternal and child nutrition and infections. He is the lead author of more than 60 international peer-reviewed papers, including the various Lancet Series on 'Childhood Diarrhea and Pneumonia', 'Maternal and Child Undernutrition', 'Newborn and Neonatal Health' and 'Stillbirths'. Dr Das has worked on various reports which have been used to influence policy both nationally and internationally. His interests are related to the use of evidence in policy and programs, including estimates of burden of disease, the development of research capacity, and the strengthening of public health.

Saskia de Pee

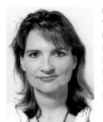

Nutrition Division, World Food Programme, Rome, Italy. Friedman School of Nutrition Science and Policy, Tufts University, Boston, MA, USA

Dr Saskia de Pee has worked in public health nutrition for more than 20 years, focusing on science as well as practical applications, policies and strategies. Her areas of expertise include complementary feeding, micronutrients, fortification, food and nutrient security, nutrition in the context of social protection, HIV/AIDS and tuberculosis, and 'evidence for nutrition'. She is co-editor of the third edition of Nutrition and Health in a Developing World (in press). Prior to joining WFP in 2007, Dr de Pee worked for Helen Keller International in the Asia Pacific region for 10 years. She has co-authored more than 150 scientific publications and holds a PhD in Nutrition from Wageningen University, the Netherlands.

Prof. Richard J Deckelbaum

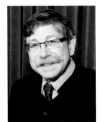

Director of the Institute of Human Nutrition at Columbia University, New York, NY, USA; Professor of nutrition, pediatrics and epidemiology

In addition to his basic research in cell biology of lipids and issues of human nutrition, Dr Richard Deckelbaum has been active in translating basic science into practical applications in diverse populations. He has chaired task forces for the American Heart Association and the March of Dimes, and has served on advisory committees of the WHO, NIH, RAND, and the US National Academy of Sciences, and has received a substantial number of honors. He helped initiate the Columbia University side of the Medical School for International Health (MSIH), a 'novel' medical school for training global health practitioners at Ben-Gurion University of the Negev in Israel in affiliation with Columbia University Medical Center. Dr Deckelbaum has led working groups in 'econutrition' to integrate research and programming in human health and nutrition with agriculture and ecology. He received his undergraduate and medical degrees from McGill University, Montreal, Canada. Currently he continues to work on projects related to health and science, bridging different populations in the Mideast, Africa, and Asia.

Prof. Glenn Denning

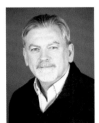

Professor of Professional Practice at Columbia University's School of International and Public Affairs (SIPA) and Senior Policy Advisor at the Sustainable Development Solutions Network

Dr Glenn Denning joined SIPA in 2009 as founding Director of the Master of Public Administration in Development Practice, a joint undertaking of SIPA with Columbia University's Earth Institute. In 2014, he received the Columbia University Presidential Award for Outstanding Teaching. Prior to joining Columbia University, Dr Denning held senior management positions in the International Rice Research Institute and the World Agroforestry Centre. From 2004 to 2006, he served on the UN Millennium Project Hunger Task Force. He also served on the Senior Steering Group of the UN High Level Task Force on the Global Food Security Crisis, and the Technical Advisory Committee of the Global Agriculture and Food Security Program. Dr Denning is a founding board member of the Institute of African Leadership for Sustainable Development (UONGOZI Institute).

347 ## Prof. Achim Dobermann

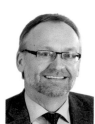

Director &
Chief Executive
of Rothamsted
Research

At Rothamsted Research, Dr Achim Dobermann provides leadership for a wide range of research programs that aim to develop solutions for the sustainable intensification of agricultural systems. He has over 30 years of field research experience from all world regions. Dr Dobermann received a MSc in tropical agriculture and a PhD in soil science from the University of Leipzig in Germany. In 1992 he joined the International Rice Research Institute (IRRI) as a soil scientist, followed by an appointment as Professor at the University of Nebraska-Lincoln from 2000 to 2007. From 2008 to 2014 he served as Deputy Director General at the International Rice Research Institute (IRRI), where he also led the Global Rice Science Partnership (GRiSP). As a member of the Leadership Council of the Sustainable Development Solutions Network (unsdsn.org) Dr Dobermann contributes to implementing the new Sustainable Development Goals.

Shauna Downs

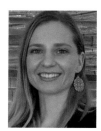

Postdoctoral
Research Fellow,
Institute of Human
Nutrition and The
Earth Institute,
Columbia University,
New York, NY USA

Dr Shauna Downs received her PhD in Public Health from the Menzies Centre for Health Policy at the University of Sydney. Her PhD work used food supply chain analysis to identify points where policy interventions could be implemented in the Indian fats supply chain to improve the quality of the food supply. She is currently an Earth Institute Postdoctoral Fellow at the Institute of Human Nutrition at Columbia University, working with Drs. Jess Fanzo, Glenn Denning, and Richard Deckelbaum. Her postdoctoral work focuses on the agriculture, nutrition and environment nexus, evidence-informed best practices regarding how to produce and consume healthy food in sustainable ways, and the use of policy for non-communicable disease prevention.

Prof. Adam Drewnowski

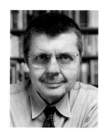

Director of the
Center for Public
Health Nutrition and
Professor of
Epidemiology at the
School of Public
Health, University of
Washington, Seattle,
WA, USA

Dr Adam Drewnowski obtained his Masters in biochemistry at Balliol College, Oxford University, UK, and PhD in psychology at The Rockefeller University in New York. His novel methods and metrics have helped consumers identify foods that are nutrient-rich, affordable, accessible, and appealing. The Nutrient Rich Foods (NRF) Index – a nutrient profiling system created by Dr Drewnowski – has been used to assess nutrients per calorie and nutrients per penny. Dr Drewnowski is a trustee of the International Life Sciences Institute (ILSI) and chair of the board of trustees of the ILSI Research Foundation. He advises governments, foundations, NGOs, and the private sector on geopolitical strategies related to diets and health. He also directs the University of Washington Center for Obesity Research, which addresses the environmental, social and economic aspects of the obesity epidemic.

Prof. Laurette Dubé

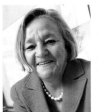

Professor, James McGill Chair of Consumer and Lifestyle Psychology and Marketing; Chair and Scientific Director, McGill Centre for the Convergence for Health and Economics; Desautels Faculty of Management, McGill University

Dr Laurette Dubé is a Full Professor and holds the James McGill Chair of consumer and lifestyle psychology and marketing at the Desautels Faculty of Management of McGill University, Canada. Her research interest bears on the study of effects and behavioral economic processes underlying consumption and lifestyle behavior, and how such knowledge can inspire more effective health and marketing communications in both real-life and technology-supported media. She is the Founding Chair and Scientific Director of the McGill Centre for the Convergence of Health and Economics. The MCCHE was created to foster partnerships among scientists and decision-makers from all sectors of society to encourage a more ambitious notion of what can be done for more effective health management and novel pathways for social and business innovation.

Prof. Manfred Eggersdorfer

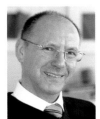

Senior Vice President, DSM Nutritional Products (Member of the Leadership Council DSM Nutritional Products); Head of DSM Nutrition Science & Advocacy, Kaiseraugst, Switzerland; Professor Healthy Ageing at the University Groningen, the Netherlands

Before joining DSM, Dr Manfred Eggersdorfer worked for BASF in various positions including Head of R&D Fine Chemicals. He studied chemistry at the Technical University, Munich, Germany and did his PhD in organic chemistry in synthesis and characterization of unusual amino acids. He undertook post-doctoral work at Stanford University, California, working with Carl Djerassi on the isolation and characterization of sterols of marine origin. Dr Eggersdorfer is a member of the Advisory Board of the Johns Hopkins Bloomberg School of Public Health; a member of the Strategy Board of the Institute of Food Science of the University Hamburg; and a Board member of the *Gesellschaft für angewandte Vitaminforschung e.V.* and the *Fraunhofer-Gesellschaft* Curatorial for Innovation. He is an Honorary Member of The Oxygen Club of California and author of numerous publications in the fields of vitamins, innovation in nutritional ingredients, and renewable resources, as well as Associate Editor of the International Journal of Vitamin and Nutrition Research.

Prof. Jess Fanzo

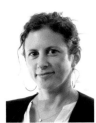

Bloomberg Distinguished Associate Professor of Global Food and Agriculture Policy and Ethics at the Berman Institute of Bioethics and the Nitze School of Advanced International Studies at the Johns Hopkins University, Baltimore, MA, USA, and Director of the Global Food Ethics and Policy Program

Prior to joining Johns Hopkins, Dr Jess Fanzo served as an Assistant Professor of Nutrition in the Institute of Human Nutrition and Department of Pediatrics and as the Senior Advisor of Nutrition Policy at the Center on Globalization and Sustainable Development within the Earth Institute at Columbia University. Prior to coming to academia, she held positions in the United Nations World Food Programme, Bioversity International, and the World Agroforestry Center. She was the first laureate of the Carasso Foundation's Sustainable Diets Prize for her work on sustainable diets for long-term human health. Dr Fanzo has a PhD in nutrition from the University of Arizona.

Prof. Habtamu Fekadu

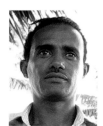

Pediatrician and nutritionist, Chief of Party at Save the Children International

Dr Habtamu Fekadu has more than 20 years' experience in child health and nutrition. He works at the Ethiopia country office of Save the Children International as a Chief of Party for a multisector nutrition project named USAID/ENGINE. Prior to this, he managed a USAID-funded nutrition and HIV project implemented by Save the Children, and a community-based nutrition project implemented by UNICEF. He leads the development of Ethiopia's first National nutrition plan of action. With an MSc in nutrition, Dr Habtamu has worked with the UN, NGOs and CBOs, as well as local government, ministries, and partners in Ethiopia to ensure that nutrition-specific and -sensitive policies and guidelines are established and evaluated. He served as Assistant Professor of pediatrics and child health and head of the pediatrics department at Jimma University, Ethiopia. He is a full member of the Society for Implementation Science in Nutrition, the Ethiopian Pediatric Society, and the Food and Nutrition Science Society of Ethiopia.

Prof. Rafael Flores-Ayala

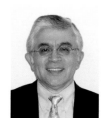

Team Lead of the International Micronutrient Malnutrition Prevention and Control Program (IMMPaCt) at the US Centers for Disease Control and Prevention

Prior to assuming his current position in 2008, Dr Rafael Flores-Ayala was a Research Associate Professor at the Rollins School of Public Health, Emory University (2001–2008), and he remains an Adjunct Associate Professor. Dr Flores-Ayala served in several distinguished positions at the International Food Policy Research Institute (IFPRI) and the Institute of Nutrition of Central America and Panama. He has extensive experience in the design, monitoring and evaluation of large-scale nutrition programs, national nutrition surveys, and surveillance systems, as well as in the development of international randomized clinical and group trials and epidemiologic studies. Currently he is Co-Chair of the Micronutrient Forum, a member of the Global Nutrition Report's Independent Expert Group, and Chair of the joint WHO/UNICEF Technical Expert Advisory Group on Nutrition Monitoring.

Prof. Michael Gibney

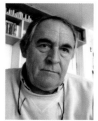

Emeritus Professor of Food and Health at University College Dublin, Institute of Food and Health

Dr Mike Gibney is a former President of the Nutrition Society. He served on the EU Scientific Committee for Food from 1985 to 1997 and then chaired the EU BSE working group from 1997 to 2000. He is a member of the scientific advisory committee of the Sackler Institute of Nutrition of the New York Academy of Sciences, a member of the Nestlé Nutrition Council, a former member of Google's Food Innovation Lab, and a Fellow of the International Union of Nutritional Sciences. He is chairman of the Food Safety Authority of Ireland. His research interests lie in metabolic and molecular nutrition, in public health nutrition, and in probabilistic risk analysis. Dr Gibney has served on the Faculties of the University of Sydney, the University of Southampton and Trinity College Dublin. He has published over 300 peer-reviewed papers and blogs at Gibneyonfood, and his most recent publication is *Ever Seen a Fat Fox* (University College Dublin Press 2016).

Jo Goosens

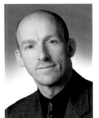

Independent strategic thinker

With a doctorate in Biology, Dr Jo Goosens is an independent strategic thinker with 30 years' experience in the agri-food industry. After 18 years as a researcher, marketing manager and business unit director in the food ingredients industry, he started the Bio-Sense consultancy in 2001, focusing on the major societal issues surrounding nutrition and health and the sustainability in the agri-food chain. Dr Goosens is particularly interested in creative processes that help to understand the underlying patterns and forces shaping markets and societies. Working together with shiftN, the Belgium-based innovative systems thinking and futures consultancy, he co-initiated and managed ground-breaking projects such as the Nutrition & Health 2020 and 2025 Fields for Food and Fuel scenario projects, as well as the first ever Nutrition & Health Open Innovation Lab in 2006. He has partnered in EU projects such as GoodFood, Food4Me and QuaLiFY.

Henry Greenberg

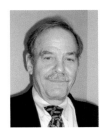

Cardiologist and faculty member at the Mailman School of Public Health and the Institute of Human Nutrition at Columbia University, New York, NY, USA

Dr Henry Greenberg is a cardiologist with an extensive background in clinical trials. Trial topics included coronary artery disease, implantable defibrillators, and congestive heart failure. He was an Associate Professor of Medicine at Columbia University's College of Physicians and Surgeons, and a Senior Physician at St. Luke's Roosevelt Hospital. Since his retirement from clinical practice in 2013, Dr Greenberg has been on the epidemiology faculty at the Mailman School of Public Health and the Institute of Human Nutrition at Columbia University. His public health focus is on global chronic diseases, and his goal is to enhance their visibility in the public health curriculum and the global donor community.

Lawrence Haddad

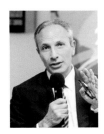

Executive Director, Global Alliance for Improved Nutrition (GAIN)

Before taking up his current position in October 2016, Dr Lawrence Haddad was a Senior Research Fellow in the International Food Policy Research Institute's Poverty Health and Nutrition Division. He was the Director of the Institute of Development Studies, Sussex, UK from 2004 to 2014. Prior to that, he was a Division Director at IFPRI and a Lecturer in Development Economics at the University of Warwick, UK. Dr Haddad is an economist, and his main research interests are at the intersection of poverty, food insecurity, and malnutrition. He is the Co-Chair of the Global Nutrition Report's Independent Expert Group.

Prof. Susan Horton

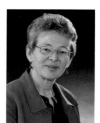

CIGI Chair in Global Health Economics, University of Waterloo, Ontario, Canada in the Balsillie School of International Affairs

In 2016 Dr Susan Horton was also Visiting Scholar in Residence at the Centre for Global Child Health at the Hospital for Sick Children, Toronto, Canada. She has worked in over 20 low- and middle-income countries and has consulted for the World Bank, the Asian Development Bank, several United Nations agencies, and the International Development Research Centre, among other organizations. Dr Horton led the paper on nutrition for the Copenhagen Consensus in 2008, when micronutrients were ranked as the top development priority. She also led the costing for global nutrition work in the Lancet 2013 series on nutrition, and for the 2009 World Bank Scaling up Nutrition book. Recent projects include the Lancet 2016 breastfeeding series, the Disease Control Priorities volumes, and work on childhood cancer in low- and middle-income countries.

Maria Elena D Jefferds

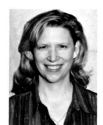

Behavioral Scientist with the International Micronutrient Malnutrition Prevention and Control Program (IMMPaCt) at the US Centers for Disease Control and Prevention (CDC)

Dr Maria Elena Jefferds has expertise in behavioral science, surveillance, monitoring and evaluation of nutrition programs. She provides technical assistance directly to countries and global partners, and leads the design and implementation of national micronutrient surveys, program monitoring systems, and national nutrition surveillance systems. She has also led the development of monitoring manuals for home fortification and biannual vitamin A supplementation, and she collaborates with WHO on the development of monitoring and evaluation indicators for micronutrient programs and other monitoring and surveillance tools. Dr Jefferds is currently a member of the WHO guideline development group for nutrition actions.

Prof. Eileen Kennedy

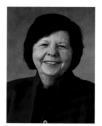

Professor of Nutrition and former Dean of the Tufts University, Friedman School of Nutrition Science and Policy, Medford, MA, USA

From 1994 to 2001 Dr Eileen Kennedy served in senior positions in the Clinton Administration. She was the founding executive director of the USDA, Center for Nutrition Policy and Planning, the organization responsible for the Dietary Guidelines for Americans and the Food Guide Pyramid. She was also Deputy Under Secretary for Research, Education and Economics, overseeing the four technical agencies within USDA. Dr Kennedy is a member of the High Level Panel of Experts on Food Security and Nutrition of the Committee on World Food Security. She has served on the United Nations' Advisory Group on Nutrition, the White House Biotechnology Council, IOM, Board on Global Health and other boards. She was the co-chair with the US Surgeon General of the National Nutrition Summit. Her research focuses on the effects of governmental and non-governmental policies and programs on health, nutrition, food security and welfare.

Lynnda Kiess

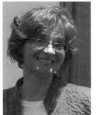

Senior Policy and Programme Advisor for Nutrition at the United Nations World Food Programme, Rome, Italy

Lynnda Kiess holds a degree in nutrition from the Purdue University, West Lafayette, IN, USA and a Master's in public health from Johns Hopkins University, Baltimore, MA, USA. She has more than 20 years' experience in nutrition programming, policy and research. Prior to joining WFP, she was the Head of Nutrition and Health at Concern Worldwide. She has worked with Helen Keller International as the Country Director in Bangladesh, Regional Advisor in Asia-Pacific, and Head of Nutrition in New York. She also worked with the World Bank, was a fellow at the US Agency for International Development, and has worked with US domestic nutrition programs. Lynnda Kiess has devoted her career to building evidence for nutrition programming and effectively linking programs, policy and research. She has experience in food systems, public health, food science and food policy.

Prof. Michael Klag

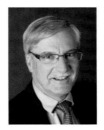

Dean of the Johns Hopkins Bloomberg School of Public Health, Baltimore, MD, USA

Dr Michael Klag is a pioneering chronic disease epidemiologist whose scientific contributions have been in the prevention and epidemiology of kidney disease, hypertension and cardiovascular disease. He was one of the earliest investigators to apply epidemiologic methods to the study of kidney disease, answering important questions about the incidence, prevalence, causes and optimal treatment of kidney disease. Dr Klag also directed one of the longest-running longitudinal studies in existence, the Precursors Study, which began in 1946, investigating risk of cardiovascular disease and other outcomes associated with characteristics in young adulthood and later life. Dr Klag was the inaugural Vice Dean for Clinical Investigation at the JHU School of Medicine, rebuilding its human research subjects protection system. Since 2005, he has served as Dean of the Johns Hopkins Bloomberg School of Public Health, the oldest, largest independent graduate school of public health with funded programs in over 100 countries.

Rolf D W Klemm

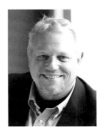

Vice President of Nutrition at Helen Keller International (HKI) and Senior Associate at the Johns Hopkins Bloomberg School of Public Health, Baltimore, MA, USA

Dr Rolf Klemm is trained as a nutritional epidemiologist and has more than 25 years of experience in international public health, with expertise that spans nutrition efficacy and effectiveness research and program design, management and evaluation. Dr Klemm served as Country Director for HKI in the Philippines, Technical Director of USAID's flagship A2Z micronutrient project, and as nutrition faculty at Johns Hopkins Bloomberg School of Public Health. He is the principal instructor of the Food and Nutrition Policy course at JHSPH. As VP Nutrition for HKI, he provides scientific and technical leadership to HKI's regional and country nutrition programs.

Prof. Richard A Kock

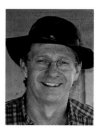

Professor of Wildlife Health & EIDs, Royal Veterinary College, London, UK

Dr Richard Kock, a wildlife veterinary scientist since 1980, worked with the Zoological Society, London until 2010 and in 2011 was appointed Professor at the Royal Veterinary College, London. Seconded to Kenya Government and African Union, 1990–2006, he researched and advised on diseases at the livestock-wildlife disease interface. In 2001 he identified the last outbreak of rinderpest globally and was awarded the FAO medal in recognition of his work. From 2006–2010 he worked from the UK on the agriculture-wildlife interface and conservation in rangelands. Currently working on antelope die-offs in Kazakhstan and global PPR virus emergence in wildlife, Dr Kock has doctoral students working on bovine tuberculosis, brucellosis, reintroduction and PPR, and supports a zoonoses project in Tanzania and a project on control of Newcastle disease in village poultry as a core element to improving childhood nutrition in Africa. He is also an educator, directing a Master's Programme in One Health.

Prof. Klaus Kraemer

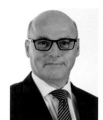

Managing Director of *Sight and Life* Foundation, and Adjunct Associate Professor in the Department of International Health of Johns Hopkins Bloomberg School of Public Health, Baltimore, MA, USA

Dr Klaus Kraemer is the Managing Director of *Sight and Life* Foundation (www.sightandlife.org), a nutrition think tank that receives its funding primarily from DSM, and Adjunct Associate Professor in the Department of International Health of Johns Hopkins Bloomberg School of Public Health, Baltimore. *Sight and Life* envisions a world free from malnutrition. The Swiss-based think tank focuses on implementation research and leadership development to empower organizations and individuals to deliver smart solutions, and strives to co-create tailored innovations through understanding of context. *Sight and Life* hosts the secretariat of the Society for Implementation Science in Nutrition. Dr Kraemer is the editor of *Sight and Life* magazine, one of the most widely read scientific magazines on micronutrient nutrition and health in the developing world. He serves several professional societies dedicated to nutrition, vitamins, and antioxidants, is a reviewer for a number of scientific journals, has published more than 120 scientific articles, reviews, and book chapters, and has co-edited 10 books.

Prof. Alain B Labrique

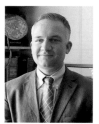

Director, Johns Hopkins University Global mHealth Initiative & Associate Professor Department of International Health/ Epidemiology (jt) Johns Hopkins Bloomberg School of Public Health Baltimore, MA, USA; Department of Community-Public Health Johns Hopkins School of Nursing (jt); Division of Health Sciences Informatics, Johns Hopkins School of Medicine (jt)

Dr Alain Labrique is Director of the Johns Hopkins University Global mHealth Initiative, a multidisciplinary Center of over 150 projects engaged in mHealth research across the Johns Hopkins system. An infectious disease epidemiologist with training in molecular biology and over a decade of field experience running large population-based research studies in low-income countries, Dr Labrique holds joint appointments at the Johns Hopkins University Schools of Public Health, Nursing and Medicine. Dr Labrique is lead investigator for research projects measuring the impact of mobile information and communications technologies on improving maternal, neonatal and infant health in resource-limited settings. He was recognized among the top mHealth Innovators in 2011 by the Rockefeller and UN Foundations and was a lead author on a Bellagio Declaration on mHealth Evidence. Dr Labrique serves as a Technical Advisor to international agencies and is the current Chair of the WHO mHealth Technical Evidence Review Group (mTERG).

Prof. J Alfredo Martínez

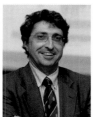

Professor of Nutrition and Chairman of the Institute of Nutrition at the University of Navarra, Spain

Dr Alfredo Martínez specializes in the nutritional control of metabolism; nutritional utilization of functional foods; evaluation of nutritional status in different populations; nutrition and immunity; obesity; cell, animal and human intervention and epidemiological studies; consumer surveys; and long-distance learning. He is Nutrigenomics Associate Director of I+D+i at INIA (Soria); a member of the Scientific Advisory Group for the 7th EU framework, ILSi, Académico Correspondiente Real Academia de Farmacia (Royal Academy of Pharmacy, Spain); a Member of the IUNS Council (2005–); President of International Union of Nutritional Sciences (2013–); and President of ISNN (2014–). Dr Martinez was Secretary of the Federation of European Nutrition Societies (FENS) from 2003–2007, and President of the Spanish Federation of Nutrition, Food and Dietetics (FESNAD) from 2005–2010. He has over 500 ISBN-registered publications to his name, over 50 published books and chapters, and has given more than 100 lectures at international and national level.

Prof. Miguel A Martinez-Gonzalez

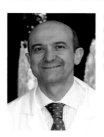

Professor and Chair of Preventive Medicine and Public Health, University of Navarra, Spain

Graduating as a Medical Doctor from the University of Granada, Spain, in 1980, Dr Miquel Martinez-Gonzalez also has a PhD in Cardiovascular Epidemiology from the University of Granada and a Master's in Public Health from the Andalusian School of Public Health (EASP), University of Granada (Spain). He became Full Professor of Preventive Medicine and Public Health at the University of Malaga, Spain, in 2005. Dr Martinez-Gonzalez is the Founder and Principal Investigator of the SUN cohort, initiated in 1999 with more than 22,500 participants and in excess of 130 scientific publications. He was a Visiting scholar at the Harvard T.H. Chan School of Public Health, Department of Nutrition in 1998, 2001 and 2004) and Coordinator of the PREDIMED Research Network funded by the Instituto de Salud Carlos III (2006–2013). An Associate Editor of the *British Journal of Nutrition*, Dr Martinez-Gonzalez has co-authored over 500 peer-reviewed articles, and his articles have been cited more than 22,000 times.

Prof. William A Masters

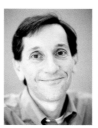

Professor at Tufts University, Medford, MA, USA in the Friedman School of Nutrition, with a secondary appointment in the Department of Economics

Dr William Masters earned his PhD in 1991 from Stanford University's Food Research Institute, then served on the faculty in Agricultural Economics at Purdue University before moving to Tufts, in 2010. Publications include an undergraduate textbook co-authored with George Norton and Jeff Alwang, *Economics of Agricultural Development: World Food Systems and Resource Use* (Routledge, 3rd ed. 2014). From 2006 through 2011 he edited Agricultural Economics, the journal of the International Association of Agricultural Economists. In 2010 he was named an International Fellow of the African Association of Agricultural Economists, and he has been awarded both the Bruce Gardner Memorial Prize for Applied Policy Analysis (2013) and the Publication of Enduring Quality Award (2014) from the Agricultural and Applied Economics Association (AAEA).

Sucheta Mehra

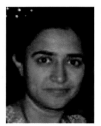

Research Associate at the Program in Human Nutrition, Department of International Health, Bloomberg School of Public Health, Baltimore, MD, USA

Sucheta Mehra is a public health nutritionist with over 18 years' experience studying the health of women and children in South Asia, having worked in India, Afghanistan and Bangladesh. Currently a Research Associate at the Program in Human Nutrition, Department of International Health, Bloomberg School of Public Health, she is also the Project Scientist at the JiVitA Research site in Bangladesh and a Co-Principal Investigator and Co-Investigator on numerous maternal and child nutritional and mobile-health interventional studies on maternal, neonatal and child health. She has a Masters in Biochemistry from M. S. University, Baroda, India and a Masters in Food Policy and Applied Nutrition from the Friedman School at Tufts University, Medford, MA, USA.

Marc Mitchell

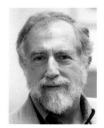

Founder and President of D-International, and Adjunct Lecturer on Global Health at Harvard T.H. Chan School of Public Health, Boston, MA, USA

Dr Marc Mitchell is a pediatrician and management specialist who has worked in over 40 countries in Africa, Asia, and Latin America on the design and delivery of healthcare services. Dr Mitchell began his career as a pediatrician in rural Tanzania and has worked at every level of the health system including Assistant Secretary of Health in Papua New Guinea and advisor to the National Family Planning Program in Indonesia. His research focuses on how mobile technology can increase access to high-quality healthcare for the poor. In 2004 this led to the founding of D-tree International, a global leader in the growing field of mHealth. Dr Mitchell holds degrees from Harvard University, Cambridge, MA, USA (BA), Boston University (MD), and MIT's Sloan School of Management, Cambridge, MA, USA (MS). He is currently living in Myanmar.

Regina Moench-Pfanner

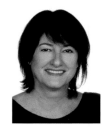

Founder and CEO of ibn360, a consulting firm specializing in food, nutrition and health, based in Singapore

Dr Regina Moench-Pfanner has 30 years' experience leading development and nutrition programs in emerging markets. She began her career with the Red Cross and Red Crescent, leading major relief operations in Africa and Eastern Europe. She then moved into development to improve nutrition through public-private-civic initiatives. Among other appointments, she worked for Helen Keller International and until 2015 for the Global Alliance for Improved Nutrition (GAIN), where she directed the organization's global nutrition programs for several years before heading the office in Singapore. She is a Fulbright Scholar, holds an MSc in International Nutrition from Michigan State University, USA and a Doctorate from the University of Bonn, Germany. Dr Moench-Pfanner has published and co-authored over 60 peer-reviewed papers and is a Board Member of the Rice Bowl Index, which monitors food security in Asia.

Mike Nunn

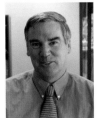

Research Program Manager (Animal Health) at the Australian Centre for International Agricultural Research (ACIAR)

Dr Mike Nunn is a veterinarian with postgraduate qualifications in tropical veterinary science, pathology, epidemiology and management. He has worked in mixed practice, field, laboratory diagnostic, research and training roles in Australia and overseas, including 13 years in Papua New Guinea. Before joining ACIAR in June 2012, he was the Principal Scientist (Animal Biosecurity) in the Australian Government Department of Agriculture, Fisheries and Forestry, providing high-level scientific advice into the formulation and implementation of policy on animal health, quarantine and biosecurity, including leading major formal import risk analyses. Dr Nunn has undertaken a range of consultancies for international organizations, including the World Organisation for Animal Health (OIE), the Food and Agriculture Organization, and the World Health Organization. He has particular interests in epidemiology, risk analysis, emerging diseases, zoonoses, nutrition-sensitive agriculture, and strategic foresight.

Prof. Jonathan Rushton

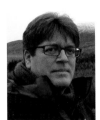

Professor in Animal Health Economics at the Royal Veterinary College, London, UK

Dr Jonathan Rushton is an agricultural economist who specializes in the economics of animal health and livestock production and food systems – interests that grew from living and working on the family dairy farm. He is currently involved in global research on One Health and food systems, and has 25 years' international experience of livestock production and the control of animal diseases in South America, Africa and Asia. Dr Rushton's principal research interests include disease impact assessment, the use of food systems analysis to understand One Health problems, and the economic analysis of health interventions. He is the professor in Animal Health Economics at the Royal Veterinary College, London, UK, holds the Norbrook endowed chair on Veterinary Business Management, and is a founding member of the Leverhulme Centre for Integrative Research on Agriculture and Health. He is also adjunct Professor in the School of Behavioral, Cognitive & Social Sciences of the University of New England, Australia.

Jonathan Steffen

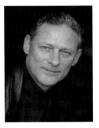

Writer, editor and communication strategist

Jonathan Steffen holds a Master's degree in English from Cambridge University, UK. During the 1990s he taught translation and interpreting at Heidelberg University, Germany and was subsequently appointed Simultaneous Interpreter to the Board of Management of the German multinational Hoechst AG. As an editor, his portfolio includes *The Road to Good Nutrition: A global perspective* (Karger, 2013); *Micro Nutrients, Macro Impact: The story of vitamins and a hungry world* (Sight and Life, 2012); and *Tomorrow's Answers Today: The history of AkzoNobel since 1646* (AkzoNobel 2008). He also edits and project-manages *Sight and Life* magazine under the direction of Dr Klaus Kraemer. Jonathan Steffen has over 150 original publications to his name in genres ranging from poetry through short stories to essays and translations. He is a member of King's College, Cambridge and St. John's College, Cambridge, as well as of the Society of Authors, the Royal Historical Society, and the Association of Business Historians.

Madeleine Thomson

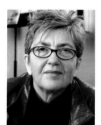

Senior Research Scientist at the International Research Institute for Climate and Society and Senior Scholar at the Mailman School of Public Health, Department of Environmental Health Sciences at Columbia University, New York, NY, USA

Dr Madeleine Thompson trained originally as a field entomologist and has spent much of her career engaged in operational research in support of large-scale health interventions, mostly in Africa. Her research focuses on the development of new data, methodologies and tools for improving climate-sensitive health interventions for infectious diseases, nutrition and public health outcomes of disasters. She has a Master's in Applied Pest Management from Imperial College London, UK (1985) and a PhD from the University of Liverpool, UK based on her field work on the vectors of *Onchocerciasis volvulus* in Sierra Leone (1989). Dr Thompson is also the Director of the IRI/PAHO-WHO Collaborating Centre (US 306) for Early Warning Systems for Malaria and Other Climate Sensitive Diseases.

Prof. Ricardo Uauy

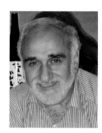

Professor of Public Health Nutrition at the Institute of Nutrition (INTA), University of Chile, and London School of Hygiene and Tropical Medicine, UK

Dr Ricardo Uauy received his MD from the University of Chile, Santiago, Chile in 1972, and his PhD in Nutritional Biochemistry from MIT, Cambridge, MA, USA in 1977. He became a full Professor an INTA in 1981, was Director of INTA from 1994 to 2002, and was President of the International Union of Nutrition Sciences from 2005 to 2009. Dr Uauy has participated in multiple WHO/FAO expert committees. He received the McCollum Lecture award ASN (USA) in 200; the Lawton Chiles International Lecturer Award NIH in 2003; the Spanish Nutrition Society Award and PAHO/WHO Abraham Horwitz award for Leadership in Inter-American Health in 2005; the Kellog's International Nutrition Award in 2006; the Rank Lecture Award/UK Nutrition Society and the British Nutrition Foundation Prize in 2008; the George Graham Lecture Award in 2010; and the National Applied Science Award from the Government of Chile 2012. Dr Uauy has written over 350 scientific journal publications and edited 10 books.

Marianne Walsh

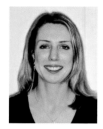

Nutrition Manager at the National Dairy Council in Ireland

Dr Marianne Walsh has a BSc in Human Nutrition from University of Ulster and a PhD in Nutritional Metabolomics from Trinity College Dublin. From 2008 to 2015 she worked at University College Dublin as a research nutritionist. She was Project Manager of Food4Me (www.food4me.org), a EUR 9 million European Commission-funded research project in personalized nutrition, which involved industry and academic partners from across 12 EU countries. She held the role of Sports Nutritionist for the UCD Ad Astra Elite Athlete Academy from 2011 to 2015, working with a wide range of elite athletes, including swimmers, footballers, short- and long-distance runners, equestrians, rowers, golfers and rugby players. Dr Walsh also engages in occasional lecturing in the area of nutrition at both University College Dublin and Trinity College Dublin. In addition, she has worked on a consultancy basis with clients from both the food industry and the public sector since 2005.

Prof. Peter Weber

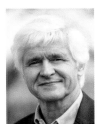

Corporate Science Fellow for Human Nutrition & Health, DSM, Kaiseraugst, Switzerland

Dr Peter Weber is a physician and also Professor of Nutrition at the University of Stuttgart-Hohenheim, Germany lecturing in Human Nutrition and Health. He received his PhD in Nutritional Sciences from the University of Bonn, Germany and his MD from the University of Münster, Germany. After working for two years at the Research Institute for Child Nutrition, Dortmund, Germany he trained in Internal Medicine with a sub-specialty in Endocrinology at the University of Mainz, Germany. He has more than 70 peer-reviewed publications in the field of iodine deficiency and goiter, thyroid diseases, metabolic syndrome, postprandial lipid metabolism, vitamin K, vitamin status of populations, and the role of vitamins and polyunsaturated fatty acids in human health, and he is a co-editor of a book on vitamins. Dr Weber's scientific interests include the role of micronutrients in the prevention of diseases, the nutritional status of at-risk groups such as the elderly, and the emerging topic of Nutrition Security.

Prof. Sera Young

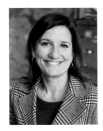

Assistant Professor of Anthropology at Northwestern University, Evanston, IL, USA

Dr Sera Young is an Assistant Professor at Northwestern University and was formerly Assistant Professor of Global Health and Nutrition, Department of Population Medicine and Diagnostic Sciences, Cornell University, Ithaca, NY, USA. The focus of her work is the reduction of maternal and child undernutrition in low-resource settings, especially subsaharan Africa. Methodologically, she draws on her training in medical anthropology (MA, University of Amsterdam) and international nutrition (PhD, Cornell) to take a biocultural approach to understanding how mothers in low-resource settings cope to preserve their health and that of their children. Her specific areas of interest include the impact of food insecurity on maternal and child health, the prevention of maternal-to-child transmission of HIV, evaluative ethnography, and pica, or non-food cravings. She has active, NIH-funded research in Tanzania, Kenya, and Uganda, and is the author of more than 50 publications, as well as the book *Craving Earth*, for which she received the 2013 Margaret Mead Award.

Index

Image credits for chapter introductions

Chapter 1

1.1: Mike Bloem

1.3: Mike Bloem

1.4: Ricardo Uauy

1.5: Mike Bloem

Chapter 2

2.1: *Sight and Life*

2.2: Mike Bloem

2.3: Friedel Amman

Chapter 3

3.1: M Kock

3.3: Mike Bloem

3.4: Institution of Mechanical Engineers

Chapter 4

4.1: Mike Bloem

4.2: *Sight and Life*

4.3: Digital Green

4.4: Mike Bloem

Chapter 5

5.1: Mike Bloem

5.2: Mike Bloem

5.4: SUN Movement Secretariat

5.5: Ministry of Planning, Development and Reform, Pakistan

5.6: Mike Bloem

5.7: Wezi Chunga, PACA Secretariat

5.8: IRRI